MEDIATORS OF CELLULAR IMMUNITY

SOME CONFERENCE PARTICIPANTS

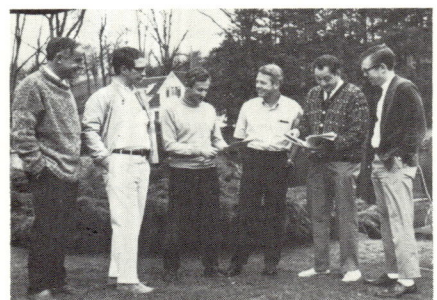

N. A. Mitchison, S. F. Schlossman,
J. R. David, R. T. Smith, R. A. Good,
G. A. Granger

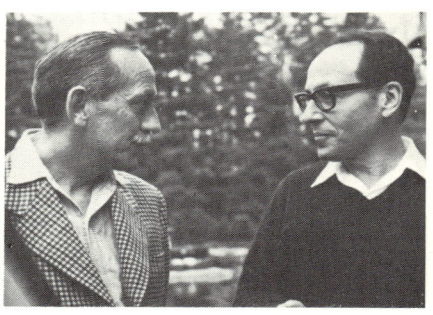

H. S. Lawrence, M. Cohn

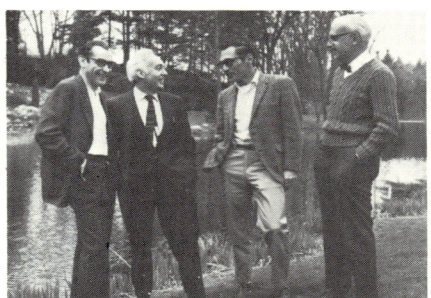

K. Hirschhorn, R. E. Billingham,
A. M. Silverstein, S. B. Salvin

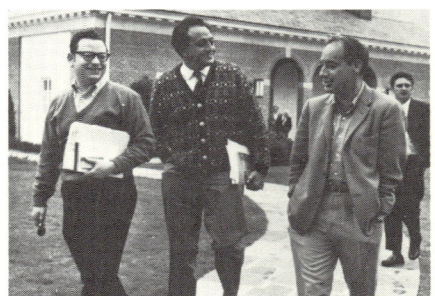

B. R. Bloom, R. A. Good, J. L. Turk

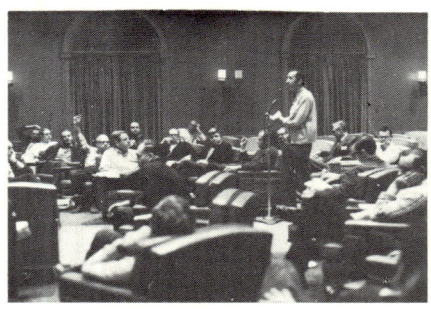

J. W. Uhr et al.

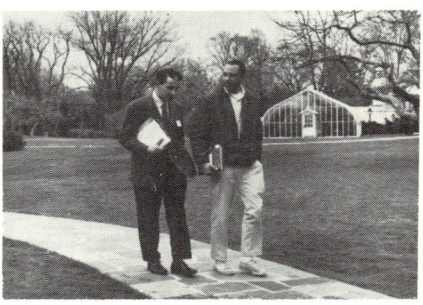

W. H. Marshall, M. W. Brandriss

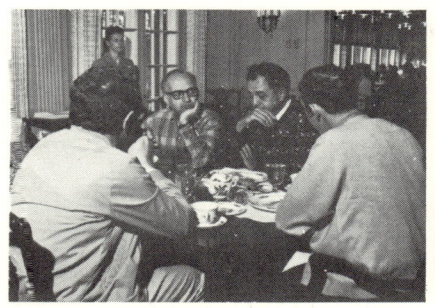
W. Braun, R. A. Good

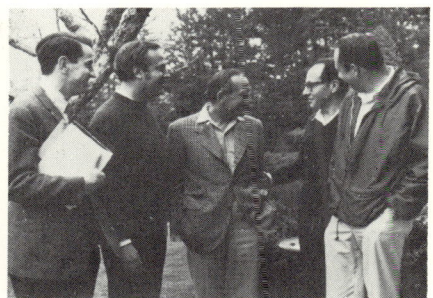
W. H. Marshall, D. E. Thor, H. S. Lawrence, M. Cohn, M. W. Brandriss

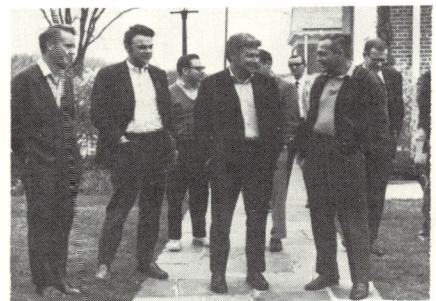
R. W. Dutton, D. B. Wilson, P. Baram, W. Rosenau

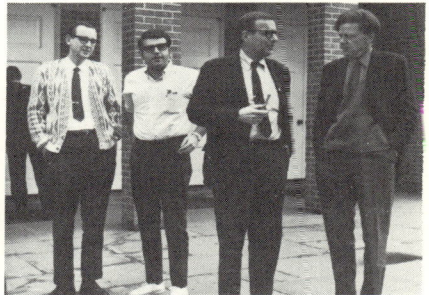
J. J. Oppenheim, L. N. Chessin, L. Thomas, P. G. H. Gell

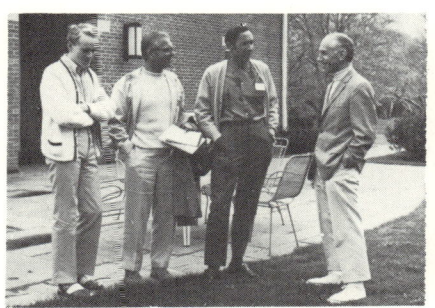
G. Moller, F. J. Dixon, J. W. Uhr, M. Landy

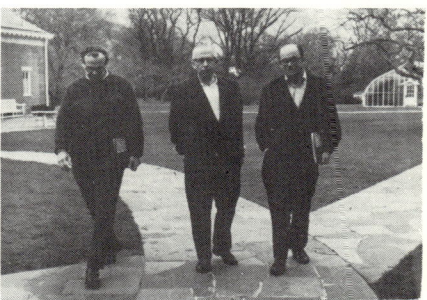
H. N. Eisen, M. W. Chase, P. Fireman

Perspectives in Immunology

A Series of Publications Based on Symposia

Maurice Landy and Werner Braun (eds.)
IMMUNOLOGICAL TOLERANCE
A Reassessment of Mechanisms of the Immune Response
1969

H. Sherwood Lawrence and Maurice Landy (eds.)
MEDIATORS OF CELLULAR IMMUNITY
1969

In preparation:

Richard T. Smith and Maurice Landy (eds.)
IMMUNOLOGICAL SURVEILLANCE
1970

Lionel A. Manson and Maurice Landy (eds.)
MEMBRANE-ASSOCIATED ANTIGENS OF
MAMMALIAN CELLS
1971

Mediators of Cellular Immunity

Edited by
H. Sherwood Lawrence New York University
School of Medicine

and
Maurice Landy National Institute of
Allergy and
Infectious Diseases

Proceedings of an International Conference
Held at Brook Lodge
Augusta, Michigan
April 28-30, 1969

Academic Press
New York • London—1969

COPYRIGHT © 1969, BY ACADEMIC PRESS, INC.
ALL RIGHTS RESERVED
NO PART OF THIS BOOK MAY BE REPRODUCED IN ANY FORM,
BY PHOTOSTAT, MICROFILM, RETRIEVAL SYSTEM, OR ANY
OTHER MEANS, WITHOUT WRITTEN PERMISSION FROM
THE PUBLISHERS.

ACADEMIC PRESS, INC.
111 Fifth Avenue, New York, New York 10003

United Kingdom Edition published by
ACADEMIC PRESS, INC. (LONDON) LTD.
Berkeley Square House, London W1X 6BA

LIBRARY OF CONGRESS CATALOG CARD NUMBER: 73-103865

PRINTED IN THE UNITED STATES OF AMERICA

CONFEREES

D. Bernard Amos, Duke University, Durham, North Carolina

Fritz H. Bach, University of Wisconsin, Madison, Wisconsin

Peter Baram, American Dental Association, Chicago, Illinois

Rupert E. Billingham, University of Pennsylvania, Philadelphia, Pennsylvania

Barry R. Bloom, Albert Einstein Medical College, Bronx, New York

Michael W. Brandriss, University of Rochester, Rochester, New York

Werner Braun, Rutgers, The State University, New Brunswick, New Jersey

Merrill W. Chase, The Rockefeller University, New York, New York

Lawrence N. Chessin, University of Rochester, Rochester, New York

Melvin Cohn, Salk Institute, La Jolla, California

John R. David, Harvard Medical School, Boston, Massachusetts

Frank J. Dixon, Scripps Clinic and Research Foundation, La Jolla, California

Richard W. Dutton, University of California, San Diego, California

Herman N. Eisen, Washington University, St. Louis, Missouri

Philip Fireman, University of Pittsburgh, Pittsburgh, Pennsylvania

Philip G. H. Gell, University of Birmingham, Birmingham, England

Robert A. Good, University of Minnesota, Minneapolis, Minnesota

Gale A. Granger, University of California, Irvine, California

Kurt Hirschhorn, Mount Sinai School of Medicine, New York, New York

Maurice Landy, National Institute of Allergy and Infectious Diseases, Bethesda, Maryland

CONFEREES

H. Sherwood Lawrence, New York University, New York, New York

George B. Mackaness, Trudeau Institute, Saranac Lake, New York

William H. Marshall, Memorial University of Newfoundland, St. Johns, Newfoundland, Canada

N. Avrion Mitchison, National Institute for Medical Research, London, England

Goran Möller, Karolinska Institutet, Stockholm, Sweden

Joost J. Oppenheim, National Institute of Dental Research, Bethesda, Maryland

Werner Rosenau, University of California, San Francisco, California

Samuel B. Salvin, University of Pittsburgh, Pittsburgh, Pennsylvania

Stuart F. Schlossman, Harvard Medical School, Boston, Massachusetts

Arthur M. Silverstein, Johns Hopkins University, Baltimore, Maryland

Richard T. Smith, University of Florida, Gainesville, Florida

Lewis Thomas, New York University, New York, New York

Daniel E. Thor, Division of Biologics Standards, NIH, Bethesda, Maryland

John L. Turk, University of London, London, England

Jonathan W. Uhr, New York University, New York, New York

Fred T. Valentine, New York University, New York, New York

Byron H. Waksman, Yale University, New Haven, Connecticut

Darcy B. Wilson, University of Pennsylvania, Philadelphia, Pennsylvania

PREFACE

Delayed-type hypersensitivity, or cellular immunity, as this class of reactions is now designated, has emerged rapidly from the ambiguity that until recently had engulfed it. Progress at the conceptual as well as the practical level suffered from the critical lack of immunologic reagents to equate with *in vivo* events—a deficit compounded by the restrictions incident to an indolent cutaneous reaction, long the sole end-point of this response. Thus matters stood locked in the past until the discovery of cellular transfer—a technique which simultaneously separated cell-mediated responses from those consequent to humoral antibody, and fortunately provided an immunologic reagent for analysis. In retrospect it was the dogged commitment of a few historic figures such as Zinsser, Landsteiner, Freund, and Dienes to this discouraging facet of immunology that kept the field viable. In the face of little understanding or encouragement, it was their perseverance that assured the survival of this field, its eventual renaissance, and finally its present emergence into a proper position in the mainstream of molecular biology.

The impediments that contributed to the static character of delayed hypersensitivity are now largely surmounted and the path ahead, although tortuous in spots, is clearly marked. The excitement and keen anticipation occasioned by this conference attest to the impact of the new *in vitro* techniques on the direction and tempo of investigative approaches to this problem. The substantial progress in the analysis of the broad repertoire of latent responses residing in sensitive lymphocyte populations, as well as the distinctive effector molecules that are triggered into production following interaction of these cells with specific antigen, are detailed in this volume.

In view of the spectre of immunoglobulin that had so long presided over investigations of cellular immunity, much as our community conscience, it is no small irony that the effector molecules themselves turn out, in fact, to be neither immunoglobulins nor specific in their diverse functions. The effector molecules so far delineated seem to be well on the way toward isolation and identification; we should soon also have an unequivocal demonstration of their relevance to *in vivo* reality.

PREFACE

Not so neat and tidy is the status of the inductive phase of cell-mediated immunity, nor its elusive corollary: the nature of the receptor site for antigen. A balance sheet has emerged from the deliberations on the receptor site with evidence presented for the recurrent postulate of an immunoglobulin receptor. While it is conceded that thymic cells do indeed have surface immunoglobulins, whether such Ig actually functions as a receptor site is still unsettled. This conflict hopefully represents the last phase of ambiguity confronting cellular immunity. Although this particular aspect of the problem is still far from resolved, the points at issue are being dissipated by experimental evidence that is now accumulating at an accelerated tempo.

This conference made clear the magnitude of the contributions arising from current *in vitro* methodology. It also underscored the extent to which these methods now limit the types of experiments that can be designed, and the rate of progress. The organization of workshops as a means of dealing with this issue was thus a natural outcome of this critical assessment. The first of a projected series of such workshops sponsored by the National Institute of Allergy and Infectious Diseases has been scheduled for later this year. Its aim will be to standardize the known effector molecules of cellular immunity and assay them interchangeably in the various *in vitro* systems currently used for their detection. The expectation is that such an interaction will lead to refinement of existing methodology and before very long the development of new and more precise *in vitro* models.

It is noteworthy that a conference primarily concerned with basic mechanisms of cellular immunity should yield a product indispensible to understanding and effectively dealing with the broad area that encompasses transplantation immunity, autoimmune disease, immunological surveillance of neoplastic cells, and recovery from intracellular microbial infections. In this field, it is now commonplace that the results of even the most esoteric and obscure investigative approaches arouse widespread interest and find prompt application to clinical investigation and treatment of disease. There may be a moral to these developments; this turn of events emerged from such unpromising beginnings that even those totally committed to this problem would not have predicted such a felicitous outcome.

PREFACE

Thus, the future looks bright. Although the tasks ahead are demanding and difficult, the goals as defined in this volume are surely attainable. The recurrent theme of these deliberations would strongly suggest that the message may be, after all, in the medium.

Scotland, Connecticut
August, 1969

H. Sherwood Lawrence
Maurice Landy

INTRODUCTORY NOTE

The increasingly urgent problems of assessing and integrating the fast-paced and diverse advances in immunology are now deeply felt by all involved in this discipline. As a meaningful adjunct to providing research grant support, the National Institute of Allergy and Infectious Diseases has sought to further facilitate the optimal development of immunolgy by a series of international conferences, planned and organized to deal imaginatively with the major issues in this field. There is at present a surfeit of meetings, both general and specialized for the conventional presentation of research reports; few indeed are primarily concerned with analysis and assessment of progress in the key areas of immunology. Accordingly, these conferences have been developed to help meet this need, with a view to exploring and interpreting the present status in significant areas of immunology, the urgent problems still unresolved, and the directions of promise; in this respect they constitute an experiment in communication.

The organization of this conference was generally similar to the preceding one on immunological tolerance. The conferees totaled 38 and represented many of the key investigators in cellular immunity and a number from related fields as well. The subject area was loosely structured into six half-day sessions. There were no formal papers or reports; the only prior assignments were for the discussion-introducers to develop in an imaginative and provocative way the background information and primary issues in their particular specialties. Their synthesis of significant information served as a springboard for uninhibited interchange among the participants under the guidance of chairmen who sought to utilize to advantage the give-and-take of free discussion for maximum development of each topic. Expert stenotyping recorded the entire dialogue and each contributor had the opportunity to edit his remarks promptly. The voluminous transcript was edited with primary emphasis on increased readability for a large and diverse audience, while seeking to retain the flavor and character of the individual contributions.

This conference, the second of a series, has served to affirm the original view of its value for dealing with challenging subject areas by utilizing a distinctive

INTRODUCTORY NOTE

format and maximal reliance on dynamic interactions among a relatively small group of experts in an ideal environment. The conference itself proved to be of unusual benefit to the participants in affording exceptional opportunities for exchange of ideas, data, and points of view. This volume, the refined product of this entire experience, brings to immunologists generally a record of progress and prospects in what has become a most exciting and important part of immunology.

Brook Lodge provided an ideal environment, contributing importantly to the success of the conference. This was reflected in the relaxed and very effective interchange among the conferees that continued well beyond the scheduled sessions. The cooperation of the Upjohn Company in again making the Brook Lodge facility available is deeply appreciated.

Bethesda, Maryland
August, 1969

Maurice Landy
Chief, Allergy and Immunology Branch
Extramural Programs, National Institute of
Allergy and Infectious Diseases

CONTENTS

CONFEREES vii
PREFACE ix
INTRODUCTORY NOTE xiii

I. Situations Leading to Lymphocyte Activation 1
   Session Chairman: Dr. Goran Möller
   Discussion Introducer: Dr. Kurt Hirschhorn

II. Basis of Induction in Cellular Immunity Contrasted with Antibody Production 71
   Session Chairman: Dr. Byron H. Waksman
   Discussion Introducer: Dr. N. Avrion Mitchison

III. Specific Recruitment of Immunocompetent Cells by Transfer Factor 143
   Session Chairman: Dr. Robert A. Good
   Discussion Introducer: Dr. H. Sherwood Lawrence

IV. Elaboration of Effector Molecules by Activated Lymphocytes 247
   Session Chairman: Dr. Rupert E. Billingham
   Discussion Introducer: Dr. Barry R. Bloom

V. Varied Effects of Lymphocyte Products Ranging from Destruction of Target Cells to Activation of Lymphocytes and Macrophages 321
   Session Chairman: Dr. Arthur M. Silverstein
   Discussion Introducer: Dr. Gale A. Granger

VI. Speculations on the Nature of Antigen Recognition by Thymic Lymphocytes and Its Consequences 407
   Session Chairman: Dr. Lewis Thomas
   Discussion Introducer: Dr. Jonathan W. Uhr

ABBREVIATIONS 455
AUTHOR INDEX 457
SUBJECT INDEX 459

I
SITUATIONS LEADING TO LYMPHOCYTE ACTIVATION

Specific versus non-specific lymphocyte stimulants — Lymphocyte stimulation as an expression of a general biological response of cells — Established lymphocytic cell lines — Reversibility of activation and the "point of no return" — Situations requiring lymphocyte-macrophage interaction for triggering a response — Obligatory requirement of immunogen for triggering signal — Stereospecific requirements of the receptor site excludes "cell-associated" antibody — Temporal sequence of events in lymphocytes immediately following uptake of antigen — Triggering of lymphocytes does not necessarily lead to cell division — Culture of murine lymphocytes; their versatility for study of cellular immunity — Distinctive capacity of normal lymphocytes for recognition of alloantigens — Low frequency of sensitized lymphocytes responding to conventional antigens — Very high frequency of normal lymphocytes responding to alloantigens — Specific activation versus amplification of lymphocyte responses.

I. LYMPHOCYTE ACTIVATION

DR. HIRSCHHORN: Much of the current progress of research in cellular immunity and the dynamic state of affairs in this field grew out of the development of <u>in vitro</u> systems for culturing small human peripheral blood lymphocytes. Accordingly, it is this basic model that seems so disarmingly simple but is actually very complex that I propose to discuss.

The response of the lymphocyte to various stimulants can be measured by any of several techniques. One of these is morphologic, involving observation by light microscopy of enlargement of such lymphocytes with the formation of new basophilic, pyroninophylic cytoplasm. A change in the nucleus is the first thing actually observable. This change is from a strongly heterochromatic nucleus to a euchromatic nucleus; one which stains diffusely with a nuclear stain such as acetic orcein. Other techniques for measuring lymphocyte response include radioactive thymidine incorporation into DNA, measured after several days in culture, and uridine incorporation into RNA, generally measured at an earlier time. Recently, in our laboratory, Waithe has developed an alternative technique for measuring the response, utilizing C_{14} leucine incorporation into microcultures. In our experience this appears to be the most reproducible and easiest technique for measuring the response of lymphocytes.

The list of agents that activate or transform lymphocytes is given in Table 1; these are so-called nonspecific stimulants, nonspecific only in reference to lymphocytes. This

---

EDITORS' FOOTNOTE: The designations "activation," "transformation," and "derepression," were used interchangeably, in a purely operational sense, to encompass the complex series of events expressed as macromolecular synthesis, transition to lymphoblasts, and subsequent cell division initiated in small lymphocytes, either by specific antigen, plant mitogens or an array of still other lymphocyte stimulators.

CELLULAR IMMUNITY

TABLE 1

Lymphocyte Stimulants

<u>Nonspecific</u>

Phytohemagglutinin, pokeweed, concanavalin A,

streptolysins, staphyloccal α-toxin,

anti-lymphocyte serum, anti-γ-globulin,

anti-allotype serum (semi-specific),

Hg^{++}, UV, ultrasound

Antigen-antibody complexes

<u>Specific</u>

Bacterial, fungal and viral antigens,

other protein and non-protein antigens,

allogeneic cells and cell products, HLA antigens

---

does not mean that they stimulate any other kind of cell. The list starts with phytohemagglutinin (PHA), originally reported by Nowell in 1960. This converts small lymphocytes into large cells, which divide about three days after the beginning of culture. More recent work has led to the recognition of several other plant mitogens, the best known of which is the pokeweed mitogen (PWM) which has the distinctive property of producing a group of cells very rich in endoplasmic reticulum. Next in this listing are certain bacterial toxins, such as the nonantigenic streptolysin S and staphylococcal alpha toxin that have been shown to be membrane-labilizing agents by Weissmann and others. Next are antilymphocyte serum (ALS) and antigamma globulins, both

I. LYMPHOCYTE ACTIVATION

specific and nonspecific ones. A rather interesting recent observation is that mercuric ion is another nonspecific stimulant; it may prove to be especially informative about some receptor sites. The last in this category are the antigen-antibody complexes; these were used by us initially to obtain some idea of just how nonspecific stimulants could be. In view of the fact that a number of these agents seem to act simply by doing something to the membrane, we decided to use immune complexes since they are known to damage membranes. They proved to be quite stimulatory for lymphocytes even when these cells were from individuals not sensitive to the antigens present in the complexes. The question of whether complement is necessary for this response is not completely settled. It seems to be necessary in our work, but the experience of our chairman has been different. It is, however, of particular interest that supernatants of precipitable antigen-antibody complexes, made in the presence of complement, are also stimulatory. This is what might be expected if we were dealing with something like anaphylatoxin.

The specific stimulants consist, of course, of antigens of various kinds, cultivated with cells derived from individuals known to be sensitive to these antigens. They include bacterial and viral products and various other antigens, both protein and non-protein. A special class of specific stimulants are allogeneic cells and, as has been recently shown, purified HLA antigens. Specific stimulants evoke a response with a somewhat different time course. The nonspecific stimulants generally result in maximal incorporation of thymidine at about three days, although antigen-antibody complexes take perhaps a bit longer. In contrast, response to specific antigens reaches a maximum at about five days, and the response to allogeneic cells is even slower, continuing to increase until about seven days.

Inhibitors of the aforementioned process of stimulation or activation are identified in Table 2. I will not discuss the various substances that interfere with RNA synthesis or protein synthesis. The list includes steroids, as would be expected in considering a lymphoid system. Chloroquine shares with steroids one particular property, namely stabilization of membranes. Ouabain is known to interfere with the ATPase controlled sodium-potassium flux at the membrane. N-acetyl-galactosamine gives another clue to the varied types of receptors that are on the cell. Amantidine, an anti-viral substance, also acts by blocking membrane receptors.

TABLE 2

Lymphocyte Inhibitors

Corticosteroids, chloroquin,

Ouabain, N-acetyl-galactosamine,

amantidine,

inhibitors of RNA and protein synthesis,

trypsin inhibitors

With this as background, I would like to delineate step by step what happens to the small lymphocyte once it meets one of these stimulants; first, what is known presently; secondly, what may be surmised; and third, what needs further work in the immediate future.

The first thing that happens is, of course, attachment of the stimulant. We know, for example, that with N-acetyl-galactosamine we can prevent attachment of PHA, in which event stimulation does not occur. Attachment implies recognition of the stimulating substance, i.e. that cells capable of responding to stimulants bear receptors. Some of these receptors may have sugar moieties, some sulfhydryl groups, and for specific antigens these receptors most probably simply represent the business end of an antibody molecule. One of the very first things that seems to happen following attachment, is a marked increase in lipid turnover and the incorporation of various moieties into phospholipids at the membrane. Recently, my wife, Dr. Rochelle Hirschhorn, in Weissmann's laboratory, has studied a number of the early events in lymphocyte stimulation. For example, she has shown that cyclic AMP, as well as dibutyryl-cyclic

I. LYMPHOCYTE ACTIVATION

AMP and theophyllin, and interestingly also adenosine, AMP and ATP, are all capable of inhibiting PHA stimulation. On the other hand, cyclic AMP, but not adenosine and the non-cyclic derivatives, is capable of inducing a small degree of stimulation of these cells in the absence of PHA. It is, therefore, possible that the membrane cyclases may be involved in the initial events. Similarly, since Ouabain is inhibitory, the ATPase pump may somehow be involved in the early events.

The next event, again shown by R. Hirschhorn, is respiration dependent pinocytosis, which occurs virtually immediately upon the addition of a stimulant. Increased neutral red uptake can be blocked by a variety of inhibitors such as cyanide, or by heating or cooling the cell. These kinds of changes have been described not only for lymphocytes, but also for the membranes of a number of other cell types that have changed from a resting to a suddenly metabolizing or dividing form. This may in fact be the very first indication that something significant is happening at the membrane.

The question that naturally arises and which I think is crucial, is what has this event to do with stimulation? Similar events apparently occur in a variety of systems besides lymphocytes. For example, in isolated liver cells studied by Jacquot that can be made to suddenly synthesize large amounts of glucose-6-phosphatase and glycogen in the presence of corticosteroids, it has been shown that these steroids attach to the membrane and very rapidly find their way into the cell. In fact, they end up in the nucleus of these cells. In other steroid-induced cells it can be shown that the intracellular steroid is incorporated into a 5S piece, and that it carries some binding material with it. Is this binding material the receptor site, and does active pinocytosis of the receptor itself represent the de-repressing or inducing stimulus for these cells? This would, of course, constitute a very neat system for specific stimulation if a specific antibody, i.e. a specific receptor site could be introduced into the cell in order to direct it and tell it what to do. In the case of nonspecific stimulation this would also fit rather nicely, because these systems that seem exceedingly variable could then all be working toward a single sequence of events.

Several other early events have been described by Mirsky's laboratory such as the phosphorylation of nucleoproteins and the acetylation of histones. An especially important early event, in my opinion, is the formation of so-called secondary lysosomes from pinocytotic vacuoles containing within them lysosomal enzymes. From the work of Dr. Z. Cohn and others, it is known that secondary lysosomes are more labile than so-called virgin lysosomes that have not been involved in digesting anything. Dr. R. Hirschhorn has found that there is a rapid shift of lysosomal enzymes from within granular fractions into the free supernatant following stimulation. Moreover, the granular fractions isolated after stimulation had a leakier membrane when exposed to labilizing agents, than did granular fractions obtained before PHA stimulation. It has been shown that the template activity for exogenous or endogenous RNA polymerase found in isolated rat liver nuclei is increased by incubation with trypsin. Lysosomes contain a trypsin-like cathepsin, and Dr. R. Hirschhorn has shown that the nuclei of unstimulated lymphocytes can be made to increase their template activity when exposed to trypsin. Similarly, the nuclei isolated from PHA-stimulated cells show greater template activity, using exogenous RNA polymerase, than do the nuclei of unstimulated lymphocytes. Stimulation can be blocked if the cells are cultured in the presence of antitrypsin agents. Template activity is measured by the incorporation of labeled RNA precursors in the presence of nuclei or chromatin and RNA polymerase. A number of workers have shown that there is, in fact, a massive increase of RNA synthesis very early following stimulation. Of particular interest is the very recent work by Dr. Cooper at the NIH in which he has studied not only the synthesis of RNA and the specific RNA moieties, but also its turnover. He has shown that the resting lymphocyte has large turnover of RNA; that almost all of this newly formed RNA is in a small pool of nuclear RNA of the polydispersed variety, while ribosomal RNA, which represents most of the RNA in the cell, turns over rather slowly, representing only two to four percent of the newly formed RNA. Within an hour, and possibly even less, after the addition of PHA, there is not only a marked increase in the net synthesis of RNA, but there is also a shift in the relative amount of synthesis between the nuclear polydispersed and the ribosomal RNA. The result is a 50 to

I. LYMPHOCYTE ACTIVATION

100-fold increase in net synthesis of ribosomal RNA, whereas there is only a small increase in the net synthesis of nuclear polydispersed RNA. Concurrently there occurs a rapid shift of RNA from nucleus to cytoplasm.

Does this mean that the resting lymphocyte is continuously making messengers which do not get out into the cytoplasm? Does it follow that upon stimulation some transport mechanism now becomes effective, so that some of this message now moves into the cytoplasm and can be used for protein synthesis? This would be aided by the marked increase in new ribosomes observed very early after stimulation has occurred. This type of increased RNA synthesis continues for about 20 hours, at which time the cell again goes into equilibrium, in that degradation now becomes equivalent to synthesis. At this time one cannot tell the difference between a stimulated lymphocyte and a HeLa cell in terms of the spectrum of RNA synthesized. This is reminiscent of other systems, such as the fertilized sea urchin egg in which stimulation of the membrane is followed by various events rather similar to those in the lymphocyte. Other examples include the regenerating liver following partial hepatectomy, the action of steroids on fetal liver cells, and the action of a variety of factors such as prolactin, corticosteroids and insulin on mammary gland cells in stimulating casein production.

The basic issue would therefore seem to be that lymphocyte stimulation is but one example of a general cell biological system, rather than a very special or unique mechanism. Just as has been well established in many other systems I think it represents a switch from a resting cell to a rapidly metabolizing cell. Following RNA synthesis, the cells begin to make proteins; Waithe has shown that within two to four hours there is a detectable rise in protein synthesis. The specificity and number of proteins that are made is just beginning to be studied. Increased activity of enzymes has also been demonstrated, although some of these may merely be activated rather than synthesized. Immunoglobulins are certainly made by these cells, there is no relative increase; however, there is an absolute increase of IgG synthesis along with many other kinds of protein. Additionally, there appears to be a host of special factors elaborated, such as the macrophage inhibitory factor, a cytotoxic factor, a cell stimulatory factor, interferon, and transfer factor. We will surely hear much more about these later on. Among the new proteins being made are the enzymes in new lysosomes that are manufactured sometime between 24 and 48 hours after stimulation. One can see a massive increase in "phase-dense" bodies that have newly synthesized acid phosphatase and a variety of other enzymes in them. As far as I know, no one has any idea about the significance of these new lysosomes. Do they leak? Do they release a nuclease or some other controlling factors that could perhaps lead to the next step, the initiation of the S period, the initiation of new DNA synthesis in preparation for division?

Generally these cells divide, although by no means all of them. Among the stimulated cells many will eventually divide, but some more rapidly than others. The question that is next asked is what the process of division means with respect to these cells. There are two kinds of systems of induction that have been studied. There are those that require at least one division before the cell becomes specialized. Such an example was reported recently by Globerson and Feldman who demonstrated that <u>in vitro</u> secondary immune responses require at least one division. Casein production by mammary cells also requires at least one division following appropriate stimulation. There are other systems, however, such as, cultured liver cells that seem ready to be turned on in the appropriate direction anytime. The stimulant simply allows the cell to make more of a particular product. Consequently the question of division becomes a very critical one. What can the cell do before it divides and in what respect does it differeniate during the time of DNA synthesis, when all the genes presumably become stripped of repressors and certain ones are likely to become active? Is it possible that delayed hypersensitivity or cellular immunity can occur in the absence of division, whereas the process of antibody synthesis or antibody secretion requires prior cell division? These are some of the questions I would pose for which we urgently need answers. Does division have yet another role in these cells? For instance, it is possible that rapid division in some of these cells eventually leads to their death. This would in effect be a control mechanism that can close down such a system when it is no longer required.

I. LYMPHOCYTE ACTIVATION

Such control could, of course, be achieved by shutting off the production of an essential component. However, it can also be accomplished by killing the cells, an event that seems to take place in plasma cells following a massive immune response.

This question of regeneration and death leads me to the basic issue of the stem cell for the variety of cells that we call small lymphocytes. I think there are some experimental data that may give us some clues as to the identity of the stem cell. Dr. Glade in our laboratory, and previously in collaboration with Dr. Chessin at NIH, developed a culture system in which lymphocyte cell lines could be established with as little as 10 ml of peripheral blood from individuals who were undergoing a lymphoproliferative phase of a disease. Originally this work was with cells from patients with infectious mononucleosis, which involves a lymphoproliferative phase with atypical lymphocytes in the circulation. What are these atypical cells? When transferred to a tissue culture environment for a few weeks, in 30-50 percent of cases they begin to divide. Two years later some of these cultures have not yet stopped dividing and still have a generation time of about 12 hours. They seem to have become permanently established, retaining their HLA specificity, retaining various genetic polymorphic markers, they remain diploid, despite their removal from in vivo homeostatic control mechanisms.

We have recently been able to duplicate the establishment of "permanent" lymphocyte lines with peripheral lymphocytes from patients with a variety of other lymphoproliferative situations such as hepatitis, mumps, herpes zoster, herpes simplex; and, interestingly, Boeck's sarcoid. One thing I have become fairly certain of is that the Epstein-Barr virus has little to do with all this. What I think has everything to do with these remarkable developments is the particular kind of cell that one encounters in the peripheral blood during these lymphoproliferative situations. I believe this cell to be a mobilized stem cell. Blood samples from such individuals immediately incubated with radioactive thymidine, yield a sizable proportion of cells that are capable of making DNA. In other words, these are cells that are in a DNA synthetic cycle at the time they are taken from the peripheral blood.

There are many and varied reasons why it would be desirable to develop the knowledge and means for establishing any given blood lymphocytes into permanent culture. Dr. Moore at Roswell Park has been successful in accomplishing this. However, his procedure requires leucocytes obtained from at least one unit (500 ml) of blood, a situation which is frequently impractical. We now are exploring the possibility that minimal stimulation of normal peripheral blood lymphocytes with suboptimal doses of PHA facilitates selection for the occasional stem cell that is presumed to get into the circulation; PHA would thus favor the establishment of this rare kind of cell. The usefulness of these developments for genetic studies, for the production of antilymphocyte sera, and for providing frozen stocks of lymphoid cells for immunologic replenishment or reconstitution in immune deficiency states are, I think, impressive. From the point of view of this conference I think that the establishment of normal blood lymphocytes in continuous culture can teach us much that is meaningful about stem cells of lymphoid lines. These cells are fully functional in that they make a variety of immunoglobulins in large quantity, they are capable of phagocytizing, they make complement components, they make interferon, and they undoubtedly make a lot of other things that perhaps will give us some clues as to what a stem cell really is.

In the foregoing I have sought to develop a framework for viewing cell stimulation in the context of general cell biology, rather than trying to restrict any commentary solely in terms of lymphocytes. Most of all I have been concerned with developing an appreciation of the key sequence of events that leads to lymphocyte activation: membrane attachment, membrane activation, pinocytosis, lysosome leakage, enzymic increase of template activity, formation of new RNA with a shift of the type of RNA, the synthesis of new proteins, the start of DNA synthesis, cell division; and then, the crucial decisive events that determine either cell death or continued growth.

CHAIRMAN MÖLLER: Now that Dr. Hirschhorn has delineated our subject area, we will seek to develop our discussion so as to explore the basic question of whether there is a difference between induction leading to cell-mediated immunity and humoral antibody synthesis, respectively. In

I. LYMPHOCYTE ACTIVATION

the latter situation, we have a good model for initiation in the Jerne-Mitchison-Cohn hypothesis. However, there is no analogous model for cell-mediated immunity. I would like to cover particularly the following points:

1. Triggering signals; both specific and nonspecific; and their kinetics.

2. Events in activated lymphocytes

3. Relation between activation and cell-mediated immunity

DR. GELL: I want to make several points about trigger mechanisms. These remarks concern anti-allotype and anti-immunoglobulin induced blast transformation, referring to work done in collaboration with Dr. Stewart Sell. These points are, I think, relevant to two aspects: one is on the effect of complexes, and the other is on the nature of the trigger, and also the point of no return, that is, irreversibility, in which we have been most interested. In the allotype system, we have a system which we can stop at any time between the initiation of an experiment and the onset of DNA synthesis. In allotype systems based on AB 4 cells, and anti-AB 4 rabbit antibody, blast transformation occurs in two or three days. If, in addition to the anti-AB 4 serum, i.e., the cell-donor's own serum AB 4 gamma globulin is added, it will block the effect.

This can be done in a time-wise fashion. We find that the blocking is virtually complete up to about 12 hours, and after that it continues with diminishing effect up to 36 hours and is no longer possible at 48 hours. Naturally, the effect varies somewhat according to the individual serum used, depending on the binding affinity of the antibodies present. One can produce the blocking effect in various ways. First of all, antiserum can be added followed by the antigen, which will block that antiserum in equivalent amounts, larger amounts, lesser amounts, and so on. The blocking is considerable up to quite a late period, and is almost complete for the first 12-24 hours.

As regards the "point of no return" i.e., irreversibility, a great many things are certainly happening in the cells in the first 8-12 hours, including the production of RNA, as Dr. Hirschhorn has told us. We have not looked for this in blocked systems, but we intend to. From all this it is a reasonable assumption that the point of no return for a given cell coincides with the onset of DNA synthesis; up to this time blast formation can be prevented or reversed by competition between free antigen and cell-receptor antigen for the stimulating anti-allotype antibody. If stimulated cells are washed free of anti-allotype serum instead of adding blocking antigen, there occurs a considerable reduction of the response up to about eight hours, though the reduction is not so marked nor so late as with active blocking with antigen. We have successfully used a whole range of different ratios of antibody to blocking antigen without finding any signs of stimulation by the complexes which must form under these conditions.

There is still another approach which is relevant to the trigger, because I think it tells us something about what is happening on the surface of the cell. The anti-allotype antibody which unites with cell receptors has allotypic markers of its own. It is thus possible to use an antiserum which does not react with the cell itself but does react with the antibody molecule attached to the cell. In these circumstances (this is what we call the "piggyback" effect) there results a striking increase in the amount of stimulation of the cells; sometimes an antiserum which on its own gives virtually no stimulation, can with this augmentation, yield marked stimulation. So it looks as if this piling of heavy, waggly material onto the surface of the cell membrane has a tendency to push that cell into blast formation.

To return to the blocking system, these experiments are performed without added complement; consequently they do not involve cytotoxic effects on the cells. Indeed, if one blocks in this way and then restimulates, that is to say, blocking of an anti-4 antibody with AB 4 antigen then washes and restimulates the same cells, one obtains the same degree of stimulation as that in the controls. What this shows is that cells are seemingly unaffected and are still able to be stimulated. Thus, the blocking process is not to be considered simply a matter of cell death.

I. LYMPHOCYTE ACTIVATION

DR. WILSON: Dr. Gell, your piling on of waggly material, the so-called "piggyback" effect, could be the effect of antigen-antibody complexes on cell membrane, rather than binding to a site already "pre-bound" to the lymphocyte. This is an important argument because it implies that a lymphocyte can acquire a receptor site by proxy, rather than by endogenous genetic control and hence become stimulatable.

DR. HIRSCHHORN: My comment is directed to Dr. Gell. As regards the "point of no return," I consider it essential, as I believe you have done, to dissect and separate the "point of no return" for RNA synthesis and that for the initiation of DNA synthesis. I believe that these two are not necessarily related events. However, if the first is permitted to go on unchecked, it will inevitably lead to the other.

DR. GELL: I am sure Dr. Hirschhorn is absolutely right on the "point of no return." I agree that RNA synthesis may have gone a long way, but blocking of DNA synthesis can nonetheless still be effected. However, we don't actually know whether it just stops or whether it reverses. I am not even certain whether you would expect this to occur or not. There are many imponderables. What happens to the messenger that is made, but then not used? The essential point is that a great many things are happening in the cell, including for example lysosome disappearance and reappearance without the cell necessarily going on into the mitotic cycle.

DR. UHR: I want to make two points regarding the triggering signal. Once antigen has encountered the hypothetical immunoglobulin antibody on the cell surface, the stereospecific event is completed. I see no need, therefore, to have the antibody-antigen complex enter the cell at this point as suggested by Dr. Hirschhorn. In other words, the specific event is like pressing a doorbell. The bell has rung. I see no need, therefore, to take the doorbell out and throw it through the window into the house to register a signal.

CELLULAR IMMUNITY

My second point concerns Dr. Gell's interesting comments about the "point of no return." The ability to reverse anti-allotype stimulation implies a need for continued stimulation by the antiserum for a period of time in order to obtain optimal differentiation. This observation bears a striking resemblance to the stimulation of antibody-forming cells by antigen where there is now considerable evidence that continued antigenic stimulation is needed to drive the antibody forming system along at an optimal rate. I think that we have here more than a suggestion of a parallel situation.

CHAIRMAN MÖLLER: With regard to both your questions, Dr. Uhr, I think the need for continuous stimulation varies with the stimulant. Specific antigen fixes firmly to the cells and additional antigen need not be present in the medium. That is to say, the cells can be washed but will respond anyway. In contrast, other stimulants such as ALS, for example, usually have to be present continuously to effect stimulation.

DR. LANDY: Following on Dr. Uhr's cogent analogy regarding the driving force of specific antigen in antibody-producing systems, I call your attention to the possible relevance of the production of a blastogenic factor by activated lymphocytes to that specific situation. Is it not possible that such a cell product then acts, in a recruiting sense, like antigen in the familiar immune system, and thus represents a means of propelling, expanding and amplifying the initial essential reaction triggered either by antigen or by the various nonspecific lymphocyte stimulating agents we are discussing? It seems to me such a factor would play a very important part in accounting for the eventual magnitude attained by the entire process. Although but few reports have appeared on this kind of lymphocyte product, I would imagine that Dr. Hirschhorn is familiar with the actual progress of the work; perhaps he could summarize it for us.

DR. HIRSCHHORN: Actually not very much has been done. Most of the work has dealt with blastogenic factors that will stimulate cells that are different in their HLA

I. LYMPHOCYTE ACTIVATION

specificity. This may simply be the production of transplantation antigens within this system, in which case I don't think the findings would be particularly relevant. There has been a report of a nonspecific blastogenic factor, and the nature of this is not at all understood.[†]

As regards Dr. Uhr's comment on entry of immune complexes into the cell, it was not my intention to imply that antigen-antibody complex is itself pinocytosed. The point I wanted to make was whether the receptor site itself must be internalized in order to turn on the rest of the system. I think this possibility ought to receive further consideration

DR. CHESSIN: I would like to present some new data relevant to the discussion on "triggering" signals. We have observed that, in contrast to protein antigens, the purified soluble specific substances, i.e., Pneumococcus Types III, VII, and XIV and Vi polysaccharides, do not display blastogenic activity against lymphocytes of individuals immunized with these antigens. However, SSS type specific immune complexes or washed, heat-killed pneumococci do induce blastogenesis in lymphocyte cultures. This suggests to me that in the case of these complex, high molecular weight polysaccharide antigens, cellular recognition probably depends on the state and form in which the antigen is presented to the lymphocytes.

In studying patients with drug induced "Lupus" syndromes, we have recently observed that heterologous DNA in the presence of the sensitizing drugs (e.g. Ampicillin, Isoniazid, Hydralazine, Butazolidine and Procaine amide) can transform the circulating lymphocytes of such patients. The observation that DNA in conjunction with the sensitizing drug can derepress resting cells is of special interest since it illustrates yet another type of specific interaction between pharmacologically active substances and macromolecular DNA. Of note are observations which

---

[†]See Discussion, Session III, for an extended discussion of blastogenic factor.

differentiate individuals with the so-called idiopathic "Lupus" syndrome from the drug-induced state, by utilizing the DNA itself. This is of interest in terms of the initiation of the blastogenic event, and furthermore, may be important in highlighting the differences between these two clinical entities.

I would suggest that we give special consideration to what I regard as a "naturally occurring" trigger event, namely, the ability of the small lymphocyte to proliferate in long term culture. We have found that in various lymphoproliferative states in man, the lymphocytes in the circulating pool have an increased potential for long term proliferation in vitro. The continuous cell line that evolves, is composed of a heterogeneous population of lymphoblastoid cells, which display a wide variety of cellular immune functions, e.g. phagocytosis, immunoglobulin synthesis, C'3 synthesis, and interferon production.

In several laboratories continuous lymphoid cell lines have been initiated from the peripheral blood leucocytes of normal individuals. It appears, however, that the proliferative potential of peripheral blood cells in such normal subjects is of a lower order to magnitude. I would estimate this at about one in 10^7 cells, whereas in lymphoproliferative states it is of the order of one in 10^4 cells. The lymphoblastoid cells seen in these cell lines resemble in many ways the blast cells so familiar to those of us working with peripheral lymphocytes stimulated in short term culture. The point is that these established lines are produced without the introduction of exogenous stimulants of any kind. In this respect they can be viewed as more closely approximating a natural situation.

DR. OPPENHEIM: I would like to comment on Dr. Uhr's concept of ringing the doorbell. Although I consider it attractive, I am not sure whether there is evidence available for it. Dr. Kay and I have been doing studies with antiserum to PHA. Considerable and specific inhibition of PHA stimulation can be obtained using such antisera. Moreover, it is possible to measure the time during which the anti-PHA still interferes with the first division cycle. It turns out that with anti-PHA we can block the first wave

I. LYMPHOCYTE ACTIVATION

of DNA synthesis for a period up to six hours after PHA stimulation of the lymphocytes. In contrast, washing the cells interferes with PHA stimulation for only a few minutes, and it binds cells in less than two hours. So perhaps the anti-PHA is a more efficient way of reversing the effect than simply washing the cells. Possibly the anti-PHA goes into some intracellular location and interferes with the PHA there; however this still remains to be proved. Alternatively it may compete with the cell for PHA, and pull it back out into the medium. I have heard some reports that antibodies can interfere with an antigen stimulated reaction for as long as 24 hours, but we have no data to offer in this regard.

DR. BLOOM: I would like answers to two simple questions. The first relates to Dr. Gell's comment about wagglier antigen being perhaps more effective brings up a rather crucial issue. How many molecules of antigen are required to fix to the cell in order to activate it? Are there any such data available? Is this a small or a very large number?

The second question is: In the discussion thus far it has been assumed that the antigen acts directly on the lymphocyte. There is, however, evidence that even in transformation with PHA, as in the case of antigen, the presence of another kind of cell is necessary in addition to the small lymphocyte. Is that the case, and if so, what does this suggest about the nature of the antigen interaction at the lymphocyte membrane?

DR. VALENTINE: Dr. Gell has shown that in the anti-allotype system, the continual presence of stimulant, in this case anti-allotype antibody, seems to be necessary. On the other hand, Dr. Möller has referred to the stimulation of lymphocytes by soluble antigen where it has been concluded that antigen does not have to be continually present for the response to be maintained. These studies were done by exposing the cell culture to antigen for brief periods of time. The cells were then washed and culture resumed in the absence of additional antigen. In Dr. Möller's case the issue is, has all of the antigen been removed? In all probability this has not been achieved. This may be relevant to the role of the macrophage in this response, as Dr. Bloom has indicated. Since antigen can be presented to the small lymphocyte via macrophages, a situation for which we do have evidence, and since this macrophage-associated antigen is probably a very small amount of the total antigen added to the culture, it then becomes difficult to establish whether one has indeed removed all of the antigen. This would also require removal of the macrophages with their associated antigen. Thus, caution is necessary in concluding that maximal lymphocyte proliferation can occur without the continued presence of antigen. We are accumulating evidence that if one employs small doses of antigen in such systems a decreased response is obtained upon removal of antigen-containing media and the lymphocytes continued in culture in the absence of additional antigen. This finding is in contrast to previously published evidence.

CHAIRMAN MOLLER: Washing the cells does not imply that antigen is not necessary. We know that there are cellular receptors that bind antigen and while few molecules may be taken up, antigen is nevertheless absolutely necessary.

DR. HIRSCHHORN: The work of Drs. Oppenheim and Hirsh, and studies of others as well, have shown fairly conclusively that phagocytic cells are a necessary requirement for stimulation of sensitized lymphocytes by specific antigen. However, the role of the macrophage in this system is not yet understood, at least not in the _in vitro_ system, although the cell-cell interaction demonstrated by Dr. MacFarland may give us some clues as to what is happening. On the other hand, there are now sufficient experiments to show that macrophages are not required for stimulation of lymphocytes by PHA. The number of macrophages that most investigators use in this system is not significantly different from the very small number of macrophages present in so-called "pure" systems. By culturing lymphocytes on a monolayer of glass-adherent macrophages, foci of agglomeration are effected which in turn increase stimulation. I believe that if one substituted antigen-coated polystyrene particles for macrophages in this situation, similar results would be obtained. The issues here are specific vs. nonspecific activation. It should be recalled that in the

I. LYMPHOCYTE ACTIVATION

local cutaneous delayed hypersensitivity response, the majority of cells are in fact not specifically sensitive. In this particular type of response the question of the necessity for the continued presence of antigen becomes a kind of secondary problem. It seems to me that the entire massive response of cellular immunity, once triggered by the interaction of the specific cell with its antigen, whether via macrophage or not, is largely a nonspecific event. This outcome may be related to the stimulation provided by antigen-antibody complexes referred to earlier.

DR. CHESSIN: While it has been persuasively argued that the in vitro transformation of small lymphocytes to blast-like cells reflects an individual's immunocompetence, the exact nature of the response in terms of either humoral or cell-mediated immunities still remains largely undefined. We should, of course, keep in mind that the pool of immunocompetent cells used for the great majority of studies is composed of a heterogeneous population of circulating lymphocytes of varied origin, fate, and function. Activation of these cells by the various categories of stimuli I have enumerated in Table 3, as well as the distinctive features regarding the initial binding processes to cell receptors, the cell types involved etc., are useful to the extent that they offer us clues as to the significance of each of these individual systems. These relate primarily to issues of the type and character of receptors on membranes, their frequency and their distribution. To account for the great heterogeneity of response in cell-mediated immunity, it should be emphasized that there are distinctive cell types in both the lymphocyte and the macrophage series that are involved in the wide spectrum of cell-mediated responses. It follows that these differences have important, and indeed major consequences as regards the inductive phase of the cellular immune response and possibly the eliciting phase as well.

DR. OPPENHEIM: My comments are directed to the broad issue developed by Dr. Chessin in Table 3, i.e., contrasting characteristics of the various agents and situations that lead to activation of lymphocytes. We have examined the effect of diphtheria and anti-diphtheria complexes, prepared

CELLULAR IMMUNITY

TABLE 3

DISTINGUISHING CHARACTERISTICS OF VARIOUS TYPES OF LYMPHOCYTE STIMULANTS[1]

Lymphocyte Stimulant	Reversibility of Interaction	Responding Lymphocytes		
		Adult		Cord
		Unseparated	Column Purified	
Phytomitogens	Binding complete within 30 minutes; irreversible.	Yes	Yes	No
Antigen	Neutralized by antiserum; binding complete by 24 hrs.	Yes	No[2]	No
Antigen-Antibody Complexes	Data unavailable	Yes	No	No
Anti-lymphocyte Sera	Reversibility;[3] critical interval not yet determined	Yes	Yes	Yes
Anti-allotype Serum	Binding reversible up to 12 hrs; partially after 36 hrs.	Yes	---	Yes
Mixed cells	Data unavailable	Yes	No	Yes

[1] Data supplied by Drs. Amos, Chessin, Hirschhorn, Gell and Oppenheim.

[2] Requires the presence of both peripheral blood lymphocytes and phagocytes. Several investigators have noted that even column purified lymphocyte suspensions contain between 0.1 - 2% phagocytic elements (which may represent the population of "phagocytic" lymphocytes capable of immunoglobulin synthesis.)

[3] The effects of rabbit ALS can be reversed; those of horse ALS apparently not. These situations probably involve different classes of immunoglobulins.

I. LYMPHOCYTE ACTIVATION

at equivalence, on column-purified human lymphocytes. Such complexes did not stimulate a lymphocyte response. This was also found to be true of whole heat-killed pneumococci types I and II as well. From such experiments I have the impression that the more immunogenic an antigen, the more rigorous one has to be in eliminating all the macrophages from the cultures in order to reduce their lymphocyte stimulating effects. Otherwise very immunogenic antigens stimulate ostensibly non-adherent lymphocytes because they have, in fact, not been entirely freed of phagocytic cells. We have also tested such complexes on cord blood cells of human newborns. The complexes that Dr. Leikin and I employed included one of the antigens also used by Dr. Hirschhorn and co-workers, namely, BSA-anti-BSA, as well as diphtheria-anti-diphtheria. These experiments were designed to determine whether complexes fulfill the criteria for nonspecificity in being able to stimulate uncommitted lymphocytes in the way that PHA and staphlylococcal filtrate stimulate cord leucocytes. The fact that cord lymphocytes manifest mixed cell reactions indicates that they are also capable of responding to histocompatibility antigens. However, as shown in Fig. 1, BSA-anti-BSA complexes did not stimulate lymphocytes of newborns; later on we found that diphtheria-anti-diphtheria complexes likewise were ineffective. With this methodology, we were able to demonstrate that the same complexes stimulated adult cells; this then served as a positive control. Moreover we found, in effect, the same enhanced reaction in adults stimulated by such complexes as Dr. Hirschhorn has described, and as seen by Dr. Möller with a variety of other ubiquitous antigens. We have also tested antigen-antibody complexes on lymphocytes of inbred guinea pigs. In this work we used tetanus-anti-tetanus complexes at equivalence. From the summary data given in Table 4, it is seen that cells of unsensitized guinea pigs did not respond; this finding is consistent with our data on the cells of newborn human infants. However, cells of sensitized guinea pigs responded much better to complexed antigen than to the same antigen alone. Furthermore, soluble complexes as well as precipitated complexes were effective, but in our experience the precipitates were much better stimulants than the soluble complexes.

TABLE 4

Mean tritiated thymidine incorporation by lymph node lymphocyte cultures from unsensitized and sensitized guinea pigs stimulated by preformed antigen-antibody complexes

IN VIVO STIMULATION		STIMULANT				
		Tetanus-Toxoid-antitetanus complexes			None	Tetanus Toxoid
	Complex	Mixture of Supernatant & precipitated complexes	Supernatant Complexes	Washed Precipitated complexes		
		CPM	CPM	CPM	CPM	CPM
1. Guinea Pigs Immunized with complete Freund's Adjuvant (CFA) only	1 Antibody excess	1,209	1,063	3,444	3,664	3,774
	2 Equivalence	1,612	1,026	3,298		
	3 Antigen excess	3,151	1,026	3,298		
	4 "	2,418	1,685	3,920		
	5 "	2,492	2,052	3,957		
2. Guinea Pigs sensitized with CFA and tetanus-antitetanus complexes	1 Antibody excess	2,407	2,407	12,655	3,882	8,152
	2 Equivalence	3,261	4,076	13,548		
	3 Antigen excess	5,357	5,202	13,742		
	4 "	5,318	7,531	12,927		
	5 "	7,880	6,716	12,617		

I. LYMPHOCYTE ACTIVATION

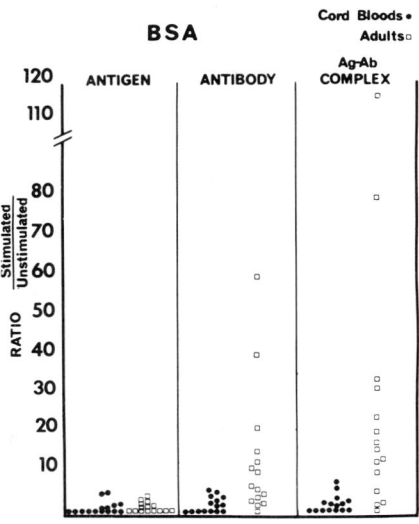

FIG. 1 Incorporation of H_3 TdR by adult and newborn human cord blood leucocyte cultures stimulated by BSA, anti BSA, and BSA-anti-BSA complexes.

By inference these observations suggest that the in vitro lymphocyte response to antigen-antibody complexes is a specific immune reaction. Complexing with antibody enhances the immunogencity of antigens. We believe that this is probably operative at the macrophage level. Complexing somehow enables the macrophage to pick up antigen and process it more readily; this is one way of facilitating the in vitro response of previously sensitized lymphocytes. We have several additional experiments substantiating this concept. With very high concentrations of BSA, we obtain a low degree of stimulation in ostensibly unsensitized adults, this is nonetheless still considerably less than that achieved by the complexed BSA. This suggests that we may be experiencing environmental sensitization or that we learn to cross react to BSA after birth. It is especially noteworthy that heat-aggregated BSA does not stimulate lymphocytes, consequently nonspecific aggregation of the antigen does not facilitate its stimulatory effects. In contrast, aggregation by antibody does facilitate stimulation and is very helpful in increasing its in vitro action as well as in vivo immunogenicity.

DR. GELL: I think it bears repeating that rabbit allotype-anti-allotype complexes are quite non-immunogenic; here we have no evidence of stimulation by complexes. The point to be made is that in considering these complexities, the species involved does make a difference. There does seem to be some evidence that human cells are rather more generally ready to react.

DR. THOR: One of the problems of major concern that has not been dealt with here relates to a progression of specific and nonspecific stimulators leading to still other events in lymphocytes. These multiple reactions require much further work in order to understand the biology of the cell at the molecular level. In considering uridine incorporation into the lymphoid cell and also the incorporation of bases into other nucleic acids, we are faced with problems for which answers may already be available in less complex systems. Spiegelman and others, using microbial cell-free systems, have already suggested some correlates of what may stimulate such kinetics and initiate the events we seek to evaluate in lymphocytes.

The progression of what is specific stimulation and what is nonspecific activation could easily be confused because many of these nonspecific stimulators may well bind to the cells in a similar manner. Specific reactions, in which we are so interested, could possibly be "turned on" by nonspecific means. To evaluate several of these lymphocyte events, we have been investigating the activities of RNA species obtained from sensitive human lymph node cells in comparison to that obtained from nonsensitive cells. Poly-U, for instance in conjunction with PHA or antigen, can change the pattern of nucleic acid synthesis. It would be helpful to re-evaluate the nonspecific and specific stimulators in terms of binding affinities, mode of attachment to cell membrane, molecular charge and size. I think that only after a much larger list of variables is investigated

I. LYMPHOCYTE ACTIVATION

would it be justifiable to view receptor sites as a kind of doorbell waiting to be rung. This viewpoint stems from recent studies in our laboratory with Poly-U specific antigenic stimulation using what we believe to be "specific" RNA extracts; the ensuing reaction was discernible in the cell much earlier than 24 hours. We now find these migration inhibition events occurring within two hours. Here too we might turn to the non-cellular models to understand what begins early in this complex reaction of getting material into the lymphocyte, since at present the macrophage only seems to complicate further this important issue.

DR. HIRSCHHORN: It would, I think, be appropriate at this point to say something about the critical nature of the medium and the particular preparation of PHA employed. In work recently completed in our laboratory by Waithe it was demonstrated that in the human system, RPMI 1640 is by far preferred among several commonly used media. He has carried out extensive fractionation of sera and also isolated a large molecule essential for cell performance in vitro; in this respect the work parallels recent findings by Adler and Smith on the culture of murine lymphocytes that will be described for us later on.

It is becoming increasingly evident that the particular PHA product used has a profound effect on the in vitro tests. In our laboratory Waithe has screened a variety of preparations including a highly purified PHA preparation recently made available by the Burroughs-Wellcome Laboratories. This refined preparation has a 25 to 1 ratio of mitogenicity vs. agglutinating potential; in this respect we have seen major differences between this purified Burroughs-Wellcome PHA and all the cruder types. In crude batches of Phaseolus vulgaris mitogen preparations there is seen a dose-related increase in stimulation followed by a plateau; with still higher concentrations, a toxic effect is evident. The more highly purified material displays the same dose-related increase; once the optimum is reached, however, even a slight further increase leads promptly to toxicity instead of a plateau. I consider this finding as being of crucial importance in considering the dissociation of RNA and DNA stimulation. While toxicity may not express itself very readily in the early events, it certainly does as regards the ability of the cells to make new DNA. It is therefore essential to establish such dose-response curves, especially when one is using a more nearly optimal system with refined mitogen.

DR. ROSENAU: We have studied the in vitro model employing nonsensitized allogeneic lymphocytes and target cells in the presence of PHA. It was, however, difficult to interpret the findings because the commercial PHA used had varied biologic activities, i.e., erythroagglutinins, leukoagglutinins, RNA and DNA synthesis-stimulating effects. Dr. Goldberg and I have, therefore, gone on to fractionate PHA with a view to obtaining preparations with only a single activity. Protein fractionation procedures yielded fractions that had several biologic activities. Subsequently we observed that the RNA-and DNA synthesis-stimulating activities resisted boiling in crude extracts and were resistant to 8 M urea, suggesting that these two activities are not proteins. It was then sought to remove the protein from PHA by means of the fractionation procedures given in Table 5. We assayed the RNA-and DNA synthesis-stimulating activities (abbreviated as RSSA and DSSA) by measuring incorporation of uridine-H_3 and thymidine-H_3 into acid-precipitable fractions of pig lymphocytes. Fraction IV, has considerably less than one percent of the original protein, and a greatly reduced content of carbohydrate; erythro-and leuko-agglutinating activates are absent. The RNA-and DNA synthesis-stimulating activities are decreased about 25% and 12% respectively. Thus we have obtained an almost deproteinized preparation and yet have retained most of the RNA- and DNA synthesis-stimulating activities. Fraction IV was then digested with pronase for 120 hours, more pronase being added at intervals. Neither treatment with RNase and DNase, effected a decrease of RNA-and DNA synthesis-stimulating activity. The two activities in fraction IV were not dialyzable; both were affected by treatment with sodium periodate, but the DNA synthesis-stimulating activity was more sensitive, suggesting that these two activities were separate entities. Accordingly, we believe that the RNA- and DNA synthesis-stimulating activities in commercial PHA are neither proteins nor large molecular nucleic acids.

I. LYMPHOCYTE ACTIVATION

TABLE 5

Purification of Nucleic Acid Stimulating Activities of Phaseolus vulgaris

Fraction	Vol. (ml)	RSSA		BSSA		Protein	Carbohydrate
		Activity/ml	Total activity ($\times 10^{-6}$)	Activity/ml	Total activity ($\times 10^{-6}$)	ug/ml	ug/ml
Crude Extract (Fraction I)	183	43,400	7.9	29,600	5.4	1500	1600
Perchloric Acid Supernatant (Fraction II)	250	33,400	8.3	22,900	5.6	830	650
Ethanol PPT (Fraction III)	183	36,300	6.6	17,000	3.1	93	37
Post-Sevag Treatment (Fraction IV)	112	32,600	3.7	26,100	2.9	2	22

The activity per ml is five times the quantity: the number of counts per minute incorporated into lymphocyte nucleic acids minus that incorporated by a control incubated with saline instead of a Phaseolus extract. Such saline control cultures incorporate about 2,200 CPM per culture into RNA and about 810 CPM per culture into DNA.

DR. LANDY: It is of course essential that we know in chemical terms the nature of the plant mitogen structures responsible for their profound effect on lymphocytes. However, I would point out that most workers have encountered great difficulties in seeking to isolate and identify the biologically active transforming moiety in PHA. In contrast, the pokeweed mitogen (PWM) has proved quite amenable to physicochemical studies and Drs. Chessin, Borjeson, Reisfeld and colleagues at the NIAID have actually achieved characterization of this particular mitogen. Dr. Chessin could provide us with the salient features of the PWM molecule.

DR. CHESSIN: I would reemphasize Dr. Landy's statement that much of the work on the purification of the PHA has encountered great difficulties. Consequently, even now rathe rather little is known regarding its chemical structure. In contrast, work by our group at NIAID (Borjeson et al., J. Exp. Med. 124, 859, 1966; Reisfeld et al., Proc. Nat. Acad. Sci., 58, 2020, 1967) resulted in the isolation and the physicochemical characterization of the pokeweed phytomitogen from Phytolacca americana. Purified PWM is a homogeneous glycoprotein containing approximately 3% of a sugar moiety, but no sialic acid; its molecular weight is 32,000. It is distinctive in its high content of cysteine and the 33 disulfide bridges in this rigid molecule. It is now a matter of record that PWM differs markedly in many of its biologic properties from the other plant lectin PHA, although its erythro-and leukagglutinating activities are of a generally similar range. Dr. Rosenau's finding that his products resisted pronase in noteworthy in view of the fact that all of the preparations thus far tested, including the ones we ourselves use in our assay systems, are all sensitive to pronase and are readily destroyed by it.

DR. HIRSCHHORN: I would again caution against measuring DNA synthesis-stimulating activity, as this is a secondary event. When one separates the two activities, one may well be stopping the cell at a particular moment due to toxic factors. In purifying PHA, one may be purifying a toxic factor as well, or else diluting out some stabilizing principle that keeps the cell membranes sufficiently integrated for survival. I personally doubt whether anyone has

I. LYMPHOCYTE ACTIVATION

in effect separated these two activities unless it can be shown that DNA synthesis can be induced by adding a DNA synthetic stimulant at the appropriate time during culture.

DR. ROSENAU: As regards the two activities that I referred to, in protein containing fractionations, it was our belief that we were dealing with adsorption of these activities to protein.

DR. AMOS: I would like to contribute some additional information on another lymphocyte stimulant, the streptococcal factor investigated in our laboratory by Janet Plate and which Dr. Hirschhorn listed as SLS. The factor is very clearly distinct from streptolysin S. It seems to be a carbohydrate; purified fractions have no detectable protein. In kinetic studies the number of cells initially responsive is probably in the order of one in 1,000 to one in 10,000. This agent, therefore, appears to be very selective in terms of the number of cells stimulated. This substance is generally considered to be a nonspecific agent, because it will stimulate fetal cord cells, but we have begun to question this. The most highly purified preparation separated by chromatography produced both immediate and delayed type of hypersensitivity reactions in a subject hyperimmunized to the parent organism but failed to do so in a subject not so sensitized. Accordingly, I wonder if the highly purified preparations of PHA or PWM are antigenic in man. As far as I know this has not yet been ascertained.

DR. OPPENHEIM: It has been demonstrated that PHA can certainly behave as an antigen in man. Dr. Astaldi and others have shown that intradermal administration of PHA usually results in typical delayed hypersensitivity reactions in man. Furthermore, when he treated some patients with aplastic anemia with homologous PHA-transformed lymphocytes, they developed antibodies to PHA.

DR. MARSHALL: I agree that the antigenicity of PHA has been clearly demonstrated, but this is not to say that the antigenic part of the molecule is the same as the mitogenic site. Presumably, since it is a molecule extracted from beans, there are many sites which are antigenic to man, even on the mitogenically active molecule, and that a coating of antibody to these sites then interferes secondarily with the function of the mitogenic site. This concept of the antigenicity of PHA is not the same as that envisioned by Dr. Amos.

Furthermore, when considering the skin reactions there are difficulties in interpreting the results in these terms. For example, stimulatory agents such as PHA which are classified as "nonspecific" could be predicted to give delayed skin reactions. Contact between randomly segregated lymphocytes and PHA at the site of injection would surely cause blast transformation and the production of all the lymphocyte factors which, in vitro, appear to be mediators of delayed hypersensitivity. These would then produce the red spot.

In fact, the picture may be even more complex since Pearmain and Lycette showed that intradermal injection of undiluted Difco PHA M produced typical immediate hypersensitivity reaction. I am unable to explain this, but have seen an immediate reaction produced in this way.

DR. TURK: There are some who have doubts about the connection between these plant products, their effects in vitro on lymphocytes, and cellular immunity. Since the question has been raised regarding the relevance of the mitogen experiments to delayed hypersensitivity I would like at this time to identify an experiment of ours which I hope would help provide such assurance. We have been studying skin-reactive factors that are produced in vitro by specifically sensitized lymphocytes interacting with antigen in the same general way Dr. Bloom has used and he will describe later on. Drs. Pick and Krejci in my laboratory have found that normal lymphocytes incubated in vitro with PHA also release into the medium a factor which when injected intradermally into guinea pigs produces skin reactions very much like delayed hypersensitivity reactions. The character of the dermal reaction is entirely similar to those produced by incubating specifically sensitized cells with antigen. Later on I will discuss this work in

I. LYMPHOCYTE ACTIVATION

greater detail. For now I would only say that it remains to be determined whether the active factor in these tests will prove to be similar to the one released by antigen from specifically-sensitized lymphocytes. The point I want to make at this juncture is that this experiment attests to the validity of the in vitro PHA-lymphocyte model and its relevance to delayed hypersensitivity, the area of our particulr concern.

CHAIRMAN MÖLLER: I think we should shift our discussion to the aspect of the specificity of the triggering signal. There is now a consensus that in cell-mediated immunity immunogenic molecules are required for elicitation as well as induction. This is in marked contrast to the situation in humoral immunity where hapten alone can suffice. Moreover, even in the extreme example where presensitized cells are examined in in vitro models, immunogenic preparations are required for elicitation of the responses we associate with cell-mediated immunity; why should this be? Can it be that there are different receptors involved, in antibody production as opposed to cell-mediated immunity, as has been suggested, or are there still other explanations? I would call on Dr. Schlossman to speak to this.

DR. SCHLOSSMAN: Clearly there is a difference in the specificity of sensitized cells and circulating antibody produced against the same chemically defined immunogen. These were previously described as carrier vs. hapten specificities in hapten-protein conjugate systems. However, if one analyzes the specificity of cells and antibody made to chemically-defined immunogens, one finds that the specificity of a cell for antigen cannot be accounted for by simply assuming the cellular receptor for antigen is cell-associated antibody with either a higher affinity or a larger binding site. First of all, antibodies are not made to the haptenic group alone. For example, numerous studies indicate that the humoral antibody has carrier specificity and that this carrier specificity involves a reasonably large area of the immunizing antigen adjacent to the haptenic group. Thus, both antibody and cells have carrier specificity, which we would like to define as the specificity for the immunogenic determinant used to induce the response.

However, the distinction is that the antibody will react with heterologous antigens containing portions of the determinant whereas the cellular receptor is stereospecific for the homologous immunogen used to induce the response. The problem is, why is it necessary to have an immunogenic molecule to turn on a cell whereas a molecule that reacts perfectly well with antibody but is not immunogenic or is a closely related but heterologous immunogen, is ineffective in turning on cells.

This requirement for an immunogen to trigger the sensitized cell leads us to believe that the initial cellular recognition of antigen is not mediated by conventional antibody but rather by another stereospecific molecule. The chemical nature of this molecule, or its distinction from a unique form of immunoglobulin, has not been resolved. The requirement for the same chemically-defined immunogen both to induce the immune response and to trigger the sensitized cell suggests that the elicitation of the many cellular immune responses recapitulates the induction process. If the latter view is correct, it is not surprising that the cellular immune response is exquisitely specific for the immunogen used to induce the response. The latter degree of specificity of cells led to the whole concept of carrier specificity.

In contrast, antibody-mediated reactions are much less specific since the preformed antibody molecule is capable of cross-reacting with related ligands to provoke immediate hypersensitivity reactions _in vivo_ or antigen-antibody reactions _in vitro_. The cellular immune reaction is a dynamic process, recapitulating the induction of the immune response, leading the production of biological mediators, e.g. MIF, LT, etc. THis latter response results from the interaction of a stereospecific receptor with immunogen and is different from the passive interaction of antibody with antigen. The major portion of binding energy of antibody ligand interaction is directed to a immunodominant group. In the DNP-oligolysine system the immunodominant group is the dinitrophenyl hapten. Thus, it is not surprising that anti-DNP-oligolysine antibody is reactive with many antigens containing the DNP group, e.g., DNP-HSA, DNP-BGG and non-immunogenic DNP-oligolysines, HSA, etc. However, cells derived from animals making DNP oligolysine antibody cannot

I. LYMPHOCYTE ACTIVATION

be stimulated by heterologous DNP containing compounds. This interaction requires the same chemically defined immunogen used to trigger the response.

Thus, the extraordinary difference in specificity of the antibody binding site and the cellular receptor for antigen has not provided any clues as to the nature of this receptor. However, I believe that we can rule out the <u>assumption</u> that the receptor for immunogen on the cell is simply cell-associated antibody. The receptor and/or the process of cellular recognition of antigen appears to be much more complex.

CHAIRMAN MÖLLER: This creates a problem. Either one postulates a new molecule for recognizing antigen, a highly unlikely possibility, or else one has to explain the findings in other terms, e.g. that some kind of interaction is involved, such as in the two receptor hypothesis, where each cell would have the same specificity as the antibody, but where the inductive processes require certain qualities of the antigen.

DR. SCHLOSSMAN: I think the specificity of the cell can be acccunted for by one stereospecific molecule complementary to the immunogen used to induce the sensitized cell. I find it difficult to conceive of two or three cells with separate specificity to the hapten and portions of carrier which recognize antigen and lead to the production of an antibody molecule with hapten-carrier specificity. This appears to me to be uneconomical in terms of antigen recognition and does not account for the fact that a single antibody has hapten-carrier specificity. There are many molecules with stereospecific receptors, e.g. enzymes, Haptoglobin, etc. We need not be committed to the assumption that the receptor molecule is either a single antibody or several antibodies with numerous specificities to different portions of the immunogen.

CHAIRMAN MÖLLER: But they are uninteresting since they have no variability. As I see it - in your work you make the point that there is a difference between the receptors involved in antibody synthesis and in cellular immunity.

DR. SCHLOSSMAN: No. That is not my point. I think the same receptor molecule is involved in the triggering of cells to make antibody, delayed hypersensitivity and other cellular immune responses. The interaction of cells with antigen is highly specific whereas the products of a triggered cell may be much less specific.

DR. SILVERSTEIN: I am disturbed by the way this issue has arisen. For thirty years we were confused by trying to compare delayed hypersensitivity with immediate hypersensitivity, a comparison that could not be made. Now wer are threatened with the same operational trap by the suggestion that the elicitation phase of delayed hypersensitivity may be different from the stimulatory or sensitizing stage. I see no reason to postulate that these are different.

DR. HIRSCHHORN: I would like to relate these remarks to a point first made in my introductory statement. This deals with the situation exemplified by fetal and adult hemoglobin. Derived from a similar stem cell, but separated potentially by a divisional event, we have a cell that makes not only fetal hemoglobin, but also fetal carbonic anhydrase and "i" antigen on its surface. This is in contrast to cells that make adult hemoglobin, also adult carbonic anhydrase and which have "I" antigen on its surface. These are two different cells, although derived from a similar stem cell. I would again stress in relating it to the immune system, that "cellular immunity" simply requires the recognition of an antigen, and that the initial event leading to antibody secretion into the circulation is preceded by one, or perhaps several divisions, thus making for a totally different cell. I don't want by this necessarily to say that these cells arise from different kinds of stem cells, as some have implied. I would not exclude that possibility, but I think that both situations could very well involve the same stem cells. The event of division, during which a specific kind of differentiation occurs, could produce quite a different cell type.

DR. BRAUN: One of the useful aspects of the preceding conference in this series that took place here a few months ago (Immunological Tolerance, Ed. Landy and Braun, Acad. Press, 1969).

I. LYMPHOCYTE ACTIVATION

1969) was the recognition that in the final detectable immune response one is dealing with the end result of a sequence of antigen-dependent events. In all probability something of a similar nature applies to cellular immunity as well. I wonder, therefore, it it wouldn't be useful to differentiate between the role of antigen in activation and the role of antigen in stimulation.

CHAIRMAN MÖLLER: Would you, for the record, define what you consider to be the difference between activation and stimulation?

DR. BRAUN: To me activation implies an antigen-dependent stimulus to the stem cell of potential antibody-forming clones. Stimulation involves antigen-dependent events required to drive a response to the production of antibody; a process which probably includes subsequent antigen-dependent events that convert memory cells into antibody-forming cells. Whether or not the antigen required in both these events must be identical in its molecular size and configuration is something that is still undecided, although I understand that Dr. Mitchison thinks it is the same.

The other point which I thought might be worthy of clarification, is one that is known to everyone here, but may not be evident to all the readers of the conference volume. I am referring to the fact that when we talk about specific triggering and nonspecific triggering, we are really talking about events involving two different cell populations. In specific triggering one turns on cells of particular clones. In nonspecific triggering one turns on all cells via a nonspecific stimulus. I think it is important to keep this distinction in mind.

Finally, coming back to Dr. Uhr's "doorbell" concept, I ask whether one should not consider the length of time during which the door must be kept open and whether there may be more than one door that has to be opened in order to yield the results that are being discussed here.

CELLULAR IMMUNITY

DR. BARAM: I wonder if we really need to consider that the triggering mechanism for nonspecific activation or stimulation has to be the same as it is for specific antigen stimulation. It is possible that antigen must be processed by the macrophage before it can be recognized by the lymphocytes. I think the possibility exists that nonspecific stimulation, on the other hand, acts directly on the lymphocytes. It may be that only macrophage-processed antigen-RNA complexes are capable of stimulating the lymphocytes that are specifically hypersensitive to the antigen. This would in part help explain the inability of pure polysaccharides to act as stimulators, since they are not readily handled by macrophages and may not complex to RNA. Yet the impure polysaccharides, containing protein moieties, can stimulate cells sensitive to polysaccharide. This may well be due to the formation of complexes consisting of polysaccharide-protein-RNA which can then interact with lymphocytes. Macrophage-processed polysaccaride-protein-RNA complexes may stimulate polysaccharide-sensitive lymphocytes. Nonspecific stimulators act directly on the lymphocyte. Pure lymphocyte cultures can be stimulated by nonspecific agents such as PHA. However, for specific soluble antigens to stimulate hypersensitive cells, macrophages must be present.

CHAIRMAN MÖLLER: Having explored the matter of triggering signals, both specific and nonspecific, and their distinguishing characteristics, we should now move on to identify the very earliest events in the series that are set in motion upon activation of lymphocytes.

DR. MITCHISON: The earliest change seems to be an increase in the uptake of uridine. This is apparently due to membrane changes.

DR. TURK: *In vivo* the earliest events that one can see in the small lymphocytes and lymph nodes is an increase in the number of cells, lymphocytes containing lysosomes and the number of lysosomes per lymphocyte.

I. LYMPHOCYTE ACTIVATION

CHAIRMAN MÖLLER: Yes. But in relative terms this would not be very early.

DR. TURK: Keeping in mind that these are *in vivo* changes, I would say they occur within two days. As many as 90% of the lymphocytes in draining lymph nodes now appear to contain lysosomes; this precedes the peak of blastogenesis by a considerable period.

DR. HIRSCHHORN: I think, Dr. Möller is right in focussing on the early events in the lymphocyte activation process. In seeking to deal systematically with his question I have assembled in Table 6 what, to the best of my knowledge, constitutes the early sequence of events thus far known to us. I would point out however that this itemized list is not necessarily complete. It is evident that a considerable number of highly significant events get under way during the very first hour. Yet, as we know all too well, the overwhelming preponderance of tests or assessments made by investigators continue to be concerned with changes that take place *after* 24-48 hours.

It must be emphasized that most of the events listed are not peculiar to lymphocytes. they have also been shown to occur in other diploid cells. I object strenuously to any discussion of biochemical changes in *E. coli* in the context that implies that such findings are relevant to diploid cells. As far as I am concerned, there is at this point no known relation between the two.

DR. SILVERSTEIN: I can't really convince myself that this is an important and central issue for our discussion. I think that what Dr. Hirschhorn has tabulated as the series of early key events is probably the normal biological sequence that takes place in any cell that becomes activated for whatever reason. But for that very reason I would suggest that it is not all that important. We are, after all, dealing with a biologic system or so one would hope.

TABLE 6

Early Sequence of Events in Lymphocyte Activation

Time elapsed after addition of transforming agent to lymphocytes	Individual events that become discernable
0 time	Attachment of activator to membrane
15 minutes	Membrane lipid turnover or synthesis Active pinocytosis Acetylation of histones Phosphorylation of nucleoproteins
1st hour	Leakage of lysosomal enzymes Increased nuclear template activity
2nd hour	Increased ribosomal synthesis (50-100x) Increased synthesis of polydisperse RNA (3-4x) Shift of RNA from nucleus to cytoplasm
4th hour	Increased protein synthesis
36 hours	New lysosomes Beginning of DNA synthesis
48 hours	Cell division

We have now spent considerable time discussing triggering signals, but I feel that much still remains to be clarified. What can those of us less expert in this aspect of the field bring away from this discussion? Would it be correct to conclude that there are multiple triggers for lymphoid cells; some of them, such as PHA, nonspecific and non-physiologic (and perhaps not having to do with real life), and others specific, involving antigenic interaction with a receptor? Would it be reasonable to gather that the nonspecific stimulants that have been described generally act on almost any lymphocyte and don't seem to be subject to any control, while the specific ones seem to work on a very few cells, perhaps with the spread of specific or nonspecific information?

I. LYMPHOCYTE ACTIVATION

I get the impression from some of the data brought forward that there seems also to be operative something I have not heard explicitly discussed, namely a feedback control over the number of cells which can be activated (or recruited). I would suggest that it would be surprising if there did not exist such a feedback control on the level of cellular proliferation, just as is the case in some of the later, productive stages of the immunologic response involving humoral antibody.

DR. GRANGER: Dr. Hirschhorn alluded several times to a point I consider extremely important for further discussion, namely not all cells which are activated to undergo protein synthesis need go on to DNA synthesis.

I would like to hear additional comment on this topic as we and others find that protein synthesis is intimately associated with the cytodestructive events observed in *in vitro* cell-mediated reactions. However, these events are not related to DNA synthesis.

DR. HIRSCHHORN: The only direct answer I can give to Dr. Granger is that in some systems specific inhibition of DNA-synthesis will still allow every one of the events that I have outline through a period of hours to continue uninterrupted. New lysosomes will be formed, protein synthesis will go on unabated; it is only the DNA synthesis that is shut off.

DR. COHN: In no biological system, even *E. coli*, do we know how DNA synthesis is triggered. An animal cell model which can be studied is therefore of interest quite independently of its relationship to the immune system. In the lymphocyte-PHA system it is theoretically possible to deal with the interaction between a characterized mitogen and a cell, which leads to DNA synthesis and division. The interaction is specific in that few substances induce cell multiplication. If I were studying this system, I would start by looking for the binding protein receptor for the PHA mitogen. In other words, it seems to me obvious that the events listed by Dr. Hirschhorn, including the "initial" one of pinocytosis, are in fact secondary events.

CHAIRMAN MÖLLER: It has been shown by Killander and Rigler that already at five minutes after addition of PHA there is a pronounced increase in the binding of acridine orange to the phosphate groups of DNA. In the mixed lymphocyte cultures Anderson et al. have shown (Fig. 2) that maximal acridine orange binding occurs after three hours. The triggering of this response was seen only in HLA incompatibilities (Fig. 3). This reaction would therefore seem to be the first sign of lymphocyte activation.

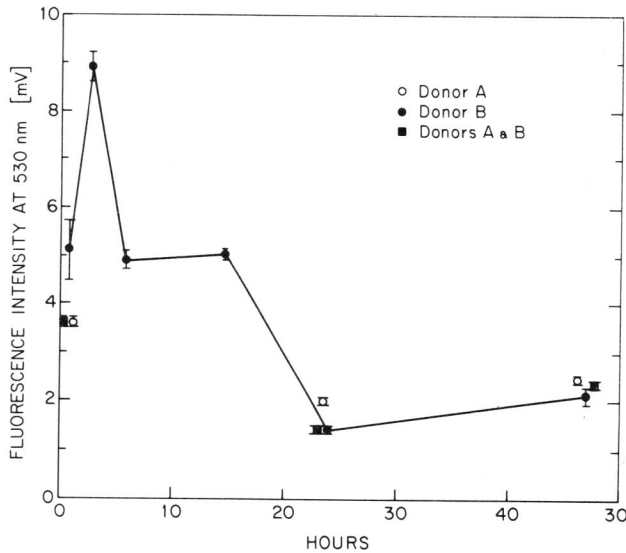

Fig. 2 Acridine orange binding by mixed allogeneic lymphocytes in culture. ·—· indicated binding intensity of mixed population. The open symbols indicate the binding in each lymphocyte population cultured alone.

I. LYMPHOCYTE ACTIVATION

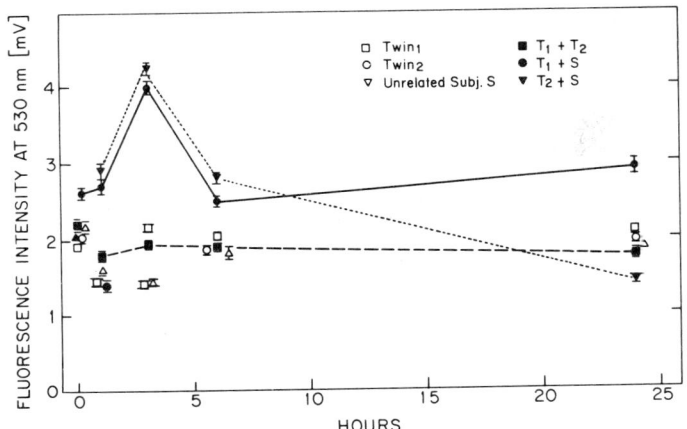

Fig. 3 Acridine orange binding in mixed lymphocyte cultures involving HLA incompatible and HLA compatible cells.

DR. BRAUN: What is known about whether the specific or non-specific triggers are signals in themselves or are merely the means for permitting something released from other cells to get into the activated, but not yet "stimulated" cell. Is there anything known about this?

CHAIRMAN MÖLLER: I think that the five-minute triggering with PHA suggests that it is an effect directly on the cell, but I know of no formal proof.

DR. LAWRENCE: Are all the cells engaged at that time?

CHAIRMAN MÖLLER: Yes, as far as can be discerned, all cells bind equally.

DR. SMITH: I would like to contribute to the identification of the sequence of events which follow lymphocyte activation by antigen, most of which lie beyond the very early phase which Dr. Hirschhorn has just summarized. To do this I must describe first a newly developed *in vitro* system for the culture of mouse lymphocytes, since this species has not been heretofore amenable to the analysis that has been possible with human, rat or rabbit lympocytes. The data I will present, obtained with Drs. Adler, Marsh and Takiguchi, indicates that this immune system provides a number of inherent advantages not shared by many other systems; it provides excellent replicate agreement and a high degree of reproducibility from day to day and from week to week.

As finally established after many trials, the system consists of RPMI 1640, an arginine-rich medium supplemented with normal human serum in a concentration of five percent. An essential requirement is that the human sera employed contain a naturally occurring antibody against mouse cells. The most suitable sera are those of low titer, whereas high titers give high background levels of reactivity. Absorption of these sera with mouse RBC renders them completely unreactive. Fresh normal human serum also contains a second component that is essential and which we designate "labile factor." It is a macromolecule (between 80 and 150 thousand molecular weight) that is resistant to exposure at 56°C for 30 minutes, but is inactivated at 60°C for one hour and does not survive storage at -20°C for one week; actually diminishing very rapidly after two or three days. Apparently what the RPMI 1640 supplies is arginine, for this amino acid is absolutely necessary for the DNA-synthesizing component of the system. Employing these conditions we found evidence of activation by PHA, by histoincompatible cells, or by antigen of mouse lymphoid cells from either spleen or lymph nodes. We see lysosome enlargement and confluence, morphologic transformation by all the criteria Dr. Hirschhorn has mentioned earlier and thymidine incorporation into DNA. Lymphoid cells in these cultures show a high degree of viability, 70 to 80% for one week, but the reation as we study it is, for all purposes, complete in 48 to 72 hours.

The time course of this reaction following PHA is illustrated in Fig. 4. This experiment shows the increase

I. LYMPHOCYTE ACTIVATION

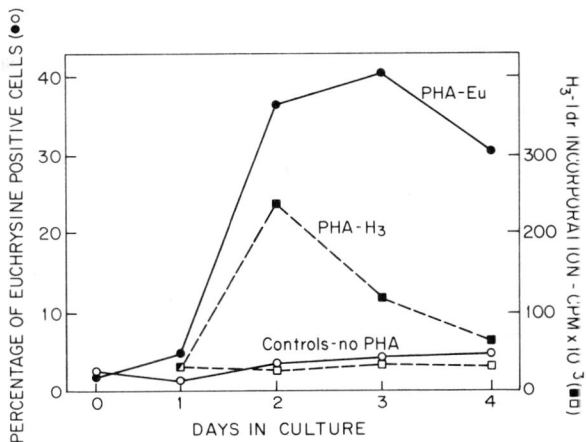

Fig. 4 Euchrysine staining compared with H_3TdR uptake by A/J cells responding to PHA.

in lysosomes as indicated by staining with Euchrysine by Allison's method, and compares this with the uptake of thymidine. Maximal stimulation of lysosomes and morphologic transformation occurs on the third day. The background remains at the indicated low levels for about five days, but rises rapidly after the sixth day. We have therefore performed all operations during the first four days. This gives high discrimination between background and stimulated cell groups. Shown in Table 7 is an experiment illustrating the arginine requirement of A/J spleen cells reacting to PHA. If the culture containing 15×10^6 spleen cells in 3 ml medium is fed additional arginine on the second day, it will incorporate additional amounts of tritiated thymidine. If additional medium isn't supplied, DNA synthesis rapidly is reduced after the second day to a very low level by the fourth day. Such feeding has no effect upon lysosome activation or morphologic transformation, suggesting that arginine probably supports only one component of the reaction. The dose-response characteristics of PHA-stimulated cells are such that it is maximal with most strains at 10 lambda PHA-M (DIFCO), but it is inhibited at high concentrations, i.e. above 50 lambda.

CELLULAR IMMUNITY

TABLE 7

Effect of Arginine Depletion on Incorporation of H_3 Tdr by PHA-Stimulated Splenocytes

Changes in the Arginine Content of 1640 Culture Medium	Stimulation over Background. H_3 Thymidine Uptake by A/J Spleen Cells CPM
Complete Medium	172,000
Ditto + Arginine 200 mg/Liter	183,000
Arginine-Free Medium	46,000
Ditto + Arginine 200 mg/liter	185,000

The primary response to a number of histocompatibility antigens has also been demonstrated. Fig. 5 shows one way stimulation of C57/BL/6 spleen cells by various numbers of mitomycin-blocked target A/J cells. The dose-response curve with one-way stimulation showed optimal stimulation by 10×10^6 cells, in tubes containing 15×10^6 reacting cells, with rapid fall off of reactivity with higher target cell doses - an approximate one to one ratio. With radiation-blocked target cells (6000 r), the responses were considerably greater than with cells exposed to mitomycin, suggesting that the high-dose inhibition has a mitomycin component. This again demonstrates the dose-response characteristics which make it necessary to explore a range of concentration especially as regards the weak-reacting systems. A variety of combinations have been explored; a few examples are shown in Table 8. H-2 differences of all types gave strong readily reproducible reactions with multiples of reactivity over syngeneic controls between four and 12, and in some combinations this multiple was as much as 50. With the congenic resistant lines, clearcut reactions only to H_2b or H_2d were strong and specific, and on the

I. LYMPHOCYTE ACTIVATION

same order of magnitude as those across the major noncongenic lines. Using a combination differing only at H-3 and H-13, smaller but highly reproducible differences were obtained.

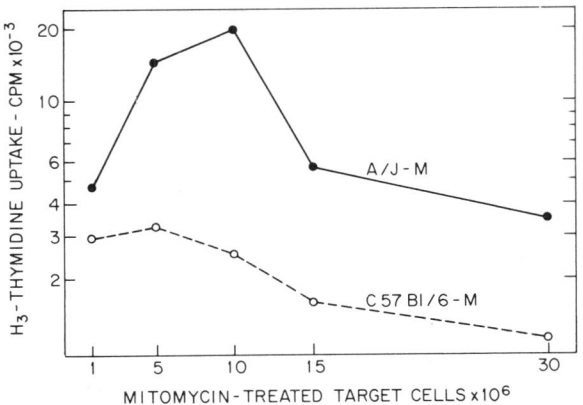

Fig. 5 One way stimulation of C57/BL/6 spleen cells by mitomycin blocked A/J cells.

This illustrates the capacity of the technique to detect weak transplantation antigens. We have preliminary evidence for recognition of tumor-specific transplantation antigens, but thus far this has not been as reproducible as the other models. Most interesting is the close parallelism between the degree of <u>in vitro</u> response and the skin graft rejection times for the tested combinations. This suggests that the method does indeed reflect some of the characteristics of the <u>in vivo</u> situation. It was next sought to determine whether one-way stimulation of F_1 hybrid cells could be elicited by mitomycin-blocked parental strain cells. Table 9 shows that this was indeed the case. Moreover, in the opposite reactions, the parental strains reacted to the semisyngeneic with about 50% of the magnitude of the reaction found with the allogeneic combination. F_1 hybrids also gave about one-half the intensity of reaction to the parental strain compared to what would be expected of the allogeneic combination. Of course, activation of F_1 hybrid by the

CELLULAR IMMUNITY

parental type, according to the classical dogma of immunology is not an immunologic response, but rather in the category of allogeneic inhibition. If it can be considered a primary response, a new set of rules will have to be developed to explain this finding. Certainly, the phenomenon will have to be considered allogeneic or hybrid <u>stimulation</u>, rather than inhibition.

TABLE 8

One-way Stimulation of H_3 Tdr Incorporation by Spleen Cells of Mice Differing by Various Histocompatibility Antigens

Reacting Cells	Mitomycin-Blocked Target Cells	Reacting Cell Stimulation* (expressed as multiples of response by syngeneic cells)
C57Bl/6	A/J CBA BALB/L C57Bl/10	4.3 11.4 2.4 1.2
B10.LP	B10.D2 C57Bl/10	8.5 1.8
B10.D2	B10.LP C57Bl/10	5.3 6.2
C57Bl/10	B10.D2 B10.LP C57Bl/6	9.2 2.1 1.5

*Average for 3 tubes

Cells from animals that had previously received spleen cell injections, were found to be several times more reactive than those exposed for the first time. Table 10 shows H_3-TdR uptake in several combinations tested in this way. Only in the case of A/J responding to CBA cells was little difference found between the immunized and non-immunized

TABLE 9

One-way Stimulation of F_1 Lymphocytes by Parental Strain Cells

Reacting Cells	Mitomycin-Blocked Target Cells	Reacting Cell Stimulation (expressed* as multiples of response by syngeneic cells)
CBA	C57Bl/6 F_1	3.4 1.8
C57Bl/6	CBA F_1	7.1 3.1
CBA x C57Bl/6	CBA C57Bl/6	2.3 2.6

*Average for 3 tubes

TABLE 10

Comparison of One-way Stimulation of Immune and Normal Mouse Spleen Cells

Target Cell	Reacting Cells	Reacting Cell Stimulation (expressed* as multiples of response by syngeneic cells)
C57Bl/6	A/J Immune A/J	4.1 11.3
A/J	C57Bl/6 Immune C57Bl/6	4.3 13.9
CBA	A/J Immune A/J	4.1 5.8
A/J	CBA Immune CBA	4.7 8.1

*Average for 3 tubes

groups; otherwise the differences were striking. We found that cells from animals that had received BCG, were highly responsive to PPD. Fig. 6 shows the time course after BCG in relation to the response to different increments of PPD. One week after receiving BCG, the animals showed practically no response, but in two and three weeks the response became impressive with a high order of difference of incorporation from the background detected at three weeks. At five weeks the reaction had waned markedly. Furthermore, the reaction showed a high degree of specificity. The dose-response curve was similar to the other system. Large amounts of PPD inhibited the response. The practical genetic and operational advantages of using the mouse should be self evident. It should simplify karyotyping, provide opportunity for determining whether in vitro reactivity is indeed equivalent to a primary response by transfer experiments and the assay of host reactivity to a variety of stimuli. These findings also provide an opportunity to control certain aspects of the reaction through the contents of the medium. Still other aspects of the reactions are taken up in Session III.

CHAIRMAN MÖLLER: We have also been extremely interested in F_1 cells responding to parental cells. I have no doubt that such reactions exist. However, as regards lymphocytes I want to report on recent studies by Lundgren, Thorsby and E. Möller. Human lymphocytes have been typed both serologically and with mixed lymphocyte cultures (MLC). The response in MCL increased with the number of HLA incompatibilities. Sensitized lymphocytes, from skin-grafted patients added to fibroblasts of various HLA types results in cytotoxicity which increases with the number of HLA antigens involved. On the other hand, in a grade B match, which is analogous to parental versus F_1 in mice, there is no response inasmuch as cells of both individuals have all the antigens. We do not know the basis for this difference but we are certain that the phenomenon is real. Allogeneic inhibition exists, of course, with tumor cells and lymphocyte-tumor cell interaction.

I. LYMPHOCYTE ACTIVATION

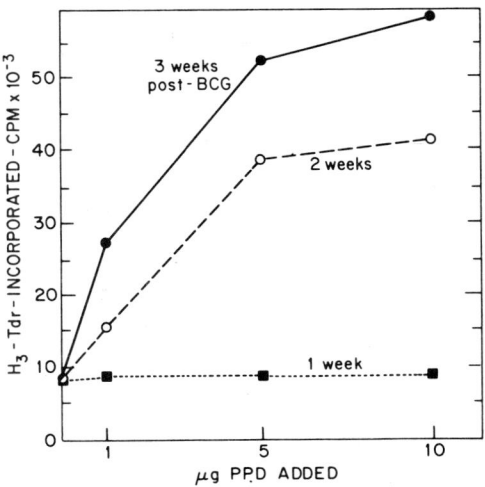

Fig. 6 Response to PPD of C57/BL/6 spleen cells after BCG immunization.

In the matter of MLC there are two remarkable findings that could now serve as the focus for our further discussions: First, what is the basis for the response in the MLC with normal cells, particularly as they have not been derived from immunized individuals? With other antigens such a response is not obtained unless the donor has been preimmunized. Secondly, how can we account for the one to two percent antigen sensitive cells in such MLC in contrast to only 0.005-0.01% in presensitized cell populations responding to any of an array of soluble antigens? I would ask Dr. Wilson to open the discussion on this intriguing and surely very important issue.

DR. WILSON: This is, of course a fundamental issue. The finding that, in certain immunologic systems involving histocompatibility differences determined by the major loci, approximately 1 lymphocyte in 50 is reactive, was originally described by Simonsen (Cold Spring Harbor Symposia on Quantitative Biology, 32, 517, 1967.) He showed that approximately one to two percent of the cells of a lymphocyte population could initiate a GVH reaction. Recently, Nowell and I arrived at a similar conclusion for the number of lymphocytes in the peripheral blood of rats which could be stimulated by histocompatibility antigens to proliferate in an MLC (J. Exp. Med., 128, 1157, 1968.) This is an awkward conclusion to accept in view of the predictions of the Clonal Selection Hypothesis as stated by Burnet.

How do we reconcile values as great as one or two percent of the cells responding to a histocompatibility antigen system with the far lesser response to other kinds of antigens? In the case of DNP, the number of reactive cells is in the range of 1 in 1,000,000, and for heterologous RBC antigens it is 1 in 100,000.

There are various possibilities which might account for the large proportion of lymphocytes reactive to major histocompatibility antigens. a) The major histocompatibility antigen system of the rat may consist of a very large number of antigenic determinants, each of which is capable of stimulating a small proportion of lymphocytes. With the frequency of reactive cells being ca. 10^{-5}, 2000 different antigens would be required to stimulate 2% of the lymphocyte population. This seems an unlikely possibility. By comparison, the H-2 antigenic system in mice consists of only about 30 different specificities that can be detected by serologic procedures. b) A second possibility is that this high proportion of reactive cells might reflect some prior experience with cross-reacting antigens, and hence proliferation in the MLC and the activity of lymphocytes in a GVH reaction is really a manifestation of a secondary immune response. This is a difficult possibility to deny; it is an unattractive one to me. Studies with animals that have been raised under pathogen and antigen-free conditions may help resolve this question.

These two possibilities have assumed that the responsive lymphocytes are unipotential. This is a point that I am sure will emerge later in these discussions. The implication of all this is rather simple: major histocompatibility antigens are recognized biologically as being "strong" simply on the basis that there are a substantial

I. LYMPHOCYTE ACTIVATION

number of cells that bear receptor sites for them, and consequently are responsive to them. Conversely, "weak" histocompatibility antigens are recognized by a much smaller proportion of the lymphocyte population.

An important prediction can be made from this argument. If, in the rat, for example, two percent of the cells are responsive to one particular strong histocompatibility antigen system, two percent to another, etc., we would soon exhaust the immune response capacity of this animal with only 50 different antigens -- assuming that these lymphocytes are unipotential with respect to their response capabilities. Consequently, I suspect that these antigens which are effectively mitogenic to presumably unsensitized populations of lymphocytes are limited to the major histocompatibility antigens of any given species. What biological purpose they might have is an extremely interesting problem, but not relevant to our discussion at this point.

DR. DUTTON: I think that there is another point to be raised in comparing these two types of frequency. On the one hand we are looking at a cell capable of responding to an antigen like sRBC and we get a frequency of 10^{-5}, while on the other hand we are looking at the cell capable of initiating an *in vitro* homograft reaction and we get a frequency of 10^{-2}. We should take into account the fact that the assay systems are quite different. In the case of the sRBC antigen we are looking at a cell that responds and eventually makes an antibody that is specific to the antigen that elicited the response. In the *in vitro* homograft response there is no evidence of specificity in the response but rather in the initiation step. The only thing we see is proliferation of cells, either as a focus on a chorioallantoic membrane; as splenomegaly; or expressed as the incorporation of thymidine. All the limiting dilution assay in the homograft experiment can tell us is that there is one component of the system that recognizes the antigen and that this is present in an effective amount on one cell in 100. This is not irreconcilable with the idea that the cell that synthesized this limiting component might have been present at a very much lower frequency, and that the product of this cell then gets distributed in such a way that one cell in 100 is sensitized to respond.

CELLULAR IMMUNITY

CHAIRMAN MÖLLER: Would not the limiting dilution technique resolve this conflict?

DR. DUTTON: The limiting dilution experiments have been done by Nisbet and Simonsen. It is a fact that one cell in 100 will indeed initiate the response. However, we don't know that the cell that <u>responded</u> in this case had made a specific immunoglobulin capable of recognizing the antigen.

DR. WAKSMAN: I want to emphasize the point made by Dr. Dutton concerning graft-versus-host (GVH) lesions. Szenberg studied GVH reactions and also estimated that in this particular model one in 50 lymphocytes was capable of initiating a response to any given histocompatibility antigen. Perhaps what one is looking at here involves the carrier function of the molecule rather than its determinant function. In looking at lesions on the chorioallantoic membrane, each initiated by a single lymphocyte, we may be looking at something comparable to the wave of mitosis seen in thymus-derived cells in the spleen during an immune response. That is quite a different phenomenon from the response of marrow-derived cells engaged in the synthesis of antibody. It may have a much lower order of specificity, i.e. one in 50 or one in 100, whereas the antibody-forming cells may have a different frequency and a finer degree of specificity.

CHAIRMAN MÖLLER: You are postulating a recognizing mechanism which does not work with immunoglobulin. There is evidence for a very high degree of specificity in the discriminative spleen assay of Simonsen. The question still remains whether there is in fact a recognition system of histocompatibility antigens which does not react via immunoglobulin receptors.

DR. WAKSMAN: Again, when you refer to the high order of specificity, you may be speaking more about the specificity of the product than that of the initial recognition. From

I. LYMPHOCYTE ACTIVATION

all the data of these laboratory groups, the latter seems to have a lower order of specificity with numbers like one in 50 rather than one in 10^5 or one in 10^6.

CHAIRMAN MÖLLER: What you are calling a lower order of specificity, is really a higher frequency of specific cells.

DR. WAKSMAN: But that also means that when two percent of the cells respond to one particular specificity, you would then be allowed only different combinations of 50 possible responses. An additional complicated issue is the fact that the H-2 antigen itself controls a whole series of antigenic specificities. You may be seeing cells responding to each of 10 or 12 different antigenic determinants in this particular case.

DR. HIRSCHHORN: As Dr. Waksman has just brought out, a histocompatibility antigen is not a single antigenic determinant, but rather a complex of antigens. Consequently, if you insist upon single recognition specificity per cell, you may have a large group of specificities that are being recognized by several cell types. Then too, who is to say that in the histocompatibility recognition system one cell may not be capable of recognizing several specificities. In that event, the number of cells required could in fact easily fit the order of magnitude we are talking about.

DR. WILSON: Dr. Waksman is quite correct. One must consider that there are numerous specificites involved. I think, however, if one can use the mouse H-2 system as a model, no two strains of mice differ at the H-2 locus by fewer than two to four nor more than 14 specificities. Preliminary evidence now emerging suggests that the rat is no different. The question of whether a given lymphocyte can respond to more than one of these histocompatibility systems is a rather awkward one to accept for genetic reasons. One can approach this with the MLC response and isogenic strains of experimental animals. With the use of lymphocytes from tolerant rats, A (tolerant of B), these will not respond to A/B F_1 hybrid cells bearing the appropriate antigen in mixed cultures, but are fully and quantitatively responsive to other antigenic systems (i.e. A/C). The response of A (tolerant of B) cells to A/C F_1 hybrid cells is identical to that of cells from normal A animals stimulated with A/C cells. This suggests that the cells which are reactive to two different histocompatibility antigen systems belong to two different lymphocyte subpopulations.

CHAIRMAN MÖLLER: I think there is evidence that we have two recognition mechanisms with regard to histocompatibility antigens. The immunological one obviously dominates, as demonstrated by the tolerance experiments. We should, however, take into account the data given earlier in this session by Dr. Smith showing that F_1 cells are stimulated by parental cells. This is analogous to allogeneic inhibition. Then too, we may be dealing with a mixture of the two.

DR. LAWRENCE: Mr. Chairman, would you restate your primary question again, since it remained unanswered?

CHAIRMAN MÖLLER: Why is it that we develop a response in mixed lymphocyte cultures despite the fact that the cells are not, to our knowledge, sensitized, whereas in all other systems they must first be sensitized?

DR. LAWRENCE: Some years ago, stimulated by the operational peculiarities of how one sensitized an individual to homografts like skin, and then tested for the presence of sensitivity, we made the suggestion (Summation in: Histocompatibility Testing, p. 141, pub. 1229, Natl. Acad. Sci. - Wash. D.C., 1965). that what had come to be accepted as an actively acquired immune response may really result from the elevation of a latent iso-immune state. This reasoning is borne out by the sort of question you asked; why should two so-called "virgin" lymphocyte populations on their first known encounter in MLC each respond as though they had prior intimate immunologic knowledge of the other?

I. LYMPHOCYTE ACTIVATION

The other circumstance which may contribute to the absence of a virgin responsiveness of immunocompetent cell populations, is the reality of the natural mammalian habitat. We do not live in an environment devoid of immunologic stimuli - quite the contrary. As isolated individual histocompatibility antigens are more highly purified they may very well be found to be sullied by prior association with a variety of bacterial, viral, fungal and mycoplasmal antigens to which, in an environmental sense, our tissues are exposed from birth. Whether this involves an intimate complexing of self-markers in a manner we have postulated by the self + X hypothesis (Physiol. Rev. 39, 811, 1959) or is as simple a circumstance as coating of cells with other antigenic determinants is not yet clear. My point is that man or other mammals may not be the private, immunologically virgin individuals, at least not in the strict histocompatibility terms, we are assuming here.

Another potent factor which complicates the assumption of an immunologically null state, is the large role that cross-reacting antigenic specificities may contribute to a baseline state of responsiveness, as exemplified by pneumococcal polysaccharides, streptococcal antigens and certain other microbial and plant constituents. In studies of skin homograft reactions in outbred human populations, Rapaport, Thomas, Converse and I (J. Clin. Invest. 41, 2166, 1962) have found that active sensitization of an individual by means of another's leucocyte fractions instead of skin homografts, resulted in the detection of cross reactivity, and a blunting of the specificity of the response. In contrast, our earlier experience in the transfer of accelerated homograft rejection, revealed transfer factor to be exquisitely individual-specific in causing a rejection only of the skin graft to which the transfer factor was sensitized and to no other graft (J. Clin. Invest. 39, 185, 1960). Thus, transfer factor is specific for the histocompatibility antigens of the sensitizing donor, whereas active sensitization brings into play a whole spectrum of cross reactivities, which appears a function of the antigenic preparation as well as the route, intensity and the duration of the sensitization procedure.

DR. UHR: Is there any reason to believe that the answer to Dr. Möller's question of why MLC interact so strongly in the absence of prior sensitization is other than a purely quantitative matter? Thus, lymphocytes from a tuberculin-negative individual are not stimulated by tuberculin in contrast to using cells from a tuberculin-positive individual. This difference could be one of degree, a quantitative one, i.e., precursor cells that can react with tuberculin are in the blood before sensitization but there are too few of them to give a detectable in vitro response.

CHAIRMAN MÖLLER: Yes, that may be so, but I am struck by the simply fantastic difference in orders of magnitude involved in this. In this respect I can't help wondering if the figures really represent what we think they do?

DR. MITCHISON: Two kinds of theories have been advanced to account for the difference in frequency of cell-cell inductions on the one hand, or antigen-cell inductions on the other. One kind are rescue operations for the clonal selection concept in which one postulates induction via abnormally low-affinity receptors, or an abnormally large number of receptors, when a response is induced by cells. The second possibility is a non-cloncal spread of the response through transfer from one cell to another.

Now, I don't think that there are data which exclude the second or "Dutton" theory, but there is a kind of experiment which places a very severe restriction on that theory, and that is this: When histoincompatible lymphocytes are adoptively transferred from an immunized donor, a state of reactivity follows against test skin grafts for example or skin allergens, according to the way that the donor was immunized. But the reactivity is transient. When the allogenic cells are rejected by the reaction of the host, that does not leave a sensitized population of lymphocytes remaining in the allogeneic host. If receptors were to spread from one site to another, one would logically expect that kind of reactivity to remain after the allogenic cells have been rejected.

I. LYMPHOCYTE ACTIVATION

DR. DUTTON: I am not pushing this explanation - rather I am merely suggesting it as a hypothesis to see of we can dispose of it. All one has to do to get around Dr. Mitchison's objection is say the recognition molecule has a rapid turnover time.

DR. COHN: If there is a lymphocyte activated to produce a product picked up by other lymphocytes, then one cell should react to different antigens.

CHAIRMAN MOLLER: I think that Dr. Mitchison's comments provide a very good bridge to lead us over to possible mechanisms of spread of reactivity and thereby to non-specific activation processes. This discussion has shown that in the course of study of the so-called nonspecific events, we have also managed to learn more about the specific mechanism of activation of lymphocytes. However, I don't think the discussion has in any way exhausted what we call the nonspecific mechanism for triggering lymphocytes; how these agents do this, and in what way this nonspecific triggering differs from the specific event, i.e., the effect of specific antigens on lymphocytes of a sensitized donor. There are three points to be considered with respect to nonspecific processes: First, how do they work? Second, what cells are actually triggered? Third, do these nonspecific activating processes have any meaningful role in what we are studying as *in vitro* correlates of delayed type hypersensitivity.

DR. WILSON: My comment is to Dr. Moller and concerns the relationship between the specific and nonspecific mitogenic events and cellular immune activities in culture. We considered that perhaps the two percent of cells that are reactive to a given strong histocompatibility system in MLC might represent (1) a rather substantial proportion that have been "recruited" by some ill-defined mechanism, and (2) a very small proportion, more in line with figures given for well known soluble antigenic models, which are specific.

To me the latter seems a little unlikely in view of the fact that karyologically marked F_1 cells cannot be "recruited" to proliferate in MLC involving parental and F_1 hybrid rat lymphocytes. Nevertheless, another way to pursue this possibility is to inquire whether lymphocytes

59

can be "recruited" out of a tolerant population. The way to ask this question would be simply to set up three-way mixed cultures using normal and isologous tolerant parental strain cells along with F_1 antigen-bearing cells. The responsive cells could be identified as to their origins with the use of sex chromosome markers. For instance.lymphocytes from a Lewis female rat tolerant of BN antigens, plus lymphocytes from a normal male Lewis animal and cells from (Lewis X BN) F_1 hybrid animals were used in an experiment that Dr. Nowell and I did. If there were a large number of recruitable lymphocytes, you might expect to find significant numbers of cells from the female tolerant donor. There might be as many as one recruited cell out of the normal animal for each recruited cell of the tolerant animal, and these would be turned on by the initiating activity of the specific few. In fact, however, this was not what we found when this experiment was performed. As judged from the metaphase plates, the overwhelming majority of the responsive cells were from the normal animal.

DR. UHR: I think this is a very significant point, but to be sure it is entirely clear to all of us. would you restate your proposition?

DR. WILSON: Let us assume that the two percent of responsive cells in mixed lymphocyte interaction consists of two subgroups: (1) a small proportion, something like one in 10,000 that are specifically responsive cells - probably possessing specific receptor sites, and (2) a majority which are recruited in some manner, by the activities of the specific few. Now, one way of testing this possibly would be to set up a mixed culture involving the three combinations of rats - A ♀ (tolerant of B) + A ♂ normal + A/B F_1. In this case we know that cells from animal A tolerant of B are not stimulatable by A/B F_1 cells. Consequently, we might presume they are devoid of specifically reactive lymphocytes. But with the three-way mixture, the question is whether we can recruit a significant number of cells out of this tolerant population by the activities of small minority of specific cells from the A normal animal. One would expect that if such a system were operative both the normal male and the tolerant female populations of parental A strain cells would supply similar numbers of "recruited" cells to the proliferating population. Because the specific A male cells

I. LYMPHOCYTE ACTIVATION

are in a small minority, the "recruited" cells of male or female origin should be roughly in a one to one proportion. We did this very experiment but could find no cells from the tolerant population that were recruited to proliferate by normal, syngeneic cells responding to homologous histocompatibility antigens.

DR. DUTTON: I would like to go back to the point of the two percent value, and make sure there isn't any confusion about it amongst us. The value of two percent comes from the Nisbet, Simonsen and Zaleski experiment (J. Exp. Med. 129, 459, 1969) in which, if I recall correctly, they injected adult fowl blood into hybrid chick embryos. The number of cells injected was either 5, 50, 500 or 5,000; the point is that they got spleen enlargement in the F_1 hybrids when they injected as few as 50 cells. In view of their findings the question of recruitment would not help here at all. It tells us that _if_ this is an immune response of the parental spleen cells against the F_1 hybrid, it has to be initiated by a component of the system which is present at a level of one cell in 50.

DR. VALENTINE: Dr. Wilson described an elegant experiment in which he sought to detect the recruitment of tolerant cells into a mixed leukocyte reaction involving two additional cell populations. This experiment might be expected to detect a nonspecific recruitment of additional cells into the response; however, if the recruitment was postulated to be antigenically specific, then the tolerant cells would not be expected to respond to the antigen stimulus. The discussion has assumed a nonspecific recruitment; one can, however, also envision a specific recruitment in which the normal cells are changed so that they respond to the antigen rather than being nonspecifically stimulated.

DR. WILSON: "Specific Recruitment" is to me a logical absurdity; either cells are non-specifically recruited, or they are specifically reactive to antigen.

DR. COHN: Dr. Dutton answered my point that one cell would express the specificities of two different antibodies, if they were passively acquired, by saying that the half life of the absorbed antibody could be short. I don't think that quite answers it, but it is not necessary further to discuss that point since the Wilson experiment appears to rule out the passive acquisition of reactivity that had been postulated by Dr. Dutton.

DR. MITCHISON: Part of the difficulty about a frequency as high as one or two percent would be removed if, in fact, this represented a presensitized population, so one needs to look rather carefully for data which point in that direction. For example, Bainbridge and Gowland, who examined the localization of small numbers of Cr_{51} labeled lymphocytes, have shown that allogeneic cells localize abnormally in a non-immunized host, indicating some presensitization. What is particularly significant is that if the allogeneic host has been rendered tolerant beforehand, the allogeneic cells then behaved like syngeneic cells. One can add, as another example, the remarkable lack of radiosensitivity of the early phase of the GVH reaction as described by Simonsen, and by Brent and Medawar in the context of the normal lymphocyte transfer test. This seems to imply a population of cells that were immunized beforehand.

DR. BRAUN: I would like to come back to the matter of nonspecific stimulators. It is worth mentioning that practically all of the nonspecific stimulators that were listed by Dr. Hirschhorn are identical with agents that produce a stimulation of antibody-forming cells in conjunction with stimulators derived from either natural or synthetic polynucleotides. I don't think that this parallel is fortuitous. I might add that in addition to the materials that were listed by Dr. Hirschhorn, we have found epinephrine and chlorpromazine to be active. It would be interesting to know whether the latter agents are also active in the cell systems under discussion here.

This brings me to a specific question. In the case of stimulation of antibody-forming cells, we know that we have

I. LYMPHOCYTE ACTIVATION

two requirements: one for altering membranes and a second to provide an actual stimulator that now has access to the cell through or within the altered membrane. Since one can suspect that any alteration of membrane does not necessarily lead to one-way events, but may lead to two-way events, I would like to know whether there is any evidence supporting the possibility that the systems under discussion may also involve events that happen, either at the membrane or in the cell, as the result of membrane alterations under the influence of materials provided by other cells.

DR. GELL: It seems to me that we are bending over backwards to postulate what I feel is a highly unbiological phenomenon, that is, the transfer of <u>primary</u> recognition from one cell to another. It seems to me it would be much simpler if we instead accept the possibility that one cell can in fact recognize two or more antigens, whether graft antigens or anything else. I think that we are allowing ourselves to be hypnotized by the dogma of unipotentiality of recognition cells, rather than really facing the facts.

DR. WILSON: In replying to Dr. Gell's point, I would like to describe an additional experiment that makes it difficult, I think, to consider that the lymphocytes in the mixed lymphocyte interaction possess multi-potential recognition capabilities. Thus, working with a high number of A/B F_1 cells to stimulate A strain parental rat lymphocytes, and thus to assure antigen excess; A strain lymphocytes reacting with A/B gives a certain number of counts per minute. Increasing the number of F_1 cells does not increase this value, and A cells, reacting to A/C also give a characteristic number of counts per minute. If B and C histocompatibility antigens are put together, as B/C F_1 hybrid lymphocytes tolerant of A, so as to assure a one-way reaction, the proliferative activity in A + B/C (tolerant of A) cultures is a summation of A+A/B and A+A/C cultures. There is a sort of philosophical control over all this. If a cell were exposed to A/B cells, would this be any different than A cells stimulated by B/B (tolerant of A, and thus A unilateral response)? In this experiment, A + B/B (tolerant of A) and A + A/B cultures responses were identical. To me, this all suggests that the proliferative response to different histocompatibility antigens involves different subpopulations of lymphocytes. Thus, the hypothetical B receptors on the A cells were saturated and it made no difference whether the antigen was presented as A/B or B/B.

DR. HIRSCHHORN: I would like to try to settle something about the numerology implicit in these discussions. For example, if one stimulates a normal peripheral blood lymphocyte culture with PHA and then performs autoradiography, in the presence of tritiated uridine, it can be shown that virtually all the cells respond by taking up the tritiated uridine. There is nuclear labeling and later cytoplasmic labeling and it seems to be incorporated. Were one to use tritiated thymidine instead, it could be shown that among these cells, all of which have responded by RNA synthesis, certainly not all of them respond by DNA synthesis. It is, therefore, quite critical to know at what interval one is measuring incorporation. I would also urge the abandoning of thymidine incorporation as a measure of stimulation. Only a minority of the cells that are activated actually go on to the S period and division. Those that do are not synchronous, so that a short thymidine pulse is not reliable. Longer pulses have the danger of nonspecificity of labelling. Alternative methods are: morphology, (which chemists don't trust); uridine incorporation into RNA; and amino acid incorporation into newly synthesized protein. RNA studies require careful prestabilization of cells and difficult isolation procedures. Protein synthesis can be measured in the first 24 hours, is linear, requires only a four-hour pulse and only 5×10^5 cells; this has been demonstrated by Waithe in our laboratory. This may, therefore, be the best, easiest and most reproducible method for quantitation of lymphocyte responses.

DR. LANDY: One issue which seems to me especially germane to this particular discussion relates to the actual number of receptors, for each of these different categories of activating agents, that are possessed by normal lymphocytes. This must differ markedly for "nonspecific" as opposed to

I. LYMPHOCYTE ACTIVATION

"specific" stimulators of lymphocytes and could have profound consequences. I know that several of the conferees, notably our chairman, have been directly concerned with this matter. I specifically recall that Dr. Gell has also made estimates of the numbers of molecules of anti-allotype required to trigger lymphocytes into blast formation. I would, therefore, like to see this kind of information brought into the general discussion.

CHAIRMAN MOLLER: There are two possibilities, (1) that cells can "sense" the number of receptors which have been triggered, and (2) that there is a recruitment process from a few triggered cells to others. There are two situations leading to activation. One, nonspecific substances such as ALS and PHA, and two, specific ones such as antigen added to sensitized cells. When nonspecific activating substances such as ALS and PHA are added in various dilutions the dose-response curve is typical. There is a peak response at a certain dilution and essentially no response at higher or lower dilutions. The difference between the low as compared to high non-activating doses in only 100 fold. Since many molecules are bound to the lymphocytes before they respond, there is a definite threshhold. If two nonspecific substances are given together they will interact in the activation process. In general, an optimal dose of one substance together with various dilutions of another substance will cause a decreased response. If suboptimal doses are used, it is generally found that two suboptimal stimulants give a synergistic effect. In these cases one can't imply recruitment of new cells, because all of the agents used attach to all of the cells. My conclusion is that in this case the lymphocytes react in accordance with the number of receptors affected.

A quite different situation pertains regarding cells responding to antigen. The slope of dose-response is very shallow; a 10,000 fold difference in antigen concentration is still capable of giving rise to stimulation. If two antigens, presumably non cross-reacting, are added in high concentrations we have consistently found a lower response than the sum of the repeated response, and usually lower than either one alone. At lower concentrations, on the other hand, there is often a clear synergistic effect.

Consequently in principle, the situation is analogous to that obtained with nonspecific stimulants. However, in this case only a few antigen-reactive cells are available, and probably different cells for each antigen. The most likely explanation for the findings with antigens is that antigens recruit cells from an "x" population to participate and magnify the response. Whatever the message for recruitment is, it seems plausible that the antagonistic or synergistic effects are exerted on this postulated "x" population.

DR. WILSON: I think it might be dangerous to generalize from soluble antigens to the cell-cell stimulating systems. With MLC I believe that one is dealing with a close-packing arrangement. The critical factor may be now many antigen-bearing cells can surround a potentially responsive cell on a three-dimensional basis. This is something likely to be very different from the number of molecules of antigen that can be visualized as having access to the cell membrane.

DR. DUTTON: I disagree with Dr. Möller's statement concerning synergism or competition by different antigens. We did a number of such experiments with two antigens some time ago. My recollection is that we found a reasonable summation of the stimulatory effect of the two antigens individually.

DR. MARSHALL: Dr. Lawrence has raised the possibility that the MLC, and by inference the homograft reaction, may actually represent a secondary response and Dr. Mitchison has brought forward some evidence in favor of this idea. I want to point out that there are two pieces of evidence that appear to be against this interpretation. First, and this is the best piece of evidence, when peritoneal cells from genetically different animals are mixed in a capillary tube, as has been done by Dr. David and others, there is no inhibition of migration. One would expect inhibition of migration if the animals were in fact presensitized. Secondly, along the same lines are the experiments of Billingham and co-workers where homografts were placed in the hamster cheek pouch and in rats onto

I. LYMPHOCYTE ACTIVATION

discs of skin deprived of lymphatic circulation. If the animals had been deliberately presensitized, the grafts in both those situations were rejected, whereas grafts remained intact if the animals had not been deliberately sensitized. Were the homograft reaction in an adult animal a secondary response, as has been suggested, then one would expect inhibition of macrophage migration and homograft rejection respectively in the two experiments cited.

CHAIRMAN MÖLLER: Can this delemma be resolved?

DR. MITCHISON: Yes, if the differences were purely quantitative rather than qualitative.

DR. MARSHALL: It seem to me that there must be a qualitative difference because the degree of lymphocyte activity in the MLC, as judged by the number of large dividing cells which develop, is equal to a rather vigorous response to antigen such as tuberculin. One would predict from the size of this response that there would be considerable inhibition of macrophage migration. It is possible that the change into lymphoblasts is a separate reaction from the release of MIF. There certainly is a difficulty here.

DR. VALENTINE: If one employs a stimulant such as PHA which involves very nearly all of the cells, and these cells then go on to divide, how can one postulate that with an additional number of stimuli that these cells can give a greater response than that induced by the PHA stimulus alone. A given cell would seem to be triggered in a threshhold fashion.

CHAIRMAN MÖLLER: That is so, but there is one especially important point you have overlooked. The nonspecific stimulants seem to trigger only one division; a situation that is in marked contrast to specific antigen, which continues to drive the reaction, resulting on continued proliferation.

CELLULAR IMMUNITY

DR. VALENTINE: I don't agree with your interpretation. Many investigators have found that PHA may induce more than one cycle of division. However, it would seem that in the case of stimulation by either PHA or antigen, any additional response which is measured must rather be due to an additional number of cells initially responding to the stimulus, than to a more rapid proliferation (within a given culture system there is no evidence for this), or to a continuation of repeated divisions for a longer time. I find it difficult to see how an individual lymphocyte would express a graded response to accumulated stimuli when the end point is division. If one obtains an additive effect, the simplest way to explain it would be that more cells are <u>initially</u> stimulated to respond.

DR. GELL: Coming back to the issue of toxicity, I feel that the fall-off, when stimulation is increased, is not necessarily a toxic effect, because the same thing occurs in the anti-allotype system. That is to say, if one uses increasing doses of stimulatory antiserum, one usually gets to an optimum or plateau and then very frequently, with an overdose, a fall-off is evident. This, however, is not a toxicity effect. One can easily control that, of course, with other systems. So it seems to me that there is, in fact, a biological phenomenon of overstimulation of the cells, or something like that which I personally find very puzzling.

DR. SMITH: Dr. Moller, would you kindly clarify for me what you meant by the lymphocyte having the capability for counting. In our system we get twice as many cells responding to the allogeneic stimulating cell, and incorporation H_3 TdR, than the number responding to the semisyngeneic or F_1 cell.

CHAIRMAN MÖLLER: In your experimental model you are dealing with a specific antigen, and the effect may be on the hypothetical "x" population from which you recruit. Obviously the cells react only when a certain number of its multiple receptors have been triggered. If, however, many of these receptors are covered, the same cell does not respond.

I. LYMPHOCYTE ACTIVATION

DR. LANDY: As this discussion draws to a close, it is evident that we have not dealt fully with the various issues raised. Any frustration should however be tempered by the recognition that we have sought to develop, in the very brief time alloted us, the extensive terrain covered by the annual Leukocyte Culture Conferences who devote several days (instead of a few hours) to a more exhaustive development of this subject. I believe, however, that despite the stringent time limitation much information has emerged that will be preparatory and especially useful for the sessions that follow.

II
BASIS OF INDUCTION IN CELLULAR IMMUNITY CONTRASTED WITH ANTIBODY PRODUCTION

Two populations of lymphocytes precommitted either to cellular or to humoral immunity — IgX, a postulated non-secretable immunoglobulin as the lymphocyte receptor for cellular immunity — Antilight chain antibody blocks lymphocyte transformation by antigen — Cooperation between thymus-dependent and marrow-dependent cells — Can thymus-independent cells achieve delayed hypersensitivity — Contributions of lymphocytes and macrophages to tissue infiltrates — Role of carrier specificity in induction and elicitation of cellular immunity — Cellular and humoral responses involve specificity to different portions of a common antigen — Diseases resulting in depressed cellular immunity in the presence of intact antibody production — Disease-associated plasma inhibitor of *in vitro* lymphocyte transformation by antigen — Variable impairment of either cellular or humoral components in immunological deficiency disease syndromes.

II. FEATURES OF CELLULAR VERSUS HUMORAL IMMUNITY

DR. MITCHISON: Cells have a wide range of options in responding to antigenic stimulation. They can choose between tolerance and immunity; if the decision is made to produce antibody, the product can belong to one or more of a range of immunoglobulin classes; they can also choose between a cellular and a humoral response. In this session we have to consider how the last of these decisions is made. In a general fashion we can imagine two alternative ways by which the decision could be made. One way would be for each antigen-sensitive cell to have the option of choosing, in which case we assume that the local environment in which stimulation occurs must influence the decision which an individual cell makes. The other way assumes that the antigen-sensitive cells are already subdivided prior to the encounter with antigen, with one population precommitted to humoral and the other to cellular immunity. The local environment in which stimulation occurs would still play a decisive role, but in this case it would do so in a selective manner, by attracting one population of cells rather than the other into encounter with antigen.

The theory of distinct populations of precommitted lymphocytes is advocated by Burnet, Good, and their respective colleagues. We shall proceed to examine the evidence for precommitment, and whether lymphocytes may reflect their commitment in other properties. We shall then inquire whether the theory can account for the efficacy of certain immunisation procedures in raising one type of response differentially. Finally we will deal with some of the difficulties raised by certain experiments with allotypes.

Two populations of lymphocytes

To start with, an indirect but powerful argument in favour of precommitment can be cited. We now have good evidence of precommitment of lymphocytes in other ways; precommitment in respect of immunoglobulin class, rather than precommitment in respect of the antigen-binding site, is particularly relevant. In a series of experiments using hapten-inhibition and antigens with different spacings of determinants, Mäkelä and his colleagues have shown that cells which produce 19S as distinct from 7S antibody are probably triggered via 19S receptors (Mäkelä et al., Proc. 4th Sanibel Conf., in Press, 1969).

The evidence of a more direct nature is brought together in Table 11. This table starts with the anatomical origin of the proposed two populations, and finishes with their respective immunological reactivities. In between are gathered the properties which may distinguish the two populations of cells, after they have emerged as lymphocytes and before they have encountered antigen. It must be emphasized that although the linkage between thymus derivation at one end and cellular immunity at the other seems to be strong and inescapable, the association with other lymphocyte characteristics is weak.

Nevertheless these weak associations deserve our attention, because they offer at present our only hope of sorting out the two populations of lymphocytes after they have emerged out of the thymus and marrow.

The first column in the table refers to (a) the classical experiments of Miller, Good, and their respective colleagues on the effects of thymectomy and bursectomy, and (b) congenital aplasia of the thymus in man, and agammaglobulinemia. In both cases the thymus appears to control cellular immunity, and effects humoral immunity in respect of only a limited array of thymus-dependent antigens.

After emerging from the thymus or bone-marrow, the two populations of lymphocytes apparently display differences in ethology, life-span, and physical characteristics, as listed in the table. Thoracic duct drainage and treatment with ALS remove selectively lymphocytes from the recirculating pool, and in doing so appear to select out thymus-derived cells. This inference is drawn from the fact that these treatments selectively deplete the thymus-dependent areas, the paracortex, of the lymph nodes and spleen (Turk and Willoughby, Lancet, $\underline{1}$, 249, 1967). As a consequence cellular immunity and the thymus-dependent

II. FEATURES OF CELLULAR VERSUS HUMORAL IMMUNITY

TABLE II

Two populations of lymphocytes, one precommitted to cellular immunity and the other to humoral immunity

Anatomical origin	Lymphocyte ethology	Lymphocyte life-span	Lymphocytes physical characteristics	Immunological competence	Molecular receptors	History	Responses
Thymus-derived	Recirculating	Long-lived	Small/large Dense/less dense	Helpers	IgX/IgG etc.	Early in phylogeny, ontogeny	Cellular
Marrow-derived	Sedentary	Short-lived	Sticky/non-sticky Antigens	Precursors	IgG, IgA, IgM	Late	Humoral
EXPERIMENTS Thymus/bursa extirpation Congenital defects	Thoracic duct drainage ALS, etc.	Auto-radiography after ALS	Columns, gradients, etc.	In vivo reconsti-tutions In vitro responses	Transformation Inhibition Protection on columns Tumours		Adoptive transfer In vitro reactions

75

responses are suppressed preferentially (Lance and Batchelor, Transplantation, 6, 490, 1968); as expected, this suppression can be counteracted by adoptive transfer of thymocytes (Martin and Miller, J. Exp. Med., 128, 855, 1968). Other treatments which selectively deplete the thymus-dependent areas include extra-corporeal irradiation, local irradiation of the spleen (Ford, Brit. J. Exp, Path., 49, 592, 1968), injection of dextran sulphate or heparinoids and polyanions (Ormai and de Clerq, Science, 163, 472, 1969), and possibly also overdosage with foreign serum proteins (Cerny et al., Folia Biologica, 15, 41, 1969). On the other hand, the recirculating pool certainly also contains lymphocytes which are precursors of antibody-producing cells (Ellis et al., Antibiot. Et Chemother., 15, 40, 1968). These cells are presumably not thymus-derived, although the point has not been tested directly; in order to reconcile the observation with the two populations theory it seems best to assume that the recirculating pool contains a majority of thymus-derived lymphocytes and a minority of marrow-derived ones.

So far as age distribution is concerned, treatment with ALS shifts the lymphocyte population towards shorter-lived cells (Denman et al., Lancet, 1, 321, 1968). But here the distinction is not absolute: long-lived lymphocytes can be found even in neonatally thymectomised rats (Rieke and Schwarz in: The Lymphocyte in Immunology and Haemopoiesis p. 229, Ed. J. M. Yoffey, Arnold, Lond. 1966).

Lymphocytes of the two populations perhaps differ from one another physically; for this reason fractionation procedures have a special interest. Adherence (Mosier, Science, 158, 1573, 1967), and gradient centrifugation (Dutton and Mishell - personal communication) have been employed to separate populations of lymphoid cells which do not respond immunologically in isolation, but which do so when recombined. The relationship of these sub-populations to the thymus and to the cells which finally secrete antibody in the experiments is not known; for this reason no assignment is made in the appropriate column of the table. Another possibility is that the two populations may bear characteristic antigens. We should be on the lookout not for antigens which are confined to thymocytes (e.g. TL), but for antigens characteristic of some but not all lympho-

II. FEATURES OF CELLULAR VERSUS HUMORAL IMMUNITY

cytes, and which may be shared in common with the thymus; a promising candidate is θ (Reif and Allen, J.Exp. Med., 120, 413, 1964).

Under the heading of immunological competence we are concerned with the cell-cell interactions involved in humoral responses to thymus-dependent antigens. The problem of interpretation raised by the in vitro response to sRBC has already been mentioned. The in vivo experiments fall into two categories. One includes the response of irradiated mice to sRBC (Davies et al., Transplantation, 5, 222, 1967; Mitchell and Miller, J. Exp. Med., 128, 821, 1968) or BSA (Smith et al., Proc. Soc. Exp. Biol. Med., 121, 1005, 1966; Taylor, Transplantation Rev., in the press, 1969), after reconstitution with combinations of thymus and bone-marrow cells. These experiments indicate that the marrow-derived cells serve as precursors of antibody-forming cells, while the thymus-derived cells serve as helpers.

The second category of in vivo reconstitution experiments have been performed with spleen cells primed against different determinants (usually hapten-specific and carrier-specific) on a macromolecule. These experiments indicate that carrier effects are the result of an act of cooperation in which one lymphocyte (the helper) picks up antigen by means of a carrier determinant, and presents it to a second cell which is thus triggered by the inducing determinant (Mitchison in "Differentiation and Immunology," 7, 29, Ed. Warren, Acad. Press, 1968); it is further believed that the helper cell may be thymus-derived (Mitchison in "Immunological Tolerance," p. 115, Eds. Landy and Braun, Acad. Press, 1969; Rajewsky et al., J. Exp. Med., 129, 1131, 1969). The argument that carrier effects can in this way be mapped onto the thymus-narrow interaction is still somewhat flimsy, and is of course prompted by a desire to bring the hapten-carrier experiments into line with the sRBC findings. If the argument is correct, cell-mediated immunity plays an important role as an antigen-concentrating mechanism in possibly a wide range of humoral responses; this in turn provides a hitherto unsuspected justification for the evolution of cell-mediated immunity, which may perhaps turn out to be as important as other justifications which have been proposed, such as combatting intracellular infections or surveillance.

What is the nature of the cellular receptor involved in recognition of antigen by lymphocytes of the cellular-immunity population? The hypothesis of a unique, non-secretable immunoglobulin class, "IgX" has been formulated (Mitchison in "Immunological Tolerance," Eds. Landy and Braun, Acad. Press, 1969; Dupuy et al., Lancet, $\underline{1}$,551,1969). The IgX hypothesis is illustrated in Fig. 7, in which the molecule is shown participating in the act of cooperation postulated in the preceding paragraph. Alternatively, these lymphocytes may bear the normal immunoglobulins but be under some physiological control which prevents their secretion. The evidence which may in the future settle this question will perhaps come from transformation experiments with anti-immunoglobulin sera, from the use of anti-receptor sera to inhibit in vitro cellular immunity, from the use of anti-receptor sera to protect lymphocytes from adsorption onto antigen-coated beads (Wigzell and Andersson,J. Exp. Med.,$\underline{129}$,23,1969;and unpublished data) or from studies on immunoglobulin-bearing, but non-secreting tumours (Klein et al., Cancer Res., $\underline{28}$, 1300, 1968).

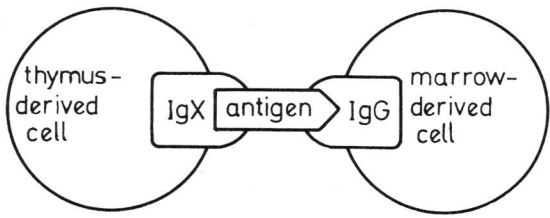

Fig. 7 Cooperation of thymus-derived and marrow-derived cells via IgX

It would of course make matters very much clearer if animals pass through a stage either in evolution or in development at which one population of lymphocytes is active but not the other. This is a matter which has been

II. FEATURES OF CELLULAR VERSUS HUMORAL IMMUNITY

debated by Good, Silverstein, Hildemann, and their respective colleagues. So far as I am aware there is no clear evidence as yet of the existence of such a stage.

Induction of cell-mediated immunity

Various circumstances are known to favour a cellular immune response in preference to a humoral one. These include use of minute doses of antigen, immunisation via the intradermal route, use of appropriate adjuvants, and presentation of a new determinant attached to a tolerated cell (the self + X hypothesis of Lawrence (Physiol. Rev., 39, 811, 1959; see also Mitchison and Dube, J. Exp. Med., 102, 179, 1955). The best established recipe for inducing delayed hypersensitivity is the use of an adjuvant which attracts a mononuclear infiltrate: Freund's complete adjuvant is the reference method, although the use of tubercle bacilli for this purpose can be traced back to the Dienes phenomenon. It is tempting to conclude from the efficacy of antigen-loaded allogeneic macrophages (Block and Nordin, Nature, 187, 434, 1960) that the homograft reaction can serve as a non-specific adjuvant in an analogous manner.

The rationale of these empirical recipes is not understood. The theory of two lymphocyte populations does at least indicate where we should seek an explanation. It suggests that the ethology of the recirculating lymphocyte may let the cell be stimulated preferentially, under the circumstances which favour induction of cellular immunity. In Cr_{51}-labelling we may have the right tool for answering this question (Lance and Taub, Immunology, 15, 633, 1968).

Some difficulties

Two studies suggest that, in the rabbit, cells which secrete immunoglobulins are derived from the thymus. (a) The rate of recovery from allotype suppression has been studied as a function of age (Dubiski, Cold Spring Harb. Symp. Quant. Biol., 32, 311, 1967). Older rabbits take longer to recover, and the relationship parallels the relationship between age and recovery from tolerance in a remarkably exact way. The latter type of recovery has been found to be thymus-dependent and it is therefore probable that recovery from allotype suppression is also thymus-dependent. Clearly the crucial experiment is lacking, and the inference is therefore indirect. (b) Upon transfer of 80×10^6 thymus cells from a 6-7 week old donor of one allotype into a newborn recipient of another allotype, a few recipients display a rapid and long-lasting increase of the donor allotype, which can be attributed to seeding out of cells into the recipient's lymph nodes and spleen (Chou et al., J. Exp. Med., 126, 305, 1967). The increase is greater than that obtained after transfer of comparable numbers of lymph node cells.

These experiments, particularly the second, present formidable difficulties for the two populations theory. I cannot see how they can be overcome, and would be glad to hear comments on this issue.

DR. GELL: In the matter of IgX - it seems to me that the key question that you raise is whether IgX is different from ordinary IgG. Moreover, if it is indeed different, just how different? Are the difficulties about the allotypes vital ones if we postulate that it is an immunoglobulin-like molecule? The odd thing about the allotypes, is of course, that all the markers, both light and heavy chains are present on all known Ig classes: if it is present on these why not also on IgX. It seems to me therefore that the presence of allotypic markers on IgX does not exclude the fact IgX might be a different sort of protein. Would you want to comment on this point?

DR. MITCHISON: I don't think your suggestion will resolve all the difficulties, because what is involved in your system is secreted immunoglobulin. When Dr. Dubiski measures allotype suppression, what he is measuring is the suppression of allotype that has been secreted into serum. It should be noted that Cinader also measured allotype that had been secreted. Consequently, we are not going to get out of the difficulties by saying that the allotype is stuck onto the membrane of the thymus-derived cell.

II. FEATURES OF CELLULAR VERSUS HUMORAL IMMUNITY

CHAIRMAN WAKSMAN: Perhaps this could be answered by showing blast transformation produced by anti-IgG, IgM, or IgA, in cells which can be proved to be thymus-derived by means of chromosome or other markers. Has anyone done that? I think this would be a useful addition to your list of desirable questions.

In Dr. Mitchison's list were suggested the use of anti-immunoglobulin to block an *in vitro* effect and identify the antibody present on sensitized cells. However, if such an antibody induces blast transformation in the sensitized cells, that process might of itself produce the *in vitro* effect and the issue would not have been resolved.

DR. MÖLLER: I think this would present no difficulty, but I would first comment about IgX which could either be an immunoglobulin or something entirely different. The latter possibility seems to me rather unlikely. I want to record some experiments done by Dr. Greaves on the effect of anti-light chain antibody on various responses (Nature, 222, 885, 1969). The systems employed were MLC, (Fig. 8) the mitogenic effect of PPD added to sensitized lymphocytes (Fig. 9) and inhibition of migration of lymphocytes from capillary tubes.

Dr. Greaves could, in fact, do just what Dr. Waksman suggested. He inhibited the mitogenic response in the PPD system as well as in MLC by means of anti-light chain antibodies, in concentrations where they themselves did not stimulate. As is shown in Fig. 10 the Fab fragment, which is not stimulatory by itself, also works in these systems.

Of course the anti-light chain antibody reacts with all immunoglobulin classes, and with IgX as well if it is, in fact, an immunoglobulin. The anti-light chain antibody will also block the inhibition of migration by specific antigen, a test considered to be a measure of cell-mediated immunity. Accordingly, from Dr. Greaves' data, it would seem that the best candidate for "IgX" is either an immunoglobulin; of the classes already known or of a new type. These findings would seem to me to exclude the possibility that "IgX" is something different.

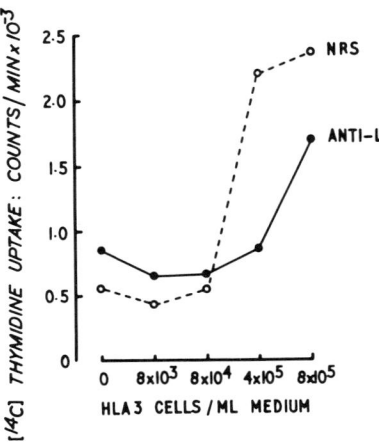

Fig. 8 Inhibition of MLC by anti-L chain antibody. Increasing doses of mitomycin treated HL-A3 cells were added to a constant number of HL-A4 cells, either with normal rabbit serum or anti-L chain antibody.

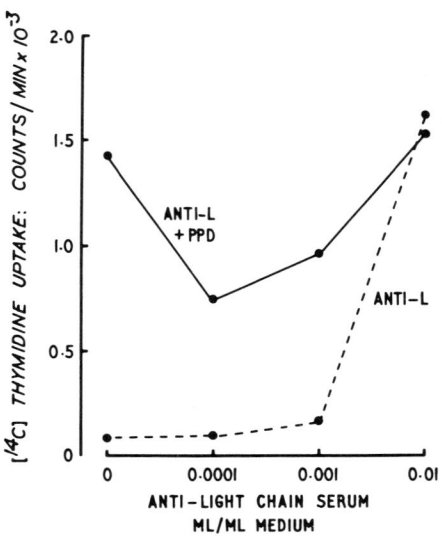

Fig. 9 Effect of various doses of anti-L chain antibody on the mitogenic response of human lymphocytes to PPD

II. FEATURES OF CELLULAR VERSUS HUMORAL IMMUNITY

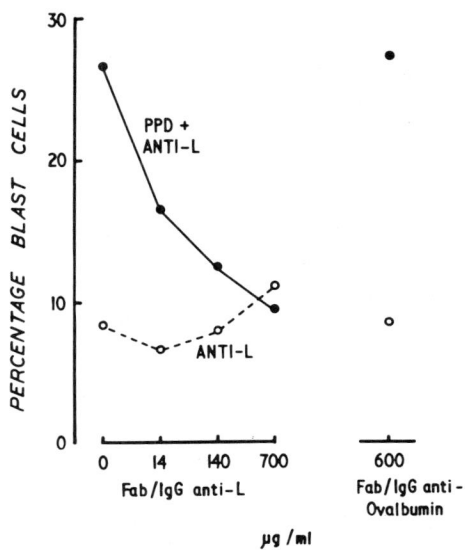

Fig. 10 Effect of the Fab fragment of anti-L chain antibody on the mitogenic response of human lymphocytes to PPD

DR. OPPENHEIM: An interesting and relevant observation has recently been made by Alm and Peterson (J. Exp. Med., 129, 1247, 1969), which illustrates the converse of what Dr. Mitchison mentioned. They bursectomized chickens, and then determined the response of their lymphocytes to anti-immunoglobulin. Bursectomy markedly reduced the response of these cells to anti-immunoglobulin, but it did not affect their reaction to PHA. The converse experiment was as mentioned by Dr. Mitchison that the lymphocytes of thymectomized chickens have a reduced response to PHA but this ablation had no effect on activation of cells by anti-immunoglcbulin. These data support the view that the two means of stimulating cells are in effect distinguishing between the humoral and cellular populations.

However, this still leaves us with the problem of why the
rabbits apparently respond well to both stimuli. My own
experience has been that rabbit lymphocytes do not respond
to PHA as well as those of man. In contrast, the anti-
immunoglobulin response in rabbits is much better than that
in man. Accordingly it may be that mammals vary significantly in the proportions of "cellular" versus "humoral"
categories of lymphocytes present in their circulation.

DR. DUTTON: I would like to speak to this second cell-
precursor cooperative effect, and decide whether it is
telling us anything about IgX. I would first want to
ascertain whether there is such a thing as IgX and if the
same IgX mediates the antigen-processing reactions that
Dr. Mitchison referred to as well as the delayed hypersensitivity response. My remarks won't really help us
resolve this, but I would like to present some information
which has at least some bearing on the question.

I have been concerned with the response of mouse spleen
cells to sRBC, a response that is depressed by neonatal
thymectomy. In this situation it is possible that whatever
it is that is affected in this system by thymectomy is the
same as is affected in cellular immunity.

The experiments we performed were with the spleen cell
cultures that respond in vitro to sRBC as antigen. We
started by separating them into "light" and "dense" cell
populations, neither of which could respond alone. We
called the light one the A band and the heavy one the D
band, and when these two cell populations were recombined,
the ability of the cells to respond to the antigen was
restored. The precursor cell is in the D band; some
second component must therefore be in the A band, helping
the precursor cells respond to antigen. The only thing I
can say about what cell type is in the A band, is that it
has the size distribution we associate with small lymphocytes, and has fewer rather than more macrophages than the
whole population.

We then did a different kind of cell separation, similar
to that described by Mosier to obtain adherent and non-
adherent cells. Adherent cells are those that stick to the

II. FEATURES OF CELLULAR VERSUS HUMORAL IMMUNITY

plastic surface of culture dishes; non-adherent cells are those that don't stick to glass beads on incubation for 60 minutes. Here again, one gets two cell populations that don't respond individually yet upon recombination they do respond. The precursor cells are in the non-adherent population and the second or helper cell is in the adherent population. It therefore seems clear, though not completely so, that these two separation procedures are functionally equivalent, inasmuch as the adherent cells will restore the D band, and the A band cells will restore the non-adherent cells (Table 12).

TABLE 12

COOPERATION BETWEEN ADHERENT CELLS AND D BAND

	(#2060)	D Band Cells		
	Cell number	20×10^6	7×10^6	3.7×10^6
	alone	8000^1	900	0
Adherent	287	13000	7700	6150
Adherent (irrad)²	0	15000	8650	5100
Whole spleen		15200		

(Combined)

[1] PFC/culture

[2] irradiation 1000R in vitro

I don't really know what type of cell is in the adherent cell population, but certainly many people would feel that this fraction is enriched for macrophages; yet here it is performing in a manner similar to the A band cells. It turns out that both these cell populations, adherent and A band, continue to function after they have been exposed to as much as 1000 r, suggesting that whatever their function, it does not require cell division. (Table 13 and 14)

TABLE 13

EFFECT OF IRRADIATION ON A BAND CELLS

(#2070)		D Band Cells		
	Cell Number	(10^7)	(3.3×10^6)	(1.7×10^6)
	Alone	[1] 320	0	0
A band	65	1600	480	280
A band (irrad.)	0	2820	180	160

combined (applies to A band and A band (irrad.) rows)

Whole spleen (1×10^7)   840

[1] PFC/culture

[2] Irradiation 1000 R *in vitro*

This led us to another experiment to determine whether we could extract a product from these "helper" cell populations that would restore the capacity of non-adherent cells to respond. We incubated the adherent cells for 24 hours, spun out all the cells at 3,000 rpm, and determined whether the supernatant would restore the non-adherent precursor cell population. In six of nine experiments we obtained restoration ranging from 20-100%. (Table 15) It is thus clear that whatever is lacking in the non-adherent cell population, it can be provided by something made by or released from the adherent cell population.

II. FEATURES OF CELLULAR VERSUS HUMORAL IMMUNITY

TABLE 14

EFFECT OF IRRADIATION ON ADHERENT CELLS

(#2056)		Non-adherent cells		
	Cell number	(8.7×10^6)	(2.9×10^6)	(1×10^6)
	Alone	225 [1]	5	8
Adherent (1×10^6)	3	820	290	154
Adherent (irrad.)	0	730	65	28

Whole spleen (1.2×10^7) 1100

[1] PFC/culture

[2] Irradiation 800 R *in vitro*

There are several possible explanations; one is that this is merely a nutritional factor that is required in culture, or, an alternative and perhaps more interesting possibility, is that it could be some sort of immunoglobulin. The only thing that one can say so far in favor of this latter possibility, is that in the two comparisons that have been made, supernatants obtained from adherent cells of immunized animals are several times more active than the supernatants from adherent cells of non-immunized animals. There is then a rather slender suggestion that this may turn out to be a product dependent upon prior exposure to the antigen, a possibility that is compatible with the idea that it is an antibody. I want, however, to point out one problem here, should this prove to be the case. In the experiments done by Mosier, he thymectomized and then irradiated the donor of the adherent and non-adherent populations. He found that in the cell populations obtained from these mice, the thymic dependent deficiency was in the non-adherent cell population. In our experiments, however, this factor comes from the adherent cells, implying that it is not made by thymic-derived cells.

TABLE 15

EFFECT OF ADHERENT CELL SUPERNATANTS ON NON-ADHERENT CELLS

(#2069)			Non-Adherent cells	
	Cell number	5×10^6	1.6×10^6	0.8×10^6
	Alone	120	0	0
Adherent cells $(2 \times 10)^6$	10	1400	258	91
				Combined
SN ^{2} from Adherent cells	-	1570	280	25
Whole Spleen		1680		

[1] PFC/culture

[2] SN= Culture supernatant from 2×10^6 cells incubated in complete medium for 24 hrs.

II. FEATURES OF CELLULAR VERSUS HUMORAL IMMUNITY

DR. TURK: Doesn't your assay for PFC reveal humoral antibody production, rather than cell-mediated immunity?

DR. DUTTON: Yes, of course. I introduced these findings primarily because Dr. Mitchison raised the possibility that the second cell in the cooperative cell-cell systems in the humoral response, may be related to the mediator of the cellular response. The point of my remark was that it really does not all quite fit together.

DR. BRAUN: I wonder whether there is one potential difficulty in the interpretation of your observations. After the Brook Lodge Symposium on Immunological Tolerance I went home to see whether it is possible to convert, with the aid of non-specific stimulators, pre-existing memory cells into antibody forming cells. We got evidence suggesting that this may indeed be possible. If you take previously primed mice, or for that matter normal controls, and give them a combination of ALS plus poly A-poly U, you get a highly significant increase in the number of spleen cells forming antibodies to sRBC, cRBC or hRBC. I am, therefore, wondering whether the increase that you are observing with your non-adherent factor may not be just that, namely, a factor that is capable of converting the already present, but non-performing memory cells, into performing antibody-forming cells. I am certain that you will agree that one has to differentiate between truly de novo initiation of committed cells and a stimulation, to performance, of existing cells.

DR. DUTTON: The data seem to be against such a possibility. If you take the whole unfractionated cell population -- and stimulate it -- you may get 1500 PFC per culture. If you take a non-adherent cell alone you get no response. If you take (in the best experiments) the non-adherent cells plus the supernatant, you get a total restoration of the response (i.e. 1500 PFC). Thus if the mechanism Dr. Braun suggests is operating, it is doing a very efficient job. Just as efficient as the complete system. There remains however the finding that the supernatant from adherent cells of an immunized donor is more effective than the supernatant from a non-immunized donor.

CELLULAR IMMUNITY

CHAIRMAN WAKSMAN: Dr. Dutton's discussion raises the implication that we are really dealing with at least three types of cells here rather than two. He didn't equate either of his cell types with the macrophage; yet, there is a good deal of evidence, both direct and indirect, that macrophages may play a role in the induction of a response.

At this point I would like to describe some work that Dr. Talmage reported in some detail recently (Fed. Proc., 1969), that shows very clearly the existence of three-cell systems, both *in vivo* and *in vitro*. There have also been reports lately, suggesting that there may be as many as four.

DR. MITCHISON: I certainly don't see why you would want four cells.

CHAIRMAN WAKSMAN: There was a recent report in which six different antigens were used and combining different types of cell populations. The results clearly implied at least two separate types in the single category you have just described as marrow-derived cells.

DR. MITCHISON: I follow what you are saying, but I believe, there are no more than three cell types.

CHAIRMAN WAKSMAN: Before moving on it may be useful to provide some further information on the Talmage experiment. Talmage used the appearance of PFC as an indicator of the immune response. In lethally irradiated animals or in tissue culture, unprimed or primed spleen cells in increasing doses, gave rise to the formation of more PFC. On the other hand, if an excess of bone-marrow was given to the recipient or bone marrow-derived cells were added to the tissue culture, this resulted in a constant number of plaques, no matter how many spleen cells were added. This then was clear evidence that two cell types were participating. In the *in vivo* system both of these sources of cell populations could be passed through a glass bead column, which presumably removed the macrophages, yet a response

90

II. FEATURES OF CELLULAR VERSUS HUMORAL IMMUNITY

occurred in the recipient. In the <u>in vitro</u> system there was no response if the two cell suspensions were passed through a glass bead column unless an additional source of macrophages was added. This was quite clearly a three-cell experiment.

DR. MÖLLER: We have used Dutton's system for separation of cells with the same results as he reported, but we also used the GVH assay to study the localization of the cells responsible for cell-mediated immunity. We found that they are in the bottom fractions and not in the top ones. I would make another point about cellular interactions between thymus and bone marrow-derived cells. This concept is derived mostly from work with a single antigenic model, i. e. sRBC. We don't know how many other antigens will be shown to be thymus-dependent, but I know at least one antigen which Anderson in Stockholm is working on which is entirely non-thymus-dependent, namely PVP (Polyvinyl-pyrrolidone). My question is, what would happen with such an antigen in delayed hypersensitivity responses. Can it induce such reactions?

Dr. Braun suggested that more than antigen alone, interacting with the cells, is required to trigger them. The additional steps could be either another specific cell or it could be an entirely non-specific event. What is needed for expression of immunity is cell division in the case of antibody synthesis, or transformation into a cytotoxic state in cell-mediated immunity. I would think that there must be additional factors which are needed for the secondary events, such as cell division or transformation in these opposing forms of the immune response.

DR. TURK: Would Dr. Möller provide us with some of the details on the experiment with the PVP and non-thymus dependent cells.

DR. MÖLLER: Bone-marrow cells were transferred into lethally-irradiated thymectomized animals and 14 days later they were immunized with PVP and they responded normally. The response was assayed in terms of humoral antibody.

Supplementation with thymus cells did not add to the effect, i. e. it was a pure bone-marrow response.

CHAIRMAN WAKSMAN: As this point it may be pertinent to ask whether there is in fact <u>any</u> non-thymus dependent system in which one can achieve delayed hypersensitivity? It seems to me that a partial answer is available in the fact that a number of carbohydrate antigens have been shown to induce non-thymus dependent antibody formation, and that generally these do not give delayed hypersensitivity. A single example of the induction of delayed hypersensitivity with a carbohydrate was reported by Battisto (Fed. Proc., 1968) which involved sensitization by dextran in the Abyssinian strain of guinea pigs. In relation to this antigen and the delayed response, guinea pigs of this strain are "responders". They provide an interesting possible point of attack on the problems we are discussing.

As regards to Dr. Möller's second question: I would in turn ask whether there is evidence that the thymus-derived cell's contribution could be simply release of a non-specific substance comparable to interfereon, MIF or chemotactic factor, which activates the bone marrow-derived cell so that it can go about its business?

DR. MÖLLER: I think that the cells need something more than a specific interaction: this could be a variety of things, such as soluble factors, other cells, or complement. Something surely is needed for triggering of the secondary manifestations of the initial reaction.

DR. BRAUN: May I suggest that you do not phrase your question the way you just did, because I don't think one should ask whether the thymus cell produces only a non-specific factor, but whether in addition to its other tasks, it may also provide a non-specific factor that is required to drive the response in a certain direction.

II. FEATURES OF CELLULAR VERSUS HUMORAL IMMUNITY

DR. MITCHISON: Thymus-derived cells may make a non-specific contribution as well, but Dr. Möller you wouldn't question that they make a specific contribution? Otherwise you couldn't have a tolerant population of cells obtained from the thymus in the experiments of Waksman and of Taylor.

DR. MÖLLER: The basic question is whether the thymocytes produce a specific product or acquire cytophilic antibodies produced elsewhere. If tolerance is developed, no response could be induced in either case, and this would not contribute to an understanding of the role of the thymus.

DR. MITCHISON: In the Taylor experiment, the mice are injected with protein, and only 24 hours later, cells are taken out of the thymus and now display altered reactivity in reconstitution experiements. In an experiment of this kind it is very hard to suggest that the cells in the thymus are getting something from the marrow, wouldn't you say?

DR. THOR: The preceding dialogue has gotten rather involved. Could it be clarified before we proceed further.

CHAIRMAN WAKSMAN: To briefly recapitulate: The suggestion has been raised that the role of the thymus-derived cell, in a situation in which the effector cell making antibody is a marrow-derived cell, may be to react to antigen specifically. This interaction then leads to release of something which is not specific, but which is needed for the marrow-derived cell to perform its task.

Dr. Möller was saying that possibly even the thymus-derived cell's activity may not be specific in terms of what this cell brings to the scene. It may be acting for example, because of an adsorbed antibody of some kind, obtained elsewhere. If I understood Dr. Mitchison's answer correctly, since tolerance can be induced specifically in these cells while they are in the thymus, at a time when one presumes they have not been exposed to cytophilic antibody, they then must have a specificity of their own. It seems to me, however, if I may insert my own opinion, that the thymus-derived cell's participation could still be via release of a non-specific mediator, even though its initial reaction with antigen is quite specific.

DR. COHN: Why would you want to ignore the contribution of the bone-marrow cell?

CHAIRMAN WAKSMAN: Because the bone marrow-derived cell must also react with the antigen, but cannot go about its business without the assistance of a component that is released.

DR. COHN: But, then you have to add still another element — one more hypothesis.

DR. DUTTON: Going back to the question of whether the thymus cells really synthesize the antigen-specific molecules in the tolerance experiment, there have been some recent experiments by Drs. Treadwell and Lennox, in which they took irradiated mice and reconstituted them with bone-marrow and peritoneal cells, rather than with bone-marrow and thymus. They found that the peritoneal cells from immune donors were more effective than those from non-immunized donors. Furthermore, by keeping the peritoneal cells at 45°C for 30 minutes, they could obtain a supernatant which had partial activity in facilitating the restoration of competence by bone-marrow cells in the irradiated recipient.

DR. COHN: Dr. Mitchison, you have given us such an informative summary of this situation, that I hesitate to raise a point of clarification, as well as what may prove to be a semantic issue. According to this model you would not expect in the delayed hypersensitivity situation, a two-cell interaction involving thymus and bone marrow-derived cells. Is that correct?

DR. MITCHISON: There is nothing in this scheme to exclude precisely the same helper function for a thymus-derived cell in facilitating the induction of another thymus-

II. FEATURES OF CELLULAR VERSUS HUMORAL IMMUNITY

derived cell or a marrow-derived cell. We are, after all, familiar with carrier effects in the context of delayed hypersensitivity. This is where attention was first drawn to the carrier, through the work of Dr. Gell and his collaborators. But you are, of course, quite right in saying that in this scheme especially in relation to the induction of delayed type hypersensitivity, there is no interaction between the thymus-derived and marrow-derived cell.

DR. COHN: So that raises the question of these experiments of yours on thymus and bone-marrow interaction and delayed hypersensitivity.

CHAIRMAN WAKSMAN: That is a perfectly proper question. Let me remind you that the situation there is the exact reverse of what we are talking about. All of our discussion has been: how do you induce the formation of an effector cell? We have not talked very much about the possibility that the actual sensitized cell of delayed sensitivity, which is the effector cell, is itself the thymus-derived cell. As far as I know, there has been no published evidence on this.

DR. COHN: Didn't you find that in addition to the thymus, the bone-marrow cell was responsible for the delayed hypersensitivity reaction?

CHAIRMAN WAKSMAN: No. The delayed reaction is initiated by a sensitized cell but the infiltrate is largely made up by cells of another type, bone marrow-derived monocyte or macrophage, as shown last year by Lubaroff in our laboratory. The macrophage is really a secondary participant and not the primary effector cell.

One of our students Mr. Williams, is trying to use Lubaroff's labeling method, to establish whether the sensitized cell of delayed sensitivity is actually a thymus-derived cell. His preliminary results are shown in Fig. 11. Lewis rats were thymectomized, irradiated, restored with syngeneic bone-marrow, and given a graft of (Lewis x BN) F_1

thymus. When these animals were tuberculin-sensitized and later tested with PPD, the proportion of cells arriving at the local reaction site which were clearly thymus-derived (estimated by indirect immunofluorescent staining with anti-BN antiserum) rose to nearly 20%. These cells were most numerous in the first 8 to 16 hours of the evolution of the reaction. The numbers correspond closely to the numbers of sensitized cells as estimated by Lubaroff.

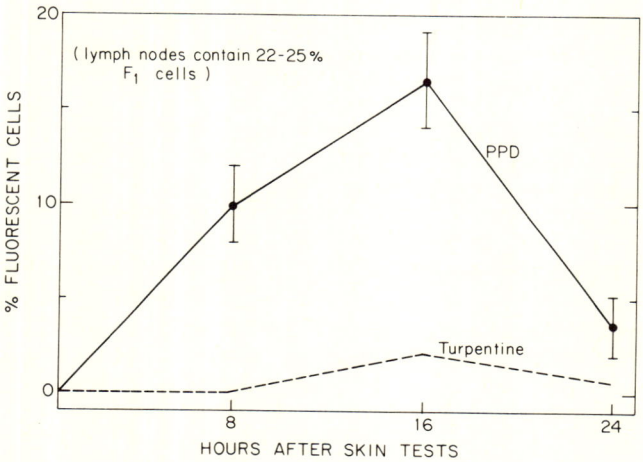

Fig. 11 Thymus-derived cells in delayed skin reactions

Accordingly it seems probable, although further control studies are needed, that the sensitized cell itself is a thymus-derived cell. I would draw a parallel between its interaction with the bone marrow-derived monocyte at the peripheral site and the interaction demonstrated by Claman, and Mitchell and Miller in the spleen and lymph nodes, where a marrow-derived cell goes on to become an antibody-forming cell. I don't know if that answers your question.

II. FEATURES OF CELLULAR VERSUS HUMORAL IMMUNITY

DR. COHN: I am not sure either. I want to make the second point, the question which might be reduced to semantics. Dr. Mitchison, you described the carrier antibody as an antigen-concentrating mechanism. You pictured one cell picking up the antigen by a reaction with one determinant, and feeding it to another cell which is an antigen-sensitive cell. If this were the only role of carrier-antibody, a non-specific mechanism that would fix the antigen and concentrate it for the bone-marrow cell, that mechanism should in principle lead to a response. Therefore, the so called IgX, or what I have been calling carrier-antibody, is not a part of the induction mechanism itself, but is instead merely a transport or concentration device. Now the point is whether there is a semantic difference between us, or a real difference in the way we are looking at carrier-antibody?

DR. MITCHISON: No, it is a real difference.

DR. SILVERSTEIN: I want to address the same point Dr. Cohn brought up about protein carriers. I think Dr. Mitchison has been guilty of being too highly selective about the data that he has chosen to support his concept. Among the many points I object to in his formulation, I will only discuss the helper-cell carrier-cell hypothesis.

I might say parenthetically that there is a tendency to treat the hapten coupled to a protein carrier as forming a qualitatively different kind of determinant than the normal antigenic determinant that pre-existed on that protein surface. I don't think this is so. Many of the ad hoc assumptions, like the helper-carrier cells, have been brought in to try to cope with this presumed difference.

There is a critical experiement that Dr. Gell and I published some years ago (J. Exp. Med., 115, 1037, 1962) with respect to the hapten-carrier issue. That work refers not only to Mitchison's helper cell, but also to the helper molecule that Cohn postulated in the recent past. I think that the observation is significant enough to warrant somebody else repeating it. We took a given hapten and coupled it by different chemical manipulations, to the tyrosine of a carrier protein with a diazonium group or onto the same carrier protein via an epsilon amino group. Guinea pigs sensitized to either of these conjugates did not recognize the same hapten placed on the same carrier, but at another locus.

This is very significant, because if the helper cell or the helper molecule is working as an anti-carrier, then the "anti-hapten" cell in this guinea pig should have been able to function, no matter what the position of the hapten on the carrier protein. In these experiments, the carrier was guinea pig albumin and the haptens used were paraminobenzoate, paranitrobenzene, and I think we also used sulfanilic acid. These data support the notion that the determinant must include the small haptenic focus as well as a portion of the neighboring carrier protein surface.

DR. WILSON: I have a question for you, Dr. Waksman: What evidence have you that these infiltrating cells of bone-marrow origin are, in fact, serving as effector cells?

CHAIRMAN WAKSMAN: I wouldn't use the term effector cell in relation to them. I didn't mean to imply that. To me the effector cell is the thymus-derived cell which becomes the sensitized cell. The macrophages are simply additional participants or secondary invaders, if you like, brought in unusually large numbers after the trigger events which occur locally.

DR. TURK: I would like to bring up a question of x-irradiation of guinea pigs in relation to the delayed phenomena, that may help us in the interpretation of whether marrow-derived cells are involved in delayed hypersensitivity reaction. There are a number of experiments in which it has been found that delayed sensitivity is not as sensitive to x-irradiation as is antibody production. I have observed similar phenomena in contact sensitivity. We could block antibody production with lethal irradiation and not block the manifestations of contact sensitivity or delayed sensitivity. Does this information help at all with eliminating the necessary participation of marrow-derived

II. FEATURES OF CELLULAR VERSUS HUMORAL IMMUNITY

cells, since the marrow-derived cell is more radio-sensitive than the thymus-derived cell?

DR. MÖLLER: It has been shown that if you irradiate the animal, you can't evoke delayed hypersensitivity or homograft reactivity.

DR. TURK: In guinea pigs you can, however, elicit delayed sensitivity in the lethally irradiated animal.

CHAIRMAN WAKSMAN: There are some interesting points here. It seems to me two separate issues are at stake. One has to do with the induction of delayed sensitivity, the actual immunization process. That is considerably more radio-resistant than the induction of antibody formation. We certainly lack information about which particular cell is doing what at any given time. The other side of the coin is that the elicitation of delayed sensitivity may be strikingly reduced by a dose of X-ray that wipes out the bone marrow-derived participants. This was shown best by Dr. Feldman in his passive transfer studies.

We will now turn to the matter of specificity of the response, whether of the delayed or antibody type, in relation to specific determinants and carrier portions of the antigen molecule.

DR. SILVERSTEIN: There are two major questions that might be posed and considered. The first question would be, is there a difference between the antigenic determinant required to stimulate the cell for delayed hypersensitivity and that required to stimulate a cell for antibody formation? The second question would be, is there a difference between the determinant required to elicit a delayed hypersensitivity reaction (and this is not necessarily different from the sensitization step) and the antigenic determinant with which antibodies can react?

I think that we know enough from the varied studies on carrier specificity to indicate that the general consensus, with one or two notable exceptions, is that the immunogen required to induce and elicit delayed hypersensitivity is identical to the immunogen required to induce antibody formation. However, it appears to be different from the antigen required to react with the antibody subsequently produced. One should be aware, however, that antibodies possessing carrier-plus-hapten specificity have been reported frequently (Borek and Silverstein, Nature, 205, 299, 1965). The exception that might be considered concerns the data of Leskowitz and others referring primarily to a restricted group of antigenic determinants (arsanilic acid, etc.) which do not seem to fit in with this system.†

---

† Afterthought: One aspect of the specificity of the lymphocyte receptor molecule figured importantly in hallway discussions, and might profitably be introduced here. It was shown by Silverstein and Borek (J. Immunol, 96, 953, 1966) that desensitization of delayed hypersensitivity to BSA in the guinea pig could be effected in a stepwise manner by intravenous administration of graded doses of I_{131}-BSA, so that final circulating concentrations of the antigen could be assessed. These studies pointed out that in the presence of a given concentration of antigen in the blood, a positive though diminished skin test response could still be evoked using an estimated five-fold molar concentration of antigen in the skin. This suggests: 1) that there is probably a distribution of association constants (K_A) for the lymphocyte receptor comparable in heterogeneity to that found for antibodies; 2) that a normal range of apparent K_A's is involved in the receptor recognition site, since responses did not disappear until {Ag} >10^{-7} $\underline{M}$ or so; 3) that very high affinity is not an obligatory characteristic of the lymphocyte receptor, thus highlighting the problem of what carrier specificity contributes to the trigger event; but posing the paradox that; 4) as little as 10^{-12} $\underline{M}$ antigen may evoke a partial skin reaction, so that if only the high K_A end of a normal distribution curve of energies were reacting at this low antigen concentration, only an extremely small number of reactive cells (many orders of magnitude smaller than the maximum figure of one-to-two percent we have previously discussed) are adequate to mediate the delayed skin reaction.

II. FEATURES OF CELLULAR VERSUS HUMORAL IMMUNITY

CHAIRMAN WAKSMAN: According to Dr. Mitchison's scheme, there are thymus-derived cells that react with antigen and bone marrow-derived cells that mature to become antibody-forming cells. In the case of immune responses to conjugates studied by Gell and Benacerraf years ago, it appeared that any delayed sensitivity elicited was directed largely at the carrier molecule, while antibody was formed against both the carrier and the haptenic determinant.

We have considered the possiblity that the thymus-derived cell reacts to the carrier only, but releases some substance that may be necessary to permit bone marrow-derived cells to fulfill their mission. The bone-marrow cells, nevertheless, are responding to the specific stimulus of antigen. Why can't one be a bone marrow-derived cell, that has a suitable receptor for the hapten, and the other a bone marrow-derived cell that has a suitable receptor for the carrier. Both must be appropriately situated and aided by the thymus cell to go on to make antibody. The thymus-derived cell, meanwhile, goes over to being the effector cell of delayed sensitivity.

DR. SILVERSTEIN: I have previously given one of the reasons that makes me think there is no obligatory participation of two types of cells, at least on this level. Further, I am not the right person to speak with authority on thymus-derived versus bone marrow-derived cells, because I don't yet fully believe in them. I do not think that there is, as yet, enough critical and compelling data to warrant the approach that has been taken with respect to these putative cell systems.

DR. SCHLOSSMAN: Although more than one cell type may be required to initiate the immune response, I am not sure that there is any compelling evidence to support the view that each of these cells recognizes different portions of the immunogenic determinant. In this regard, it may be worthwhile to consider the specificity of the cellular receptor for antigen and the possible role of two cells in recognizing a single antigenic determinant. I would like to briefly describe a series of experiments using the α, DNP-oligolysine system. In this system we can evaluate the chemical requirements necessary to induce the immune response as well as those required to elicit the cellular immune response either in vivo or in vitro. Further, one can compare the specificity of the cellular response to the specificity of circulating antibody produced to the same chemically defined antigen. The α, DNP-oligolysines all have a single DNP group on the N terminal α, amino group and differ from one another in lysine chain length.

α, DNP-oligo-L-lysines containing fewer than seven L-lysines, i. e. α, DNP-Lys$_{3-6}$, are not immunogenic in guinea pigs, i. e. they can not induce the formation of delayed hypersensitivity or circulating antibody. In contrast, α, DNP-oligolysines equal to or larger in size than the heptamer can induce the formation of both delayed hypersensitivity and circulating antibody. The basis for this sharp cutoff between immunogenicity and nonimmunogenicity in the guinea pig has still not been resolved. Nonetheless, we can test an animal sensitized to α, DNP-Lys$_9$ with the various α, DNP-oligolysine peptides. Intradermal injections of α, DNP-Lys$_3$ to α, DNP-Lys$_6$ provoke only an Arthus-type reaction but no delayed skin reaction, anamnestic response or in vitro cellular immune response (incorporation of thymidine-2-^{14}C or production of macrophage inhibiting factor). In contrast, peptides equal to or larger in size than the heptamer provoke the Arthus-type, delayed and anamnestic response in vivo and the cellular immune reactions in vitro. Similarly, a nonimmunogenic stereoisomer of α, DNP-nona-L-lysine, i. e. α, DNP-L$_4$DL$_4$, can only elicit the antibody mediated Arthus-type response but no cellular immune response. The latter observation is consistent with the view that minimal chain length, while necessary, is not sufficient to trigger an immunologically competent cell. Further, these observations indicate that the cellular immune responses and antibody dependent reactions reflect specificity to different portions of a common immunizing antigen. Although the cellular immune response is more specific than antibody mediated responses and may require a larger portion of the immunizing antigen to elicit the response (carrier specificity), it was clear that the distinguishing characteristic of antigen was not size alone but the capacity of the determinant to induce the immune response. That is, precisely the same chemical requirements for antigen exist for immunogenicity as are required to trigger the sensitized cell. Furthermore, it

II. FEATURES OF CELLULAR VERSUS HUMORAL IMMUNITY

appears that the "carrier specificity" found in more complex hapten protein conjugates reflected not on the size of the carrier but on the immunogenicity and uniqueness of the multiple determinants found in each hapten conjugate used to induce the response.

The obvious question was whether the binding characteristics of antibody to α, DNP-Lys$_9$ could distinguish between the heptamer and the hexamer. If, for example, there was a marked increase in affinity or specificity for the heptamer, one could attribute the observed differences in behavior of immunogenic and nonimmunogenic peptides to antibody affinity or specificity. Anti-α, DNP-Lys$_9$ antibody was studied by the techniques of quantitative precipitin, fluorescence quenching and equilibrium dialysis (with labeled peptides). The antibody binding site was maximally inhibited, bound or quenched on a molar basis by α, DNP-Lys$_7$; thus, indicating that the upper limit in size of the binding site was complementary in size to that of the heptamer. Furthermore, it could be shown that the hexamer contributed a minimum of 96% of the binding energy of the heptamer. Despite this, the heptamer but not the hexamer provoked the delayed skin reaction <u>in vivo</u> and <u>in vitro</u> thymidine-2-^{14}C incorporation and production of MIF (studies with Dr. John David). In addition, a 1000-fold molar excess of α, DNP-Lys$_{5-6}$ <u>in vitro</u> could not inhibit the stimulatory effect of α, DNP-Lys$_9$.

These studies suggest that the receptor on the sensitized lymphoid cell requires "something extra" in its interaction with antigen than does the simple interaction of antigen with antibody <u>in vitro</u>. The specificity of the cellular immune response could not simply be attributed to larger binding site or higher affinity of a cell fixed antibody. Within the confines of the two cell hypothesis it remains a theoretical possibility that a minimum of seven lysines are required by the carrier specific cell; fewer than seven lysyl residues are not recognized. In addition, the carrier specific cell has to be exquisitely specific since it obviously can not recognize the nonalysine if it has a single D-lysine at the 5th lysine position. In order to shed some further light on the specificity of the cellular receptor for antigen, Dr. Yaron and I prepared a series of six different nonalysines, each differing from one another in the position of the DNP group or a D-lysine residue. Cells from animals sensitized to these compounds exhibited an extraordinary degree of specificity and can readily discriminate among compounds differing from one another only in the position of the DNP group or D-lysine residue on an identical oligolysine backbone. For example, in cultures derived from animals sensitized to 5, ε, DNP-nonalysine the homologous antigen provoked a 25-fold increase in thymidine-2-^{14}C incorporation. In contrast, heterologous DNP-analysines, for example 9, ε, DNP-nonalysine containing the same nonalysine but with the ε, DNP group on a different residue, α, DNP-nonalysine or Lys$_9$ without the DNP group provoked no cross-stimulation. The antibodies from these animals, however, cross-react extensively as a consequence of specificity for a common DNP group. Similarly 9, ε, DNP-nonalysine cells do not cross-react with 5, ε, nonalysine, α, DNP-nonalysine or nonalysine without the DNP group. In contrast, cell cultures derived from animals sensitized to α, DNP-nonalysine behave somewhat differently than the above cultures since they cross-react partially with other immunogenic DNP-nonalysines. However, the crucial observation is that these cells react in an identical fashion with nonalysine without the DNP group as well as they do with heterologous DNP-nonalysines. It is believed that the latter cross-reactions result from a separate oligolysine sensitive population of cells and not as a direct result of the interaction of the α, DNP-nonalysine cell receptor with other heterologous DNP-nonalysines. The exquisite specificity of the cellular receptor for the total immunogenic determinant does not support the hypothesis outlined by Dr. Mitchison and is not compatible with the assumption that the cellular receptor for antigen is conventional cell associated antibody irrespective of its affinity or binding site size. The nature of the receptor, its distinction from an unique form of immunoglobulin obviously has still not been resolved.

DR. COHN: Which compound did not cause stimulation of the cells?

DR. SCHLOSSMAN: If we sensitized an animal to 5, ε, DNP-nonalysine there is no cross reaction with α, DNP-nonalysine, 9, ε, DNP-nonalysine or nonalysine. If we

II. FEATURES OF CELLULAR VERSUS HUMORAL IMMUNITY

sensitize with 9, ε, DNP-nonalysine there is no cross reaction to 5, ε, DNP-nonalysine, α, DNP-nonalysine or nonalysine. However, when you immunize with α, DNP-nonalysine, these cells will react with many compounds containing 7 L-lysines.

DR. CHASE: How many dinitrophenyl groups on that compound?

DR. SCHLOSSMAN: One. It should be noted that α, DNP-Lys$_9$ sensitized cells cannot be triggered to incorporate thymidine 2^{14}C or produce M.I.F. with non-immunogenic D Lysine containing nonalysines or α, DNP-Lys$_{3-6}$.

If we stimulate α, DNP-Lys$_9$ cells with 5, ε, DNP-nonalysine or 9, ε, DNP-nonalysine, we do get a cross-reaction, but the important point is that the same cross-reaction occurs with Lys$_9$ without the DNP group. Thus in this particular instance we are seeing a minimum of two populations of cells, induced by α, DNP-Lys$_9$; one population is specific for the oligolysine, and the second specific for α, DNP-Lys$_9$. We cannot separate the carrier specificity from hapten specificity. It thus becomes difficult to reconcile this with two different cells, one with specificity to the carrier, and one with specificity to the hapten.

DR CHASE: Dr. Schlossman, what was the sensitization routine you used with these various compounds all containing only one DNP group? Also how did you test the animals?

DR. SCHLOSSMAN: We used the Difco adjuvant. Immunogenic peptides could sensitize 100% of strain 2 guinea pigs, no strain 13 guinea pigs and about 70 percent of Hartley guinea pigs.

DR. CHASE: A single dinitrophenol providing you had 9 lysine residues?

DR. SCHLOSSMAN: That is correct. The other kinds of compounds are single dinitrophenol group in other positions on the molecule, and by the Merrifield stepwise synthesis procedure Dr. Yaron and I have prepared a number of D lysine containing stereoisomers of these compounds.

DR. MITCHISON: The compounds which Dr. Schlossman used, can be drawn in a different way. (Fig. 12). According to the view I have suggested in this figure, his data provide beautiful evidence of carrier-specific immunity which can be interpreted in terms of the two-cell theory. The carrier antibody would be directed against different configurations of the lysine chain which are stabilized by the different DNP-substitutions, although they do not include the DNP group itself. The prediction is that antibodies should be produced against these configurations. He should be able to detect them by measuring the binding of radioactive DNP-oligolysines, if necessary using non-radioactive DNP-lysine to inhibit binding by DNP-directed antibodies.

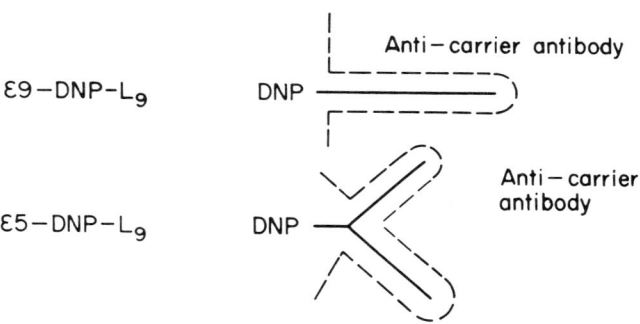

Fig. 12 Alternative configurations of the lysine chain on DNP; influence on binding of carrier antibody.

DR. SCHLOSSMAN: I think I lost you but perhaps it would be clearer if I said that in a thousand-fold molar excess the α, DNP-pentalysine which cannot trigger also cannot block the stimulating effect of immunogenic DNP oligolysines.

II. FEATURES OF CELLULAR VERSUS HUMORAL IMMUNITY

DR. MITCHISON: That is quite alright. When you add the DNP-pentalysine, you are trying to block the DNP directed sites, but not the sites directed towards DNP-stabilized determinants in the lysine chain.

DR. SCHLOSSMAN: I thought you required two cells to function together. In this case we clearly block the hapten-specific cell and should thus inhibit stimulation by DNP-oligolysine. Can you draw the molecules of DNP-BSA which you use?

DR. MITCHISON: No, I can't.

DR. MÖLLER: There is one point here that I think is very important, and which suggests that the receptor is really different: that would be the blocking experiments.

DR. SCHLOSSMAN: I am not quite sure. We don't get blocking. You can inhibit antibodies rapidly with DNP-pentalysine. However, DNP-pentalysines neither stimulate the cell nor inhibit the stimulatory effect of immunogenic DNP-nonalysine.

DR. MÖLLER: I would like to determine whether there is a model system in which you can show that it is very easy to inhibit stimulation in an analogous system.

DR. OPPENHEIM: In reply to Dr. Möller's query, we have this kind of control in another system. In studies using a conjugate of orthanilic acid as the hapten with guinea pig albumen as a carrier at approximate ratios of 15 to 1 hapten to hapten conjugate, we consistently saw partial inhibition by the haptens of the hapten carrier stimulation of _in vitro_ guinea pig lymph node lymphocyte-transformation.

DR. EISEN: Dr. Schlossman's elegant experiments certainly seem to show a remarkable lack of cross reactivity between α, DNP-octalysine and α, DNP-hexalysine. These very similar ligands would surely be expected to cross-react extensively with the vast majority of conventional anti-DNP antibodies. Nevertheless, I question whether this difference is a sufficient basis for postulating that the antigen-recognition substance on antigen-sensitive lymphocytes is qualitatively different than conventional immunoglobulins.

We know that the ability to discriminate between a pair of related ligands is not the same for all antibodies of a given specificity. In fact, discriminating-ability varies widely -- not only from antibody to antibody, but even with the same antibody under different assay conditions. I should not be at all surprised, therefore, if some sets of conventional anti-DNP antibody could be found that distinguish just as sharply between α-DNP-hexa- and heptalysines as Dr. Schlossman's Ag sensitive lymphocytes do. One experimental example that comes to mind of a changing level of discrimination deals not with delayed hypersensitivity but with the use of DNP proteins to induce a secondary response in intact animals. It was shown long ago, by Ovary and Benacerraf, that when they induced a primary immune response with DNP on one protein, say bovine gammaglobulin, and then challenged the animals 16 days later with DNP on ovalbumin, they did not get a secondary response, a clear example of carrier specificity. But subsequently, it turned out that under other conditions, with a longer interval between first and second injections, it is easy to show that carrier specificity can be overcome and that secondary responses are readily evoked with the hapten on a variety of different protein carriers; i.e. specificity was much less pronounced.

Dr. Schlossman's antigen-sensitive cells seem now to exhibit almost perfect specificity. It would not surprise me if, with slight variations in experimental conditions, they would show much more extensive cross-reactions. Delayed type hypersensitive skin reactions seem, in general, to show fewer cross reactions than conventional serum antibodies. Nevertheless, cross reactions can also be demonstrated in these reactions. Perhaps Dr. Chase could speak to this; he has far more experience in this area than anyone else.

II. FEATURES OF CELLULAR VERSUS HUMORAL IMMUNITY

DR. CHASE: The subject is not strictly relevant to the present topic. First, if animals have been sensitized by applying dinitrochlorobenzene (DNCB) or picryl chloride (TNCB) to their skin epicutaneously, a process in which self-coupling occurs and the animals are subsequently tested with the same haptenic grouping coupled to various different carriers, of course you will find that the hapten-protein conjugates made in the laboratory do not give good skin reactions, although the free allergen applied in a contact test will give good skin reactions.

But if the animals have been sensitized with preformed hapten-protein conjugates, for example, a TNP-protein rendered insoluble, as by combining it with alumina, comparative tests may be made with TNP-conjugates where the carrier varies from soluble epithelial protein of the guinea pig, guinea pig serum albumin, bovine albumin, and chicken albumin. When 8 or 10 guinea pigs sensitized, say, by means of the picrylated epithelial protein material, are tested with such a battery of products, all pigs invariably react strongly to the sensitizing product itself. But you will find much variation in the capacity to react with these other hapten-carrier products. Some animals will react significantly to the chicken complex, in which the TNP-grouping is the predominant portion of the recognized structure, and perhaps they will react also to some (but usually not all) of the other hapten-carrier structures. Other individuals will fail to recognize the chicken complex but will recognize the bovine carrier complex, and so on. Thus, you can find a series of responses by individual guinea pigs.

The same principle holds, of course, when rabbits are injected with dinitrophenyl- or trinitrophenyl- proteins. Only a small portion of the total antibody which is synthesized is capable of precipitating hapten-carrier complexes where the carrier differs markedly from the one used to stimulate antibody formation. This portion of antibody which can precipitate with, for example, chicken serum albumin complexes is perhaps not over 8 to 12 percent of the total antibody formed. The remainder of the antibody recognizes only the hapten-carrier complex which was used to stimulate the antibody, that is, it is "hapten-carrier" specific.

DR. GELL: It seems to me that the operational difference one is considering in these two situations which has to be taken into account, may be the accessibility of the antibody. When one is dealing with the free antibody, it is freely accessible -- when one is dealing with a cell, accessibility may not be so perfect.

DR. COHN: It was really pretentious for me to rise to defend Dr. Mitchison, but I would like to comment on Dr. Schlossman's question: Can Dr. Mitchison draw the conformation of DNP-BSA? The implication of that remark was that because DNP-BSA is such a heterogeneous system you can't draw any conclusions by working with it. Therefore, I would like to ask Dr. Schlossman whether he can draw the conformation of ε, DNP-lysine$_9$ and whether the antibody response to ε-DNP-lysine$_9$ is a homogenous one.

DR. SCHLOSSMAN: I would like to reply to Dr. Eisen's comments since this was the very point we were trying to make. It has been convenient to assume that antigen recognition requires the participation of cell-fixed antibody and postulate that the differences in specificity of cells and antibody can be accounted for by an antibody with a larger combining site or higher affinity. However, when you study both the specificity of cells and antibody it becomes increasingly difficult to ascribe the specificity of the sensitized cell to that of conventional cell-fixed antibody. That is all we are trying to say. We are not trying to say that ours is an absolutely homogeneous system, that there is no cross reactivity among cells, but that the cross reactivity that is detected in the α, DNP-oligolysine system can not be simply accounted for on the basis of postulating an antibody receptor with a different sized combining site or affinity. This does not mean that antibody is not on the cell surface and that it is not the receptor for antigen. It may well be, but to draw a parallel at the present time between the <u>in vitro</u> behavior of antibody and suggest that this is what is occurring on the cell surface can not be done. The cell surface receptor-antigen interaction requires something extra to trigger the sensitized cell; that something extra can not be ascribed to known behavior of conventional serum antibody. Under

II. FEATURES OF CELLULAR VERSUS HUMORAL IMMUNITY

such circumstances, it is reasonable to consider the existence of a totally different type of receptor system, despite our unwillingness to complicate matters. In point of fact, α, DNP-Lys$_9$ cells cross react with heterologous immunogenic DNP-nonalysines. However, the basis for this cross reaction is not as a consequence of the immunodominant haptenic group, but appears due to specificity for the oligolysine carrier. I believe the concept of immunodominance in antigen-antibody reactions is too well founded to be discarded when one deals with "cell-associated antibody".

The other point is in reply to Dr. Cohn. Clearly I can't draw a model of DNP-nonalysine but neither can Dr. Mitchison. However, I can make a closer guess to its structure than he can with a DNP-protein conjugate. We have not had enough antibody from a single guinea pig to study the homogeneity of these antibodies and most of our studies are done with serum pools. The antibody appears heterogeneous by Sips plot but it is still not known whether this is a consequence of the serum pools we use. The K_o of the antibody for the heptamer, octamer and nonamer is approximately 1×10^7 whereas the affinity for α, DNP-Lys$_3$ is about 5×10^6. The K_o for α, DNP-Lys$_{4-6}$ falls between that found for the trimer and heptamer.

CHAIRMAN WAKSMAN: We should now turn to a consideration of instances, both natural and experimental, in which delayed sensitivity and antibody formation appear to be separated. This includes Sarcoidosis and Hodgkin's disease, where in effect, antigens induce one kind of response rather than the other. Since Dr. Lawrence has dealt with examples of both kinds, he might comment first.

DR. LAWRENCE: As Dr. Waksman had indicated, there are models in acquired human disease where cellular immunity may be sharply separated from serum antibody formation, coincident with or as a consequence of the disease process. Putting aside for the moment the congenitally acquired diseases in this category, like agammaglobulinemia and DiGeorge's Syndrome. I would like to begin with consideration of Boeck's sarcoid. This is a granulomatous disease characterized by a loss of delayed allergy to tuberculin and a variety of other antigens reflected in cutaneous anergy and depressed lymphocyte responsiveness to PHA as well as to specific antigens, in the face of unimpaired immunoglobulin synthesis.

Such patients generally have no difficulty in antibody production and are apt to exhibit a chronic hyperglobulinemia, comprised in large part of functional immunoglobulin molecules.

There is thus presented a curious acquired dichotomy of immune response not only associated with the loss of prior cellular immune responses but also characterized by an inability to develop tuberculin sensitivity following active immunization with BCG. Such patients also fail to respond to sensitization with dinitrochlorobenzine (DNCB) with the acquisition of contact sensitivity.

Sarcoid patients have no trouble in handling those diseases that require serum antibody for recovery, such as pneumococcal pneumonia. They do have difficulty and are more susceptible to diseases requiring intact cellular immune mechanisms that are characterized by intracellular parasitism as exemplified by tuberculosis. For example, corticosteroid therapy is known to result in disseminated tuberculosis in many of these patients; it is therefore routine practise to add antimicrobial therapy to any such regimen.

Here then, is an acquired disease syndrome that results in a variable impairment of cellular immunity with intact immunoglobulin synthesis; and invariably associated with the impaired cellular immunity there is a positive indolent, cutaneous reaction to the Kveim antigen. It appears that the deficiency detected results from a suspension of cell-mediated immunity, rather than complete abolition; since tuberculin negativity and Kveim-positivity may fluctuate, and when the Kveim test becomes negative, tuberculin sensitivity usually reappears.

Since cellular or subcellular transfer in man is not a "passive" transfer and requires a contribution on the part of the recipient to the transaction, transfer factor affords a precise analytical tool to delineate the locus of the derangement in congenital or acquired immune deficiency

II. FEATURES OF CELLULAR VERSUS HUMORAL IMMUNITY

disease. We therefore studied the response of seven well-documented, either Kveim Test and/or lymph node biopsy positive, Sarcoid patients to intradermal injections of dialysable transfer factor (Lawrence and Zweiman, Trans. Assoc. Amer. Phys., 81, 240, 1968). The patients were repeatedly negative when tested with tuberculin (PPD-5 µg.) on various occasions.

In Fig. 13 is illustrated our earlier experience with viable cell transfer in normal tuberculin-negative humans, showing intradermal depots of tuberculin-sensitive leucocytes following injection with tuberculin, develop marked tuberculin reactions in the local cell site and also in remote unprepared skin sites in which simultaneous tuberculin tests were placed.

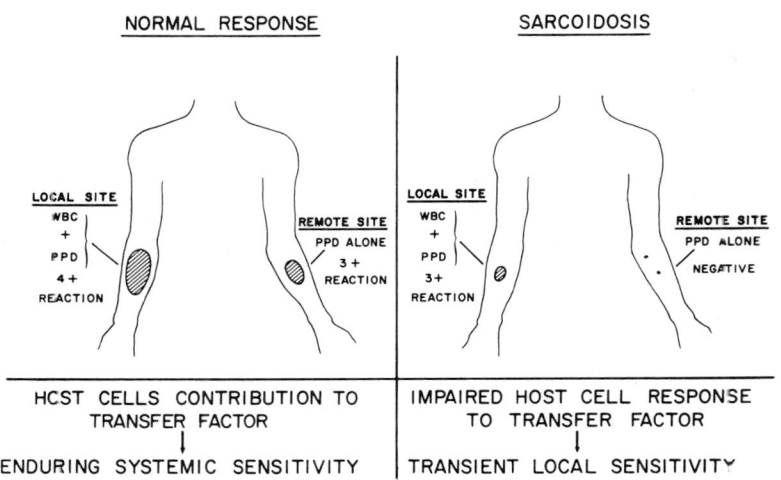

Fig. 13 Comparison of response of normal individuals to that of Sarcoid patients following local transfer by means of viable cells. (With permission of Transactions Association American Physicians.)

Thus in normals, individuals possessed of immunocompetent cells capable of being engaged by transfer factor, enduring systemic sensitivity is the expected and usual result. Using intact cells and applying this technique, Urbach et al. (N. Eng. J. Med., 247, 794, 1952) found tuberculin-negative Sarcoid patients develop only local tuberculin sensitivity and not systemic sensitivity and the local reaction is evanescent in these patients. This result was in contrast to their experience as well as ours in normal individuals where systemic sensitization is an inescapable consequence of transfer and the transferred sensitivity is enduring.

Thus where the host cell response to transfer factor is impaired, only transient local sensitivity can result.

In Fig. 14 is illustrated the protocol used in our study to evaluate the response of Sarcoid patients to equivalent aliquots of dialyzable transfer factor prepared from the same tuberculin-positive donor with a well-documented and potent capacity for transfer. Since dialyzable transfer factor is not antigenic in rabbits or man, and since human transplantation antigens remains inside the dialysis sac, dialysate can be injected repeatedly intradermally without causing any local reaction or detectable immune response.

In the absence of systemic sensitization, this situation affords an internally controlled *in vivo* assay of transfer factor, where the host in effect is loaning his skin and a few responsive lymphocytes plus a few macrophages to reveal the interaction between specific antigen and transfer factor.

In this type of experiment, the leucocyte extract resulted in a 3+ tuberculin reaction; the dialysate resulted in a 3+ tuberculin reaction; no reaction was transferred by dialysate heated at 56°C for 30 minutes or 100°C for 30 minutes. Depending on whether a (1:1) ratio of inside:outside contents of the dialysis sac is used for dialysis, one may still detect transfer factor in the non-dialyzed sediment.

II. FEATURES OF CELLULAR VERSUS HUMORAL IMMUNITY

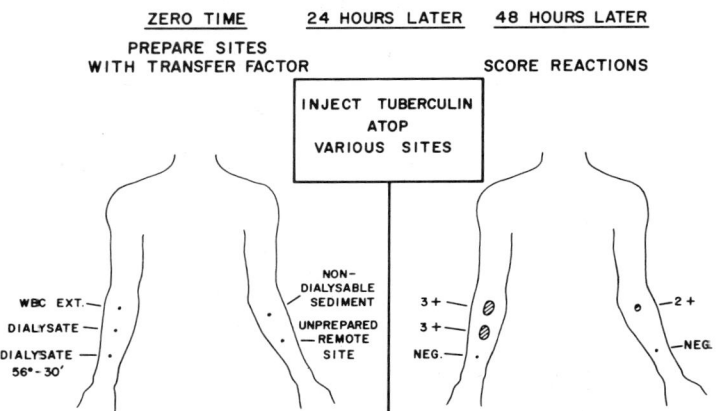

Fig. 14 Protocol for local transfer to Sarcoid patients of tuberculin sensitivity by means of dialysable transfer factor. (With permission of Transactions Association American Physicians)

We found that one could leach out into the dialysate more transfer factor from the contents of the dialysis sac. This type of result raises a question with regard to how much of the transfer factor detected inside the bag remains behind as a result of an equilibrium established with the amount of transfer factor outside of the bag.

In Table 16 are summarized the results achieved, showing that normal recipients of tuberculin-positive dialysate develop intense local reactions and simultaneous systemic tuberculin sensitivity as well.

CELLULAR IMMUNITY

TABLE 16

LOCAL TRANSFER OF TUBERCULIN SENSITIVITY TO SARCOID PATIENTS WITH TRANSFER FACTOR FROM A SINGLE DONOR

SARCOID PATIENT	TUBERCULIN REACTION AT SITES OF TRANSFER FACTOR INJECTION - 24 HRS.			UNPREPARED REMOTE SKIN SITE
	DIALYSATE	NON-DIALYSABLE SEDIMENT	DIALYSATE 56°C - 30'	
A l.	3+	3+	1+	1+
McG.	2+	3+	0	1+
Ko.	2+	1+	0	0
Wi.	2+	0	0	0
Bu.	1+	▨	▨	0
Sm.	0	▨	▨	0
Wa.	0	▨	▨	0
NORMAL RECIPIENTS	3+	▨	▨	3+

DIALYSATE ⇌ 40 MILLION WBC - INSIDE/OUTSIDE RATIO = (1:1)
3+ = 30 x 35 mm. INDURATION AND ERYTHEMA

(Data reproduced with permission of Transactions of Association of American Physicians.)

As may be seen five of the seven Kveim-positive, tuberculin-negative Sarcoid recipients of dialysate developed strong to moderate degrees of local but not systemic tuberculin reactivity, while two recipients developed neither local or systemic sensitivity. However, two of the seven patients did develop systemic sensitization of a mild degree. Note also that heating the dialysate (56°C - 30 min.) did not inactivate transfer factor nor block the transfer of sensitivity locally. The sediment inside the dialysis sac may retain a variable amount of activity depending on the ratio of dialysis fluid inside to outside.

We conclude that dialysable transfer factor is capable of prompt local transfer, within 18 to 24 hours, in normal individuals and in patients with sarcoidosis. The local transfer is inactivated by heat and unaffected by pancreatic RNAse.

II. FEATURES OF CELLULAR VERSUS HUMORAL IMMUNITY

Systemic transfer may reflect increased dose of transfer factor or an increased responsiveness of the patient's lymphocytes. We suggest on the basis of this data that the anergy of sarcoidosis results from the impaired production or function of the patient's own transfer factors for common delayed allergies. The local transfer excludes anticutins and other periperhal inhibitors of delayed cutaneous reactions. The systemic unresponsiveness to transfer factor suggests an impairment of host cells processing such immunological information. The occasional transfer of systemic sensitivity suggests the immunologic deficit is not absolute. If one looks at the anergy of Sarcoidosis in relation to the Kveim antigen, the recent reports of the cellular transfer of delayed cutaneous reactivity to Kveim antigen by means of blood leucocytes obtained from Kveim-positive sarcoid patients, is of great significance. These observations were originally reported by Lebacq and Verhaegen (Rev. Franc Etudes Clin et Biol, $\underline{8}$, 377, 1963; Int. Arch. Allergy, $\underline{24}$, 208, 1969) and have been recently confirmed by Behrend et al. (Klin. Wschr., $\underline{18}$, 1010, 1968). The transfer of Kveim reactivity was determined by biopsy of recipient nodules and a histologic picture of epitheliod granuloma characteristic of the Kveim reaction. The impaired response of sarcoid patients to tuberculin transfer factor, taken together with the capacity of their leucocytes to transfer skin reactivity to Kveim antigen, suggests the possibility that antigenic competition with Kveim antigen may pre-empt production or function of transfer factors for other delayed reactions in such patients and result in the anergy encountered. This constant preoccupation with Kveim antigen may be expressed by the Sarcoid patient's amnesia for prior cell-mediated immunologic experiences and his feeble recognition of the immunologic memories of the donor conveyed by transfer factor.

This study in addition to yielding information about transfer factor and delineating the type of immunologic defect in Sarcoidosis is a preliminary step towards the application of transfer factor in reconstitution therapy of acquired cellular immune deficiency states that are complicated by disseminated viral, mycobacterial or fungal infection.

CELLULAR IMMUNITY

To turn to this consequence of cellular immune deficiency states, there are a number of frequently lethal infections in this category, all caused by preferential intracellular microorganisms (for example: miliary tuberculosis, histoplasmosis, candidiasis, moniliasis, and disseminated vaccinia). Impaired delayed sensitivity or anergy to the infecting microbe is the usual concomitant of dissemination in each of these diseases and cutaneous anergy signals a bleak outlook for recovery from the infection, despite the invariable presence of normal or high serum antibody titers specific for the infecting microbe. Moreover, in each instance, acquisition of delayed skin sensitivity is usually associated with a good prognosis and ultimate recovery of most patients.

The detection of congenital cellular immune deficiency states and the production of similar secondary immunologic derangements by associated disease (e. g. Sarcoidosis, Hodgkins, Cancer, Leprosy) or by immunosuppressive therapy (steroids, 6-MP, ALS) has also afforded indirect evidence for a beneficial role of cell-mediated immunity and its association with heightened resistance to or recovery from preferential intracellular microbial infections.

More positive and more direct evidence has been forthcoming from the use of the transfer factor in the treatment of such disseminated infections. The first application of transfer factor in this situation was that of Kempe (Pediatrics, _26_, 176, 1960), who treated a child with progressive generalized vaccinia despite the presence of a high-titer circulating antibody directed against vaccinia virus. The progressive dissemination of this disease was not interrupted by administration of hyperimmune vaccinial gammaglobulin. However, local and systemic transfer of specifically sensitive blood and lymph node leucocytes resulted in prompt and dramatic regression of the vaccinia lesions with recovery from an otherwise fatal infection. The patient's recovery was coincident with the appearance of transferred delayed cutaneous sensitivity to vaccinia virus.

This type of successful therapeutic application of transfer factor has been confirmed in other cases of progressive vaccinia (O'Connell et al., Ann. Int. Med., _60_, 282, 1964; Hathaway et al., N. Eng. J. Med., _273_, 953,

II. FEATURES OF CELLULAR VERSUS HUMORAL IMMUNITY

1965), in the face of cutaneous anergy and high titer circulating antibody. It has also proved effective in disseminated moniliasis using parental marrow lymphocytes for transfer (Buckley et al., Clin. Exp. Immunol., 3, 153, 1968). The coincidence of high titers of specific circulating antibody in these patients and the ineffectiveness of administered specific anti-vaccinial or anti-monilial gammaglobulin in checking dissemination of the infection suggest an "enhancing" effect of antibody, perhaps brought about by camouflaging microbial antigenic determinants to blunt or dissipate a sustained cellular immune response.

We have suggested elsewhere (cf. Editorial, Transfer Factor and Leprosy, New Eng. J. Med., 278, 333, 1968), that transfer factor may be adapted to immunologic reconstitution of patients afflicted with lepromatous leprosy and convert them to the more benign tuberculoid type of disease. The lepromatous type of disease goes virtually unchecked by the host and despite a high titer of serum antibody bathing his tissues and his macrophages laden with bacilli, there is no inflammatory reaction to lepra bacilli or their products in his skin or elsewhere. This as Bullock (New Eng. J. Med., 278, 1968) and others have shown is associated with a loss of previously established cellular-immunologic memories as well as a diminished capacity for active sensitization (DNCB). In contrast the tuberculoid type of leprosy is characterized by a benign self-limited course, few lepra bacilli detected in cells or tissues, little or no serum antibody response and positive delayed cutaneous reactions to tuberculin and lepromin. Following our suggestion, Paradise et al.(New Eng. J. Med., 280, 859, 1969) have reported that both lepromin (Fernandez Reaction read at 48 hrs) sensitivity and tuberculin sensitivity can indeed be transferred to patients with lepromatous leprosy and the transferred sensitivity persisted in two patients for approximately one year. It remains to be determined what beneficial effects, if any, immunologic reconstitution with transfer factor effects in this specific situation.

Transfer of viable immunocompetent cells to some hosts incapable of rejecting them via a homograft response can result in a graft vs. host syndrome resembling runt disease (Hathaway et al., New Eng. J. Med., 273, 953, 1965; Hong et al., Lancet, 1969). To avoid this hazard we have suggested elsewhere (Adv. in Immunology, 1969) that dialysable transfer factor affords a safer and more effective immune reagent to attempt reconstitution of cellular immune deficiency disease. The advantages of dialysable transfer factor for this purpose are 1) it is not antigenic in animals or man and can therefore be given repeatedly from the same or pooled immune donors to the same recipient, repeatedly without immune response of any kind except intensification of the delayed reactivity transferred; and 2) it is freed of all macromolecular cell constituents including transplantation antigens and cannot therefore react against the host.

In our experience, the only detectable consequence of giving transfer factor from the same donor to the same recipient has been an increase in the intensity and duration of transferred tuberculin sensitivity. It should be emphasized that to date the dosage of transfer factor employed by ourselves or others are miniscule yet sufficient for the study of the mechanism of the delayed response in normal individuals. We have recommended therefore for treatment, much higher dosages of transfer factor be administered and repeated over a prolonged period of time if sensitivity wanes or reversion to a negative state occurs. The means for increasing the dose of transfer factor (dialysis concentration, lyophilization) and its safety on repeated administration has been demonstrated repeatedly (Advances in Immunology, 1969). The application of dialysable transfer factor has therefore proved of value in the reconstitution of those cellular immune deficiency states where the defect of the small, circulating, thymus-dependent lymphocyte is an acquired rather than a congenital deficiency.

CHAIRMAN WAKSMAN: It seems to me that we are dealing with two separate issues. As I understand it, in diseases like leprosy, there is a greater suppression of reactivity to antigens of M. lepra itself, than to other infectious agents or agents that cause delayed sensitivity. We should therefore distinguish specific inhibition from a generalized or non-specific suppression which may also be present.

II. FEATURES OF CELLULAR VERSUS HUMORAL IMMUNITY

In connection with specific inhibition, one again has to concern himself with two alternative possibilities. The individual in question may have tolerance to the antigen, tolerance, that is to say, of the split sort in which delayed sensitivity is suppressed while antibody formation continues or is increased. Alternatively, there may be a feedback inhibition of delayed sensitivity by the antibody, a well-known mechanism in some experimental cases involving tumors, as Drs. Allison and Gerson have recently showed. This is apparently a more widespread mechanism than has been recognized in recent years. Dr. Turk has done important work in this area and can no doubt add to our information.

DR. TURK: I have been studying leprosy for the last year or so, and thought it might interest you to give you a diagram of the immunological state of leprosy, and which is a spectral disease, although it originally was thought a polar disease. Basically the difference between the two manifestations is that in tuberculoid leprosy there are large plaques in the skin which look like delayed sensitivity lesions while in lepromatous leprosy there are granulomatous nodules, consisting of macrophages packed full of lepra bacilli. There are very few lepra bacilli seen in the lesions of the tuberculoid patients.

Being a spectral disease, patients can swing right across the spectrum toward one direction or towards the other. To further emphasize this fact histological sections, can be subclassified into "LL" for lepromatous and "TT" for tuberculoid. Between these extremes there is a designation of borderline leprosy "BB" which is located between the two polar forms in between which you get "BL" in one direction and "BT" in the other.

These are artificial categories because the patients swing across the spectrum, although some do remain fixed in the LL or TT positions. When lepromatous patients are treated with sulphones they can shift towards borderline leprosy. The lepromin test that is used to determine their cellular immunity is always positive in TT and BT parts of the spectrum but negative in BB, BL and LL. This test acts as an indicator of the cell-mediated immunity and correlates well with the lymphocytic infiltration of the lesions. This

THE SPECTRUM OF LEPROSY

	TUBERCULOID		BORDERLINE (DIMORPHOUS)			LEPROMATOUS	
	TT	BT	BB	BI		LI	LL
LEPROMIN	+++ ++ +	+ −	−	−		−	−
DNCB (% Positive Reactors)	100%		75%			50%	
HEMOCYANIN	100%		100%			100%	
ERYTHEMA NODOSUM LEPROSUM	−		+ −			+++	
PLASMA CELLS IN LYMPHOID TISSUE	+ −		+			+++	
ANTIMYCOBACTERIAL ANTIBODIES (% patients with precipitins in serum)	11%	28%		82%			95%
AUTOANTIBODIES (% patients with autoantibodies in serum)	3 − 11%					30 − 50%	

II. FEATURES OF CELLULAR VERSUS HUMORAL IMMUNITY

is an indication of specific cell-mediated immunity against the lepra bacillus. However, in LL there is often a non-specific loss of cell-mediated immunity, this can be tested in a number of ways.

The standard way used is to attempt sensitization to DNCB. Fifty percent of patients at the lepromatous end of the spectrum cannot be actively sensitized to DNCB. However, if another antigen is employed, such as KLH, the 50 percent that cannot be sensitized with DNCB, can be sensitized with KLH. There is thus not a complete absence of cell-mediated immunity, but a relative deficiency.

These people are not more susceptible to other infectious diseases. We have seen DNCB-negative old people, who have had leprosy for many years, and inability to be sensitized does not appear to affect this lifespan. When patients are treated with sulphones, some can swing across the spectrum and regain their cell-mediated immunity. A certain proportion never regain immunity and they have to continue to be treated for the rest of their lives.

The antibody against mycobacteria is very scanty at the tuberculoid end of the scale, but in very high concentration in lepromatous leprosy. At the lepromatous end of the spectrum there is a very high incidence of autoantibodies: such patients exhibit very strongly positive reactions to anti-nuclear factor; rheumatoid factor; and thyroglobulin autoantibodies; and they have lupus erythematosus cells in the circulation. They behave in the same way as an animal who has been given massive doses of Freund's adjuvant.

It has been reported that these patients, especially those with lepromatous leprosy, have lymphocytes which cannot be transformed with PHA; a proportion of the tuberculoid leprosy patients lymphocytes also can't be transformed with PHA.

As shown in Fig. 15 the lymph nodes from patients with tuberculoid leprosy possess paracortical areas that are packed full of lymphocytes, and normally developed. They also contain immunoblasts to a greater extent than one would see in normal lymph nodes. (Fig. 15a, b, c)

CELLULAR IMMUNITY

In the lepromatous end of the scale, one gets a completely different picture, the paracortical areas are depleted of small lymphocytes, but there are large germinal centers with a normal cuff of small lymphocytes which are probably bone marrow-derived (Fig. 15d). There are large numbers of plasma cells in the medulla, whereas the paracortical area is depleted of small lymphocytes (Fig. 15e). Their appearance is just like that of lymph nodes of guinea pigs treated with antilymphocyte serum, or those of neonatally thymectomised mice. The paracortical areas are replaced by histiocytic cells which are markedly phagocytic (Fig. 15f). In lepromatous leprosy these cells can be seen to have phagocytosed many mycobacteria. (15g) However, mycobacteria are not seen in the germinal centers or in relation to the marginal cuff of small lymphocytes.

Upon treatment these patients regain their cell-mediated immunity and tend to get lymphocyte infiltration of their lesions and the bacillary index in their lesions drop. In one or two of these cases, we have looked at lymph nodes and it can be seen that small lymphocytes begin to repopulate the paracortical area round the postcapillary venules (Fig. 15h).

The situation in lepromatous leprosy is that there is a familial incidence of this disease, and the children of patients with leprosy cannot be sensitized with mycobacteria to be made tuberculin-positive as well as normal people, and so one would say that they are possibly subthymic. In addition, the patients with lepromatous leprosy begin to get a massive infiltration of their tissues with the organisms, and they then begin to develop tolerance, in respect to cellular immunity against the mycobacteria. This begins a vicious circle and in the end they get massive replacement of their paracortical areas, so that they develop a non-specific inability to show cell-mediated immunity to other antigens. In fact, a certain proportion of them will also accept skin grafts as well.

DR. SILVERSTEIN: Did the patients with lepromatous leprosy have a significant lymphopenia?

DR. TURK: No.

II. FEATURES OF CELLULAR VERSUS HUMORAL IMMUNITY

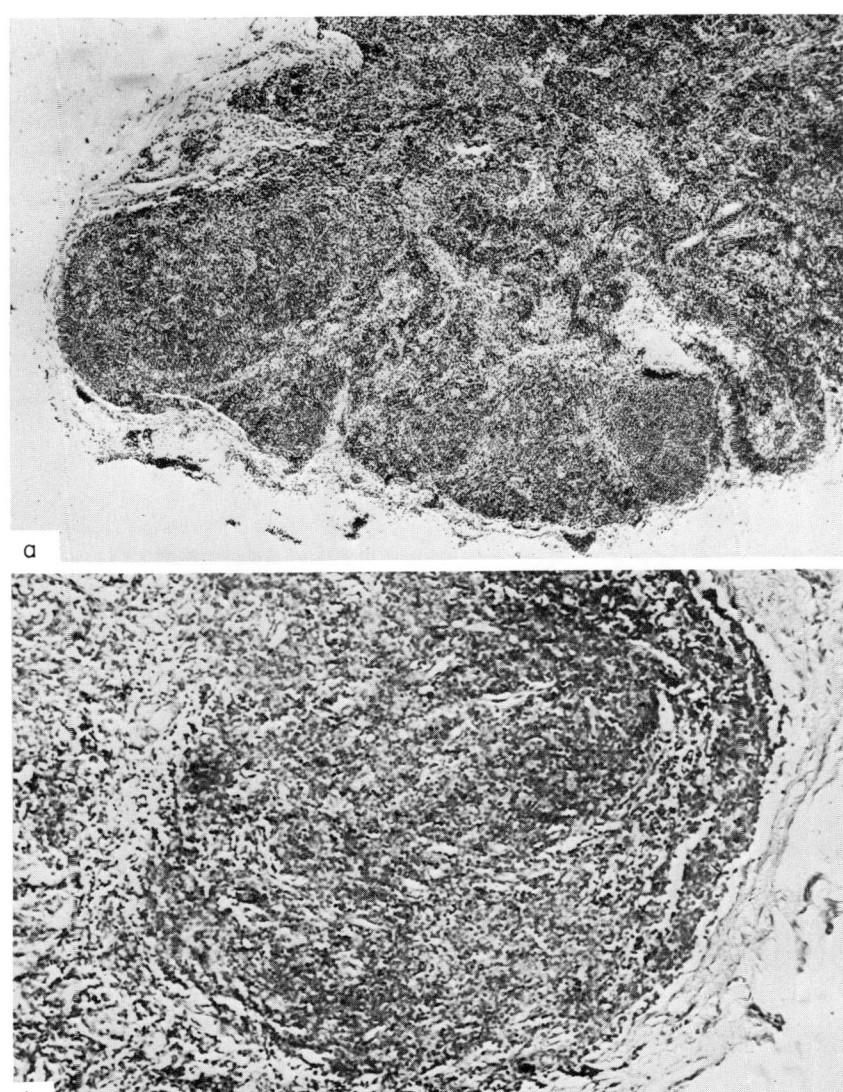

Fig. 15 Lymph nodes in leprosy, a) <u>Tuberculoid leprosy</u> x 30. Note well developed paracortical areas. (Haematoxylin eosin). b) <u>Tuberculoid leprosy</u> x 75 Paracortical area. Paracortical areas well populated with lymphocytes (Methyl-green pyronin).

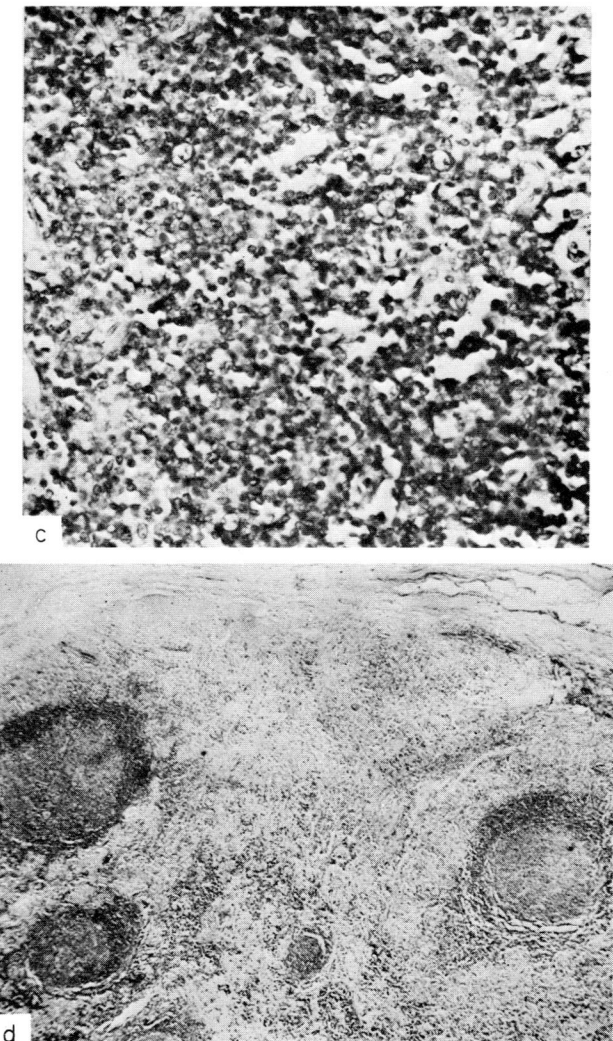

Fig. 15 c) <u>Tuberculoid leprosy</u> x 188. Occasional large pyroninophilic cells in paracortical area. (Methylgreen pyronin). d) <u>Lepromatous leprosy</u> x 30. Depleted paracortical area. Well developed germinal centres. (Methylgreen pyronin).

II. FEATURES OF CELLULAR VERSUS HUMORAL IMMUNITY

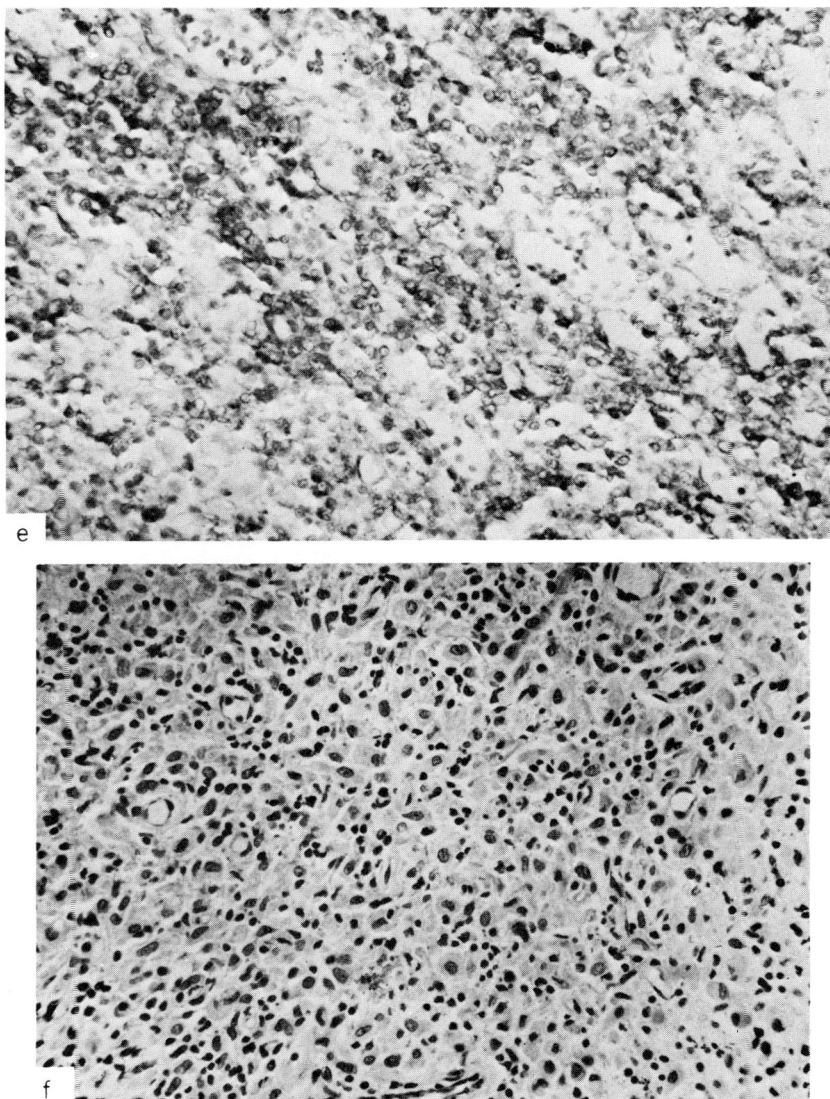

Fig. 15 e) <u>Lepromatous leprosy</u> x 75 plasma cells in medulla. (Methylgreen pyronin). f) <u>Lepromatous leprosy</u> x 75. Histiocytes in paracortical area replacing lymphocytes. (Haematoxylin eosin).

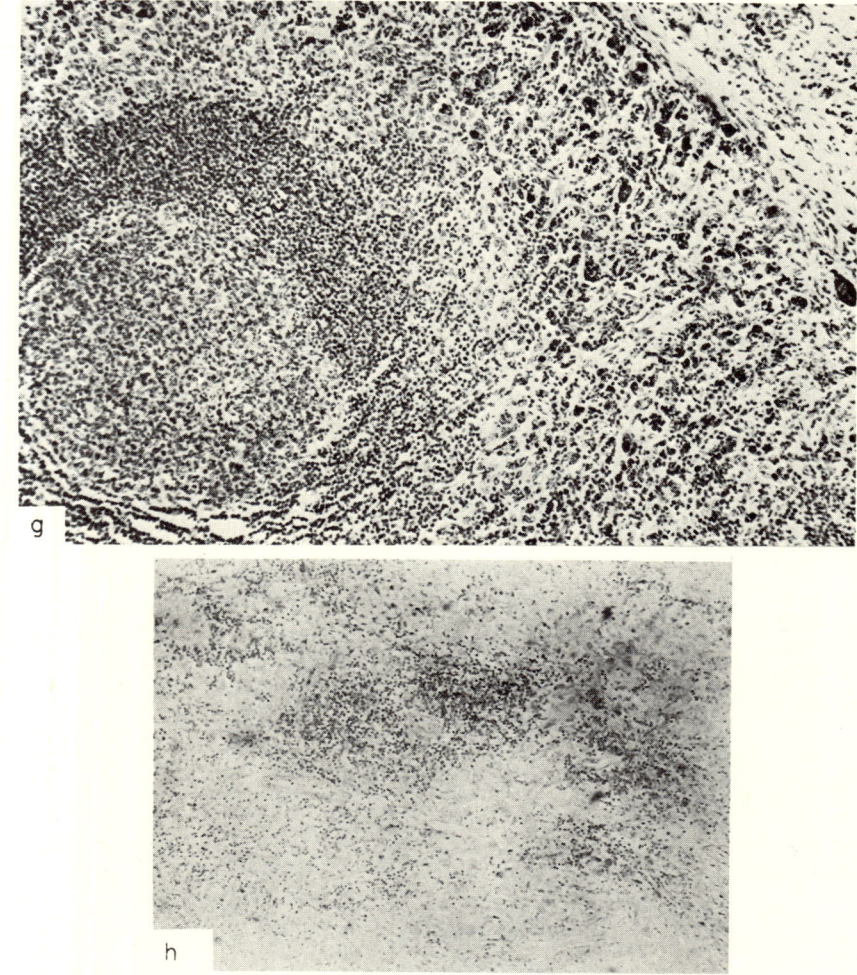

Fig. 15 g) <u>Lepromatous leprosy</u> x 75. Histiocytes in paracortical area with ingested clumps of mycobacteria. Germinal centre and marginal cuff of small lymphocytes unaffected. (Ziehl Nielsen). h) <u>Borderline leprosy</u> x 75. Postcapillary venule in depleted paracortical area surrounded by small lymphocytes. (Methylgreen pyronin).

II. FEATURES OF CELLULAR VERSUS HUMORAL IMMUNITY

DR. OPPENHEIM: One would perhaps predict that these patients may have a serum inhibiting factor or something toxic to lymphoid cells in their circulation. Have you been able to demonstrate anything along that line?

DR. TURK: Dr. Bullock has deomonstrated and described a factor at the recent International Congress on Leprosy, that inhibits the transformation of normal lymphocytes by streptolysin-O, but does not inhibit their transformation by PHA.

DR. LANDY: In this connection I recall relevant findings by Drs. Heilman and MacFarland to the effect that patients with clinical manifestations of tuberculosis have in their plasma a component that markedly suppresses transformation of the patient's peripheral cells by PPD. The same cells upon washing reacted well with the antigen.

DR. TURK: We have, in fact, found a serum factor in patients with secondary syphilis that produces a depression of normal lymphocyte transformation by PHA. Patients with primary syphilis don't have this factor and they have large pyroninophilic cells in the paracortical area of their lymph nodes.

In secondary syphilis, there are found areas of relative depletion of lymphocytes from the paracortical areas. This might explain why in this phase of syphilis, there is a sudden and rapid dissemination of the organisms throughout the body.

DR. HIRSCHHORN: We have previously reported that lymphocytes from patients with sarcoidosis are hyporeactive to PHA and other non-specific stimulants. They are responsive to Kveim antigen in tissue culture but they are not responsive to PPD, in most of the patients studied. This agrees quite well with some of the things that Dr. Lawrence has just said, but I begin to wonder what the explanation is. I also wonder whether there is not some induced stoppage of differentiation at one particular point in the natural development of these cells.

The reason I bring this up relates to what Dr. Mitchison was saying earlier. The concept of bone marrow-derived and thymus-derived cells may lead to confusion. I wonder whether we have the right to call these "derived" rather than "dependent". There is really no solid evidence that these organs are their point of origin. I think they probably all originate from a similar stem cell; there are different directions of differentiation or different sequences of differentiation.

The sarcoid situation may give a clue to this dilemma. The leprosy situation may also be relevant, in that there may be blocks in differentiation. With reference to this, I would repeat my earlier comment, that one can isolate from the blood of some patients with sarcoidosis, cells which behave like stem cells; in other words, they are readily established in culture as continuing cell lines.

CHAIRMAN WAKSMAN: I must take issue with you, on the matter of using terms like "thymus-derived" and bone marrow-derived", since I believe they have a fairly specific meaning. Certainly "thymus-derived cell" is a term which is being used for cells which have been shown by adequate marker techniques to travel from the thymus to the periphery

DR. HIRSCHHORN: True - but, where does it come from?

CHAIRMAN WAKSMAN: The fact that they originate in the bone-marrow does not lessen the fact that they sojourn in the thymus and there undergo an important differentiation. The term "bone marrow-derived" is used for other cells that do not pass through the thymus. This class may have sub-categories, as we said before. I don't think these terms should _yet_ be abandoned, since they serve a useful function.

DR. SALVIN: My question is directed to Dr. Lawrence. It is known that patients with localized acute moniliasis or histoplasmosis have lymph node cells or peripheral blood cells which react to specific antigen, either by migration or by blastogenesis. Do you know whether lymph node cells

II. FEATURES OF CELLULAR VERSUS HUMORAL IMMUNITY

or blood lymphocytes of patients who have developed a disseminated mycotic disease are defective in their <u>in vitro</u> responses with regard to migration inhibition or blastogenesis?

DR. LAWRENCE: No, I don't, except for studies on Sarcoidosis where such a deficient response to PHA or tuberculin has been shown. The only information on histoplasmosis or coccidioidomycosis for example, is the cutaneous anergy detected in patients coincident with dissemination of the infection.

DR. THOR: In a study of four patients, three with miliary tuberculosis and one with severe open cavitary tuberculosis I found that none of them demonstrated migration inhibition with PPD in their migrating lymphocyte cultures.

They did, however, show some radioactive incorporation with tritiated thymidine, but not considered significant for what we expected in humans who had known tuberculosis contact or who were thought to be sensitive PPD. None of these people had positive skin tests with intermediate strength (0.01 μg.) of PPD. We have not looked at severe histoplasmosis or coccidioidomycosis.

DR. VALENTINE: The blast transformation of human blood lymphocytes <u>in vitro</u> has been achieved with coccidicidin, histoplasmin, and candida and cryptococcal antigens. In one study the response to histoplasmin <u>in vitro</u> was decreased in patients with chronic pulmonary or mucocutaneous histoplasmosis as compared with patients with acute histoplasmosis or histoplasmin-positive normal individuals. The patients with chronic disease had positive skin tests, and their decreased responsiveness <u>in vitro</u> was not correlated with the presence or absence of detectable antibody. In general, however, this study found that even the response of histoplasmin-positive normals was decreased by culturing in media containing antibody to histoplasmin. (Newberry, <u>et al</u>., J. Immun. <u>100</u>, 436, 1968).

CELLULAR IMMUNITY

DR. LANDY: It has become widely accepted and I suppose considered entirely appropriate to assess the functional capability or performance *in vitro* of lymphocytes by determining their activation or transformation by PHA. The correlation of this potential with cell-mediated immunities is now considered so solid that this *in vitro* criterion is extensively utilized by clinicians as a very convenient overall index of cell-mediated immunity in man. However, in the absence of PHA transformation, I can't help wondering, if in some instances at least, we may instead be discerning cells that are innately capable of functioning but which are non-reactive primarily because they lack the blood group-like membrane receptors for PHA. In other words, lack of transformation by PHA can also reflect a deficit in receptors, rather than a deficit in the capacity of the cell to perform in the subsequent events.

If we seriously entertain this possibility, we should be seeking still other ways to assess lymphocyte performance. To my way of thinking, it does not necessarily follow that these receptors for PHA and PWM are stable, uniform, and indefinitely persisting characteristics of blood lymphocytes. It is this assumption that we are constantly making; we seem to persist in taking this for granted.

CHAIRMAN WAKSMAN: That is a good point you have raised. Dr. Good and his group have taken the number of peripheral lymphocytes responding to PHA as a measure of the availability of thymus-derived lymphocytes, in a particular patient. They have studied a variety of immune deficiency states using this parameter to derive conclusions. I think you are quite right that it would be desirable to further document this assumption.

DR. VALENTINE: A brief elaboration on an earlier remark of Dr. Landy's, concerning patients with clinically severe tuberculosis, whose lymphocytes have been found by several groups to be unresponsive to PPD in culture. Heilman and MacFarland showed this to be due to a serum factor which inhibited the response; the factor also inhibited the usual transformation response of lymphocytes from other tuberculin-sensitive, but non-tuberculous patients. If the cells

II. FEATURES OF CELLULAR VERSUS HUMORAL IMMUNITY

of the tuberculous patients were put in normal medium with serum, they then were capable of responding. Thus the role of inhibitory serum factors should be excluded by those who describe an inability of lumphocytes from an immunized individual to be stimulated by antigen.

CHAIRMAN WAKSMAN: Was this serum component identified as an antibody by any other criterion?

DR. VALENTINE: No, it was not. However, the fact that it was an antigen-specific substance in the serum, certainly suggests that it could be antibody.

DR. BRANDRISS: With respect to the point Dr. Valentine has made, Dr. Bullock reported (Clin. Res., 16, 328, 1968) that the defect in in vitro reactivity to streptolysin O of cells from lepromatous patients was evident only in autologous plasma. When the cells were grown in normal homologous plasm their reactivity was normal. Moreover, plasma from patients with leprosy suppressed the in vitro reactivity of "normal" cells to streptolysin O and to PPD; suggesting that both cellular and humoral factors could be important. Although these effects of lepromatous sera apparently did not extend to PHA stimulation, it is evident that, similar to the situation in tuberculosis, one should not conclude a cellular defect is present before taking into account the possible inhibitory role of humoral factors.

DR. DAVID: I would like to extend this discussion in another direction. This involves three patients Dr. Rocklin and I have been studying in collaboration with Drs. Chilgren and Good. These three children had chronic cutaneous candidiasis, with negative delayed cutaneous reactions to Candida. On three repeated occasions each one of them failed to make any macrophage inhibiting factor in vitro, using the method of Thor and Dray. In two of these, we tried to transfer delayed sensitivity using dialysable transfer factor prepared from normal people with positive Candida skin tests. Each of the patients had been skin tested many times previously for Candida and had been negative.

CELLULAR IMMUNITY

One patient had slight erythema when tested intradermally with Candida 24 hours after transfer. At this time the patient's lymphocytes produced no MIF when stimualted by Candida. However, she gave a positive skin test 20 x 15 mm. with erythema and induration 6 days after transfer. At this time, as well as 8 days post transfer, her lymphocytes produced MIF *in vitro* in response to Candida. The transfer appears to have been transient since she reverted to a negative skin test two weeks after transfer. It is still too early to evaluate the effect of transfer factor on her clinical course. It is noteworthy that this patient had intermittently positive lymphocyte response to PHA and Candida prior to transfer, at a time when her skin test and MIF production were negative. The second patient with more generalized candidiasis, who also did not respond to PHA *in vitro*, did not become skin test positive via transfer factor. In collaboration with Dr. Fred Rosen, we are studying still another anergic child whose lymphocytes respond normally to PHA but do not produce MIF.

DR. BLOOM: In trying to relate the present discussion to the models that were described earlier, there are two areas that perplex me.

One, is that if one had a "clean" lymphocyte in transformation, I don't understand at what stage in development the switch occurs that would determine whether or not a given cell activated by antigen makes circulating antibodies on the one hand, or a mediator of delayed hypersensitivity on the other. Dr. Mitchison's model, would require entirely separate cell lines, with fixed capabilities, either destined towards antibody formation or towards cellular hypersensitivity.

If that were the case, then the present discussion makes me wonder whether there is some immunological deficiency disease in man in which there is a total absence of cellular immunity, while antibody production remains as a separate intact entity?

II. FEATURES OF CELLULAR VERSUS HUMORAL IMMUNITY

CHAIRMAN WAKSMAN: There have indeed been reported cases where there appears to be an isolated defect in cellular sensitization.

DR. LAWRENCE: Among a number, there is the patient studied by Gitlin, Rosen and Janeway with a cellular immune deficiency state. This could not be reconstituted following cell transfer, but only subsequent to a thymic transplant. (Pediatrics, 33, 711, 1964)

DR. DAVID: There are problems even in some of the syndromes of "pure delayed hypersensitivity deficiency", such as the DiGeorge Syndrome. Although these patients can produce some antibodies, it is still not definitely determined whether their plasma cells are maternally derived or are their own. This might be determined by identifying the allotypes of their immunoglobulins.

DR. LAWRENCE: I would make the point here that we distinguish between congenital immunologic deficiency syndromes and acquired deficiencies of cellular immunity. Diseases like Sarcoidosis, Hodgkins or Leprosy represent an acquired spectrum of lymphoid and reticular cell involvement which happens to depress functions of immunocompetent cell populations primarily concerned with cell-mediated immunity and yet may involve other immune responses also to a greater or lesser degree. The resultant immune deficiency state will therefore be conditioned by variables such as the extent, duration, tempo and strategic cellular and tissue location of the disease process.

CHAIRMAN WAKSMAN: If I may say so, I am a little out of sympathy with your last comment. It seems to me that the phrase "experiment of nature" includes certain instances which are absolutely clearcut and where there is no fussiness about what one is dealing with. In the so-called DiGeorge Syndrome, there is no thymus in the individual at all, yet he is busily making immunoglobulin. That tells us something and is not a borderline situation.

DR. LAWRENCE: Nevertheless, I would maintain that acquired cellular immune deficiency differs from inherited congenital immunological deficiency disease. Moreover, even sickle cell disease or hemophilia, two examples of a "one-gene, one-enzyme" type of inborn error of metabolism, had to be broadened to include variants of the classical disease entity as laboratory techniques became more refined and genetic variables came to be better understood.

DR. OPPENHEIM: I would like to add another variant to the list of the "experiments of nature". These are the Wiskott-Aldrich patients. They have a combined deficiency of cellular immunity and some reduction in antibody production which is most noticeable with carbohydrate antigens, but also detectable with soluble protein antigens to some extent. They have a marked deficit of their delayed hypersensitivity reactions to DNCB as well as to PPD and the usual fungal extracts. Their transplant rejection time is also prolonged. In five patients of this type that Drs. Blaese, Waldman and I have studied, as has been reported by others, their response to the non-specific stimulant, namely PHA, was normal. This was also true of their lymphocyte response to the pokeweed mitogen and staphylococcal filtrate. With the proper trigger their lymphocytes can therefore function very adequately. However, their responses to specific antigens such as streptolysin O, Vaccinia, diphtheria and tetanus toxoids as well as MLC, were all markedly diminished.

In this instance we have an immunological deficiency due to some type of genetic, sex-linked, recessive defect, which apparently is somehow interfering with the way the lymphocyte obtains its information; because if given the proper stimulus, the lymphocyte can respond. I would, therefore, like to add this condition to the list of abnormal situation to be studied further as a means of understanding the steps in the normal immune response.

DR. CHESSIN: My question is directed to Dr. Lawrence. In your experience of following patients with Boeck's Sarcoid, do they retain their anergy throughout life or does this change with the natural history of the disease?

II. FEATURES OF CELLULAR VERSUS HUMORAL IMMUNITY

DR. LAWRENCE: Yes, anergy changes with the activity and tempo of the disease in any one individual patient. The so-called "burned out" sarcoid patients during the active phase of their disease are likely to have been tuberculin negative and Kveim test positive, and when retested months or years later during a quiescent phase, have been found to revert to tuberculin positive and Kveim test negative states. (Siltzbach, JAMA, 178, 476, 1961). Buckley et al. (Ann. Int. Med., 64, 508, 1966) have shown a depressed response of sarcoid patient's blood lymphocytes to PHA during exacerbation of the disease with return toward a normal response during remissions. With regard to two of the seven Sarcoid patients to whom we transferred systemic sensitivity, the reactivity, although feeble (10 x 10 mm.), persisted for at least a year following transfer (Trans. Assoc. Amer. Phys., 81, 240, 1968).

DR. SCHLOSSMAN: I would like to speak to the issue of antibody production in patients with the DiGeorge Syndrome and Hodgkins' Disease. I think it is clear that many patients with Hodgkins disease are anergic and it is true they do make a normal antibody response. But there was a report by Aisenberg and Leskowitz a number of years ago which pointed out that the antibody response in Hodgkin's disease is not quite normal. Normal individuals when injected with pneumococcal polysaccharide antigens make antibody for years. However, many of the Hodgkin's patients no longer have significant antibody titer about six months after injection of pneumococcal polysaccharide.

Another point of considerable interest is found in the DiGeorge Syndrome. It is true that they have cellular anergy. However, their antibody response is not entirely normal either. Dr. Fred Rosen has shown that these patients also do not sustain their antibody titers as normals do. What this does is complicate the issue a bit, preventing one from completely separating cellular immune response from antibody production.

I personally believe that we will have to study antibody response more thoroughly in patients with disorders of cellular immunity and reputedly normal antibody. The antibody should be characterized in terms of the combining site, affinity, etc. I think we will find many deficiencies in kind and degree of antibody production in such individuals. I suspect that the DiGeorge and Hodgkins syndromes are indicative of a lack of clearcut separation but rather a more complex disorder of both cell and antibody-mediated immunity.

CHAIRMAN WAKSMAN: You are raising an extremely interesting issue that really was here from the beginning. Dr. Mitchison did not say that delayed sensitivity is completely separate from antibody formation; quite the contrary. A relevant subject, that was not mentioned even once thus far, is whether the memory cell, in appropriate situations related to humoral antibody, is the same cell as the thymus-derived cell of delayed sensitivity, as it may well be. It seems to me that the case that you describe would sustain such an interpretation.

DR. UHR: In looking for a common denominator between these various conditions that affect the lymphoreticular system, I think it is apparent that there is quite a variety of pathological conditions that give rise to a variety of immunologic deficiency disorders. Several examples were given already as genetic defects giving rise to different patterns in responsiveness, and I wonder if this doesn't simply indicate that there are many steps missing in the sequence of events which are under a different genetic control.

CHAIRMAN WAKSMAN: This is precisely why I made my comment. Many of the cases arising in nature are very fuzzy. Only cases where an appropriate organ is missing can be accepted as clearcut and shedding light on unknown mechanisms in the immune response. For all the others, we have to try to find an explanation. They don't really help us.

DR. HIRSCHHORN: Dr. Oppenheim briefly discussed the Wiscott-Aldrich syndrome. Recent experiments from our laboratory may give another clue to this disease. Two brothers with this syndrome were compared as regards the

II. FEATURES OF CELLULAR VERSUS HUMORAL IMMUNITY

PHA response to their normal brother and to their mother, who was heterozygous for the gene. We found that cells from the affected individuals responded far better to PHA than did those of the normal brother or the mother.

Does this mean that perhaps the response of this cell is not being affected by the presence of, or events at, other receptor sites, and that in this disease, a lot of non-specific receptor sites are now more readily available coupled with some kind of inability to handle a variety of other types of stimuli?

DR. SILVERSTEIN: I want to second Dr. Schlossman's cautions about the interpretation of some of these so-called experiments of nature. I think that nature is a very bad experimentalist that varies simultaneously far too many parameters. Were we to experiment as poorly as she does, I think most of us would not be around very long.

DR. LAWRENCE: Would you mean to include conception also? I consider that a pretty good experiment, although admittedly an uncontrolled one, which has kept the species around a very long time indeed.

DR. FIREMAN: I did want to call attention to another human disease, measles, in which delayed or cellular immunity is suppressed. Clinical measles will not satisfy Dr. Bloom's search for a clinical situation where there is absolutely no expression of delayed hypersensitivity since natural measles or attenuated measles virus suppresses but does not totally abolish delayed hypersensitivity. However, this observation led us to a series of clinical investigations (Pediatrics, 1969). We found that upon receipt of attenuated measles virus, 80 or 90 percent of normal individuals have a significant suppression of pre-existing cutaneous delayed hypersensitivity to a variety of antigens, including tuberculin, Candida, Vaccinia and diphtheria toxoid. In vitro responsiveness of these patient's lymphocytes to PHA was not affected, despite suppression of their in vitro responsiveness to specific antigen, i. e., tuberculin and Candida. Similar data have been reported by

Smithwick and Berkovich as well as Zweiman and Hildreth; when measles virus was incubated with sensitive lymphocytes in vitro, the lymphocytes did not respond to the specific antigen. None of the patients with thymic immunologic deficiency syndromes studied in Pittsburgh in the past four years have demonstrated a total dichotomy of cellular (delayed) hypersensitivity and humoral antibody synthesis. Even those patients who had immunoglobulin synthesis in the presence of thymic dysfunction and absent cellular (delayed) hypersensitivity could not develop good antibody responses to several antigens.

DR. COHN: Dr. Mitchison presented a very clear model in which he proposed that a thymus-derived cell was a precursor of the delayed hypersensitive cell and that for delayed hypersensitivity reactions there was an antigen-mediated interaction between two thymus-derived cells, one recognizing one antigenic determinant and the other recognizing another determinant. This predicts that if there is found a single authenticated case of an individual that cannot give a delayed hypersensitive response but does respond with antibody production, then this hypothesis is untenable. I therefore think that instead of listening to anecdotal medicine, we need one such case.

CHAIRMAN WAKSMAN: I think you overlooked the fact that there is a whole set of antibody responses which are not thymus dependent.

DR. COHN: That is my point.

DR. MITCHISON: I would like to make a comment on Dr. Cohn's pronouncement. With reference to Dr. Fireman's contribution, I would like to remind you of the Liacopoulos phenomenon, in which large doses of antigen induce a transient state of general unresponsiveness. This has also been recently examined by Cernyi and his colleagues, and the lymph node histology there looks very much like the picture that Dr. Turk showed us in lepromatous leprosy, that is, depletion in the paracortical area. I can't help wondering whether this

II. FEATURES OF CELLULAR VERSUS HUMORAL IMMUNITY

kind of high dose of virus might be working through the same mechanism.

III
SPECIFIC RECRUITMENT OF IMMUNOCOMPETENT CELLS BY TRANSFER FACTOR

Biological activities in leucocyte extracts — Physico chemical properties of dialysable transfer factor — Effects of dialysate on lymphocytes *in vitro* — Relationship of antigen-liberated transfer factor to non-dialysable lymphocyte transforming activity — Clonal proliferation *in vitro* of antigen-stimulated circulating lymphocytes — Does transfer factor elevate latent sensitivity or confer it *de novo* — Evidence for transfer in the absence of overt prior exposure to antigen — Properties of dialysable transfer factor compared to non-dialysable lymphocyte transforming activity — Possible contribution of cross-reacting antigens in recipients of transfer factor — Failure of transfer factor to confer contact sensitivity — Estimate of frequency of antigen-responsive lymphocytes — Quantitative variables governing the effectiveness of transfer factor — Transfer factor viewed as an unusual immunogen — Tuberculin sensitivity conferred on murine lymphocytes by dialysable human transfer factor — Human transfer factor preparations induce antigen responsiveness to primate and guinea pig lymphocytes.

III. TRANSFER FACTOR

DR. LAWRENCE: Our work on transfer factor over the past two decades has had as its major goals the chemical identification of this biologically potent material and an elucidation of its mechanism of action. Since our original demonstration of the cellular transfer of tuberculin sensitivity in man (Proc. Soc. Exp. Biol. Med., 71, 516, 1949) the general applicability and uniform reproducibility of the findings has been subjected to extensive confirmation. The ease with which delayed hypersensitivity has been transferred in humans to a variety of bacterial, fungal, viral, denatured serum protein and transplantation antigens underlines the unusual responsiveness of man to this system. This conclusion is reinforced by our own cumulative experience, notable for the regularity of transfer successfully achieved in 143 of 152 consecutive attempts in normal subjects; an incidence of 94% success. These observations led to the finding that extracts of frozen and thawed leukocyte are as effective as viable cells and that the active principle is not destroyed by treatment with desoxyribonuclease, ribonuclease (J. Clin. Invest. 34, 219, 1955) or trypsin (In: Cellular and Humoral Aspects of Hypersensitive States, Ed. Lawrence, Hoeber, 1959). The transferred delayed sensitivity is immunologically specific and appears promptly in the recipient - as early as four hours and is generally present when tested at 18 hours after transfer. Sensitivity is systemic in distribution and it usually persists for months to 2 years. Transfer of delayed allergy to diphtheria toxoid showed that human blood leukocytes do not transfer the capacity for a serum antibody response (Lawrence and Pappenheimer, J. Exp. Med. 104, 221, 1956.) Therefore, recipients of transfer factor are neither immunized by it as if it were antigen, nor is the capacity to respond to antigen by production of serum antibody transferred along with delayed sensitivity. Hence, recipients of tranfer factor express delayed sensitivity without concomitant detectable serum antibody, a finding subsequently confirmed by Good in agammaglobulinemic patients as well as in normal individuals (Ann. N. Y. Acad. Sci. 64, 882, 1957.)

Our studies on the transfer of coccidioidin sensitivity suggested (J. Immunol. 84, 358, 1960) and transfer of skin homograft rejection established (J. Clin. Invest. 39, 185, 1960) that the transfer factor confers de novo sensitization and excluded the possibility that its activity depends merely upon elevation of latent sensitivity possessed by the recipient. I think we can finally agree, in the face of repeated confirmation in other laboratories, that there is no longer any question of the fact that leucocyte extracts or dialysable transfer factor do indeed transfer enduring delayed sensitivity in humans and get on with the more pressing question of how this may come about. The facts are straight forward and therefore not in question any longer. The interpretation of the available facts is of course still a matter of healthy dispute (cf. Adv. Immunol. 1969).

The type and intensity of the transferred reactions as they appear in the recipient are illustrated in Fig. 16. It should be noted that reactions in the recipient are in general qualitatively and quantitatively much like those occurring in the natively sensitive donor. When intense degrees of reactivity are transferred, we have seen the recipient develop draining lymphangitis, lymphadenopathy and fever coincident with the skin reaction to antigen. Such skin-test sites may develop a blister which then goes on to eschar formation.

Our work on transfer factor and its extension by others, has raised a number of possible interpretations - namely is it antigen in the guise of superantigen or infra-antigen; is it an immunoglobulin of known or as yet undiscovered species and properties; is it an informational molecule; or is it a derepressor of a select population of non-sensitive lymphocytes? I, therefore, intend selectively to discuss only those data old, recent and unpublished that derive from experiments yielding discrete answers and narrowing the number of possible interpretations.

In this regard, our observations demonstrating that serial transfer of delayed hypersensitivity from individual A to B to C can be accomplished using leucocyte extracts, are most instructive (J. Clin. Invest. 34, 219, 1955.) The essential details of two consecutive attempts at transfer are set out in Table 17.

III. TRANSFER FACTOR

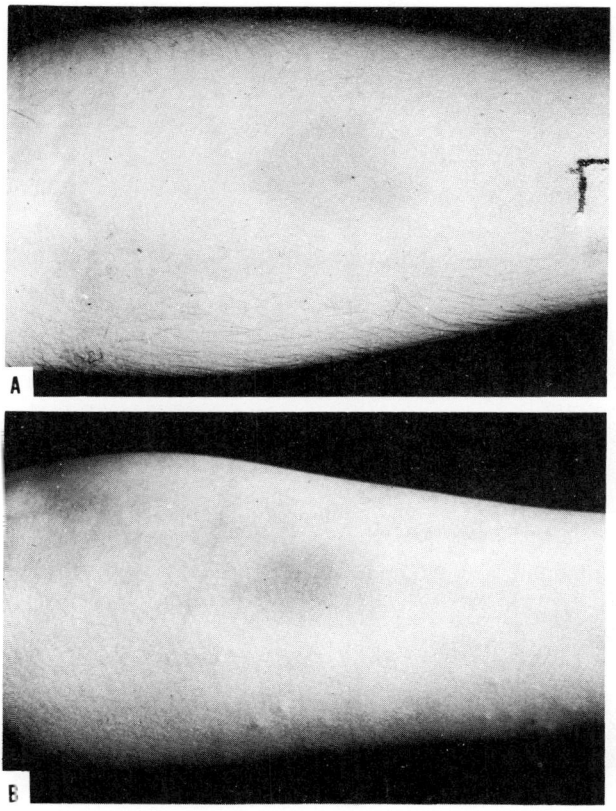

Fig. 15 A and B Similarity of intensity of delayed cutaneous reactions following systemic transfer with different preparation of transfer factor. A. Tuberculin reaction 35 x 40 mm to PPD 5γ 3 weeks post-transfer using frozen-thawed leucocyte extracts; B. tuberculin reaction 35 x 22 mm to PPD 5γ 3 months post-transfer using dialysable transfer factor.

(With permission of Journal of Pediatrics)

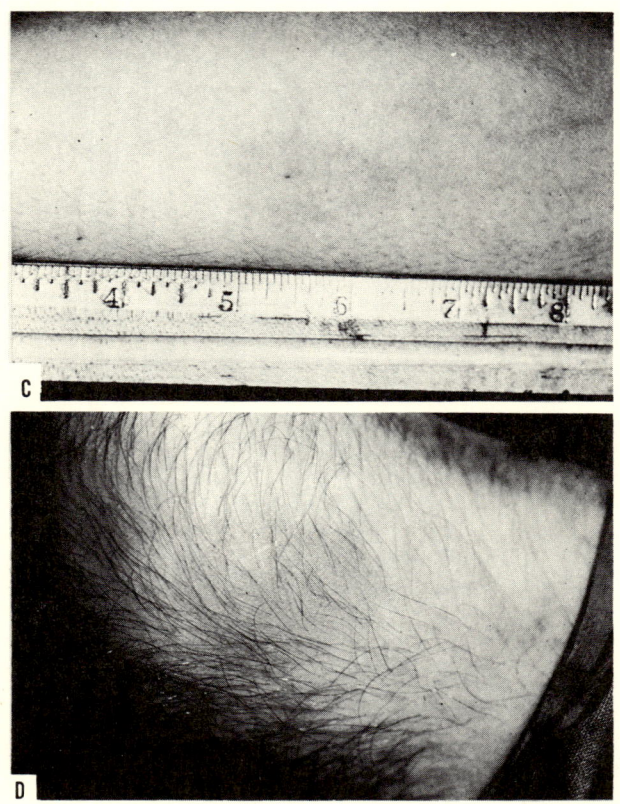

Fig. 16 C and D Similarity of intensity of delayed cutaneous reactions following systemic transfer with different preparations of transfer factor. C. Coccidioidin reaction 45 x 25 mm, 1 week post-transfer using frozen-thawed DNAse-treated leucocyte extract; D. coccidioidin reaction 35 x 45 mm, 3 months post-transfer using dialysable transfer factor. Cutaneous reactions photographed at 24 hours.

(With permission of Journal of Pediatrics)

III. TRANSFER FACTOR

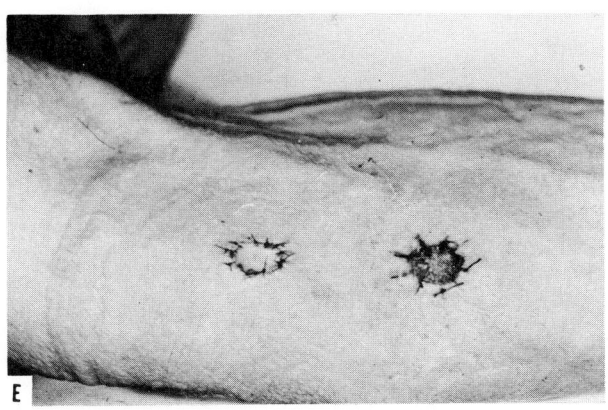

Fig. 16 E Transfer of skin homograft sensitivity (accelerated rejection) by means of transfer factor sensitized to A's skin. Photo taken 4 days after application of skin grafts and 12 days post-transfer. A-graft is black eschar; control graft from unrelated individual (B) is unaffected and survived 11 days.

(With permission of Journal of Pediatrics)

TABLE 17

SERIAL TRANSFER OF DELAYED HYPERSENSITIVITY

SENSITIVE DONOR "A"	TRANSFER FACTOR PREPARATION	1° REACTION RECIPIENT "B"	TIME BLED AFTER 1° TRANSFER	TRANSFER FACTOR PREPARATION	2° REACTION RECIPIENT "C"
Strep - M Positive 4+	Water - Lysis 0.5 ml WBC	4+	Day 3	Water - Lysis 0.5 ml WBC	2+
Tuberculin Positive 4+	Freeze - Thaw 0.2 ml WBC	4+	Week 3	Freeze - Thaw 0.5 ml WBC	2+

Each 0.1 ml packed wet WBC ca. 85 x 10⁶ cells; each (+) = 10 x 10 mm. induration and erythema.

(With permission Advances in Immunology)

III. TRANSFER FACTOR

As may be seen, the original observation was made using leucocyte extracts prepared by lysis from an individual with delayed sensitivity to streptococcal M substance. This leucocyte extract transferred delayed M-substance sensitivity to a primary negative recipient. Three days after transfer had been accomplished, leucocyte extracts obtained from the primary recipient, in turn transferred delayed M-substance sensitivity to a secondary negative recipient. This initial positive result of serial transfer was confirmed when frozen and thawed leucocyte extracts obtained from a tuberculin sensitive donor also transferred intense cutaneous sensitivity to a primary negative recipient: three weeks after transfer had been accomplished, leucocyte extracts obtained from the primary recipient transferred long-lived tuberculin sensitivity to a secondary recipient.

Since non-viable leucocyte extracts were used, these results foster the conclusion that transfer factor activates or sensitizes the circulating leucocytes of the recipient. Of particular significance is the prompt appearance of transfer factor in the M-positive recipient B's blood cells, coinciding with his positive cutaneous reaction. This occurs as early as the third day after transfer as measured by the capacity to transfer sensitivity to a secondary recipient. The presence of transfer factor in the tuberculin positive recipient B's blood cells persists as late as the third week after the initial transfer.

These results, although limited to two attempts, suggest that the expression of cutaneous sensitivity by the recipient serves as an indicator of the capacity of his cells to transfer, in turn, the same sensitivity to other individuals. It is very likely therefore that the property conferred on normal circulating leucocytes by transfer factor persists and may be detected by serial transfer for at least as long as the recipient himself expresses an intense degree of the cutaneous reactivity that was originally transferred.

On the basis of the dilutional aspects of this transaction alone it is difficult to sustain the notion that transfer factor is a potent form of antigen or antigen-RNA complex or a unique species of immunoglobulin. Since the transferred sensitivity is systemic in distribution, consider the minute quantity of leucocyte extract effective for

transfer in relation to the 1.73 sq. meter surface area of
a 70 Kilo recipient who provides an additional intra- and
extra-vascular fluid compartment of 35 liters as diluent.
The results also suggest more than mere random distribution
of transfer factor among the recipient's total cell populations (e.g. lymph nodes, spleen, marrow, blood.) Operationally, the recipient's circulating cells have promptly
acquired the same characteristics of the donor cells in
relation to the delayed sensitivity; namely, initiation of
events that result in skin reactivity and the capacity to
transfer the reactive state to another individual. From
this particular result and from our cumulative general
experience, one may deduce that recipient B's cells bear
transfer factor, as does the donor's cells, for at least
as long as cutaneous reactivity persists. However, in order
to demonstrate serial transfer successfully *in vivo* it is
obligatory that the primary recipient's (B's) own cutaneous
reaction be of marked intensity at the time his leucocytes
are obtained.

Rather than exclude the notion of replication of transfer
factor, the results of serial transfer favored such an
assumption and fostered the conclusion that the recipients'
circulating leucocytes are intimately involved in the process. These *in vivo* results, however, yielded no clue as
to whether the exact initiating event occurred in central
or peripheral lympho-reticular cells. However, as will be
shown, our current *in vitro* studies coupled with *in vivo*
transfer of sensitivity using dialysable transfer factor,
have afforded evidence that transfer factor engages a select
population of small circulating lymphocytes in the recipient's blood directly. Moreover, the intimations of
transfer factor as a replicating entity are now clarified
by our additional demonstration that it is the circulating
lymphocyte following conversion to an antigen-responsive
state by transfer factor, which undergoes transformation,
repeated cell division and clonal proliferation. It is
thus the lymphocyte engaged by transfer factor that undergoes replication in the presence of antigen.

Nevertheless, since these facts were not available at
that time (1953) the results of serial transfer led us to
consider that we were dealing either with a mammalian
equivalent of the pneumococcal transforming principle; or
transduction; or a phenomenon skin to lysogeny in phage infected bacteria. To test these, among other assumptions, the

III. TRANSFER FACTOR

leucocyte extracts were treated with DNAse, RNAse and sequentially DNAse plus trypsin in an attempt to inactivate transfer factor should it be associated with or dependent upon molecules known to have replicating potential. These specific exogenous enzymes in great exogenous enzymes in great excess had no discernible effect on transfer factor beyond that of endogenous lysosomal hydrolases released by freezing and thawing alone. These results were so uniform and reproducible that all subsequent leucocyte extracts prepared for transfer in this laboratory were routinely treated with pancreatic DNAse to facilitate handling. These data reaffirmed in a negative way that transfer factor was not likely to be either super-antigen; immunoglobulin; polymerized DNA or RNA or a trypsin susceptible protein.

It could be argued that the effects of transfer factor might result from an elevation of latent sensitivity when tuberculin, streptoccal proteins or diphtheria toxoid are used as antigens. To exclude this possibility, coccidioidin sensitivity was next selected for transfer in view of the natural restriction of this fungus to isolated areas of the far western portion of this country. The one fungal antigen with which coccidioidin may cross-react is histoplasmin and this fungus is also restricted to central and southern rural areas of the country. For our purpose leucocytes were collected from healthy sensitive donors residing in the endemic area in California, frozen and flown east. Aliquots of DNAse-treated leocucyte extracts were administered to negative recipients chosen for not having been in an area endemic for coccidioidomycosis and for having lived all or the greater part of their lives in the North Atlantic States (Rapaport et al., J. Immunol. 84, 358, 1960). Transfer of coccidiodin sensitivity was readily accomplished and persisted for as long as the recipients could be followed (i.e., 1 - 1 1/2 years). This study afforded the opportunity to observe the duration of transferred sensitivity in the absence of environmental exposure to antigen and in the absence of repeated skin tests. It was demonstrated that under these conditions the duration of transferred sensitivity was correlated with the intensity of the original skin reaction transferred when tested at the end of the first week (i.e., 6 recipients with initial transferred reactions of 1 to 2+ intensity became negative while 6 recipients with initial transferred reactions of 3 - 4+ intensity remained coccidiodin positive when finally retested 1 to 1 1/2 years after transfer). It was also noted that injection of coccidioidin-negative leucocyte extracts incubated with coccidioidin failed to transfer sensitivity, and repeated skin tests administered to such recipients did not cause delayed skin reactivity.

These results yielded suggestive but not conclusive evidence, for transfer of *de novo* sensitivity and showed that although exposure to antigen may indeed play a role in the recipient's response to transfer factor, such exposure is clearly neither the cause of the sensitive state; nor of the degree of sensitivity transferred; nor of the duration of transferred sensitivity. Moreover, indifferent mixtures of enzyme-digested leucocyte extracts and antigen are not sufficient to transfer sensitivity - an event which has an obligatory requirement for a specific pre-existent moiety only found in the leucocytes of a specifically sensitive donor. An abbreviated summary of some of the properties of transfer factor elucidated at this juncture (1949-1959) is detailed in Table 18. We next turned to the transfer of accelerated skin homograft rejection, a system which at once dispensed with screening skin tests, and excluded the spectre of elevation of latent sensitivity (J. Clin. Invest. *39*, 185, 1960). To accomplish this the donors of transfer factor had to be actively sensitized with 11 mm skin grafts, thus individual B was sensitized to A's skin on four sequential occasions. Anti-A transfer factor prepared from B's DNAse-treated leucocyte extracts was then injected into an indifferent individual C either 8 days before or 3 days after the target skin graft (A) and control skin grafts (D, E or F) were placed. Recipients of anti-A transfer factor invariably reacted to the A graft with accelerated rejection while control grafts were unaffected and accorded a first-set survival time (i.e., lived through 8-10 days.) Thus anti-A transfer factor caused individual C to respond as if he had met only A's skin before and had no effect at all on his response to control grafts from other individuals. These studies clearly demonstrated that: 1) *de novo* sensitivity is indeed transferred; 2) transfer factor exhibits a high degree of immunological specificity in selecting only the appropriate individual's histocompatibility antigens for rejection and no others; 3) the testing of recipients with antigen immediately before or just after transfer is neither responsible for, nor an obligatory requirement of the induction of the state of transferred reactivity;

TABLE 18

SOME PROPERTIES OF TRANSFER FACTOR

BIOLOGICAL	BIOCHEMICAL	IMMUNOLOGICAL
	TF Unaffected by:	
Endows recipient with specific sensitivity of donor	$25^{o}C$ or $37^{o}C$ - 6 hours	Interacts with but is not neutralized by antigen
Sensitivity is systemic	Distilled water lysis	WBC desensitized by antigen
Onset early (hrs.) Duration long (mos. → >1 yr.)	Freeze-thaw 10 cycles	Neg. WBC + antigen → no transfer
Minute dosage WBC effective:	Deep Freeze - 5 months	No detectable AB in donor WBC extract
As little as 0.01 ml → local transfer As little as 0.1 ml → systemic transfer	DNAse	No detectable AB in skin or serum of recipient of transferred sensitivity
Capacity for transfer parallels donor sensitivity and dosage WBC	RNAse	Not active sensitization early onset
Negative donors incapable	Lysosomal hydrolases	Not passive sensitization long duration
Extracts or cell-free superratants as effective as viable cells	(DNAse + trypsin)	Repeated test with antigen may increase intensity and duration of transferred sensitivity -- yet is not necessarily its cause
Does not cross species barrier *in vivo*		

(with permission CIBA Foundation Symposium on Cellular Aspects of Immunity)

4) a new transfer factor is elaborated by each individual following exposure to any other individual's tissues and its specificity is exclusively directed against that particular individual's histocompatibility antigens; 5) the corollary of the latter finding suggested to us that immunosuppressive agents in general and ALS in particular are effective in suspending the process of transplant rejection to the extent that they impair or deflect the few lymphocytes bearing a specific transfer factor produced by the recipient in response to the particular histocompatibility antigens of the organ transplant.

Our subsequent studies characterizing human histocompatibility antigens in sub-cellular leucocyte fractions, showed antigen activity to be associated with the endoplasmic reticulum and to be non-dialysable (Rapaport et al. Transplantation, 3, 490, 1965). Moreover, dialysates of leucocyte extracts containing transfer factor, do not have antigenic activity as measured by their failure to cause active sensitization to skin grafts obtained from the same leucocyte donor. Thus, in the homograft system of delayed hypersensitivity, the antigens which actively sensitize are separable and distinct from the moiety, transfer factor, that can only transfer sensitivity but cannot actively induce it. Clearly, although the cellular vehicle of transfer factor is rejected via a homograft response, transfer factor itself is not. This finding could explain the prolonged duration of transferred reactivity observed in humans (months to 2 years). The latter observation has raised questions of active sensitization, particularly when contrasted to the short duration of transferred delayed sensitivity routinely observed in outbred experimental animals (5-7 days.) Unlike transfers in outbred humans, the function of the transferred cell populations in outbred animals has been shown to be terminated in this period via a homograft rejection mechanism (Harris and Harris, Ann. N. Y. Acad. Sci. 87, 156, 1960; Warwick et al., Ann. N. Y. Acad. Sci. 99, 620, 1962.)

So much then for the phenomenological aspects of transfer factor as it occurs in complex leukocyte extracts; a slow and laborious, but necessary prelude to further attempts to identify and characterize the biochemical moiety responsible for the biological activities catalogued. Progress in the efforts at purification and identification were greatly facilitated by our finding that transfer factor is a dialysable moiety of low molecular weight (Lawrence et al. Trans. Assoc. Amer. Phys. 76, 84, 1963.) By this means transfer factor was separated from all non-dialysable cell constituents of >40,000 molecular weight, including proteins as well as transplantation antigens. We have concentrated on studies of dialysable transfer factor, since it possesses all the biological properties and activities of the parent leucocyte extract from which it is prepared. For example, the transfer of tuberculin or coccidioidin sensitivity with dialysable transfer factor appears promptly in most

III. TRANSFER FACTOR

recipients and persists for prolonged periods. Moreover, when smaller, ineffective volumes of dialysate prepared from sensitive cells were used, transfer of sensitivity did not occur post-transfer despite repeated testing of recipients with tuberculin or coccidioidin.

To evaluate the size of the constituents of the dialysate, Bence-Jones protein or papain-digested gamma globulin fragments were added to the dialysis sac as markers. Immunodiffusion studies on the dialysate revealed no albumin, alpha-2 globulin nor gamma globulin and no protein was detectable with 10% trichloroacetic acid. The dialysate gave a positive orcinol test. It was therefore concluded that the dialysate contained no protein nor immunoglobulin fragments and the materials it did contain were of <40,000 molecular weight. Passage of dialysate through Sephadex G-25 revealed 2 peaks as is shown in Figure 17.

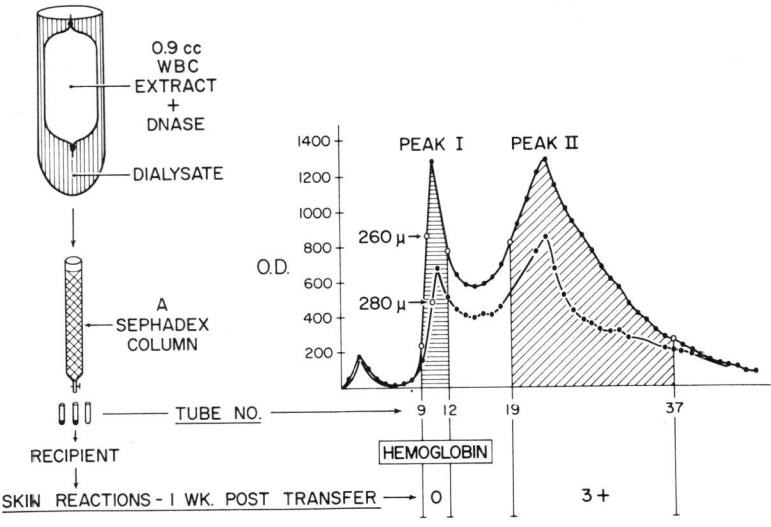

Fig. 17 Transfer of coccidioidin sensitivity with active fraction (peak II <10,000 mol. wt.) isolated from leucocyte extract dialysate after passage through Sephadex G-25

(With permission Transactions Association American Physicians)

The fraction collected under Peak I (<40,000 and >10,000 mol. wt.) failed to transfer coccidioidin sensitivity whereas the fraction collected under Peak II (<10,000 mol. wt.) transferred a marked degree (3+) of coccidioidin sensitivity. When retested two weeks after transfer the Peak I recipient developed minimal (1+) but definite sensitivity, and the Peak II recipient developed more intense (4+) sensitivity. The fraction under Peak I was contaminated with a minute but biologically effective quantity of transfer factor. It should be noted that dialysates prepared from coccidioidin negative donors and passed through Sephadex G-25, exhibit identical absorption spectra as those prepared from coccidioidin sensitive donors. This is not surprising in view of the potentially large number of transfer factors with other specificities that any one individual possesses.

We have already indicated that dialysis frees transfer factor from transplantation antigens. We also have tried without success to make specific antibody in rabbits given transfer factor injected in Freund's adjuvant. Moreover, repeated injection of pooled dialysable transfer factor in high dosage weekly in two humans over a year's interval has failed to produce specific antibody. Repeated intradermal injection of dialysable transfer factor in man from the same donor or pooled donors to the same recipient causes no cutaneous reaction, the only discernable effect being an increase in the intensity and duration of the tuberculin sensitivity that is transferred.

Dialysable transfer factor, like the parent leucocyte extract, is unaffected by 5γ, 50γ or 500γ pancreatic RNAse, despite the demonstration that in controls known RNA added to the dialysate is affected by this treatment. In other studies heating the dialysate at 56°C or 100°C for 30 minutes inactivated transfer factor. In its heat lability and insensitivity to pancreatic RNAse transfer factor shares properties unique for double-stranded RNA. If transfer factor should prove to be a polynucleotide, such properties would assume great significance (Lawrence and Zweiman, Trans. Assoc. Amer. Phys. 81, 240, 1968).

Transfer factor has thus emerged as a heat-labile, dialysable moiety of <10,000 molecular weight that is non-antigenic and certainly not an immunoglobulin. Of the

III. TRANSFER FACTOR

materials in the dialysate, the main candidates for the type of biological activity expressed by transfer factor are small polypeptides and polynucleotides. The dialysable nature of transfer factor; its low molecular weight; its absorption spectra patterns on Sephadex G-25; its polypeptide-polynucleotide composition; and the absence of immunoglobulins in the dialysate have each been rapidly confirmed in explicit detail by Baram et al. (Immunology 8, 461, 1965; J. Immunol. 97, 407, 1966); Arala-Chaves et al. (Int. Arch. Allergy 31, 353, 1967); Fireman et al. (Science, 155, 337, 1967) and by Brandriss (J. Clin. Invest. 47, 2152, 1968.)

We next turned to the development of in vitro techniques for the study of transfer factor. The macrophage migration method described by George and Vaughan (Proc. Soc. Exp. Biol. Med. 111, 514, 1962) has been studied extensively in our laboratory in collaboration with David, Al-Askari and Thomas (J. Immunol. 93, 279, 1964) and has proven a powerful tool in the investigation of mechanisms of cellular immunity, as this conference illustrates. The adaptation of this technique to human cell populations by Thor and Dray (J. Immunol. 101, 51, 1968) has confirmed the original observations and extended the scope of the operation. The transfer of the capacity to synthesize MIF to normal lymphocytes in vitro by RNA preparations made from sensitive lymphocytes by Thor and Dray (J. Immunol. 101, 469, 1968) is an observation of great interest. Moreover, using dialysable transfer factor in vivo, Rocklin et al. (Clin. Res., 1969; see II this volume) have transferred both specific delayed cutaneous sensitivity as well as the capacity to make MIF to a patient with chronic candidiasis. Observations such as these promise to clarify the relationship in humans of transfer factor as an initiator or derepressor molecule for the production of effector molecules such as MIF. Happily, in vitro studies of this type have also been successfully adapted to experimental animal models (Thor et al. Nature, 219, 753, 1968; Adler and Smith, Fed. Proc. 28, 813, 1969) and may help resolve the vexed question concerning how or why the guinea pig differs from man in the detection of transfer factor in vivo (Bloom and Chase, Progr. Allergy 10, 151, 1967.)

The availability of a relatively clean dialysable preparation of transfer factor has allowed it to be adapted to the lymphocytes transformation reaction in vitro. These studies have been undertaken in collaboration with my colleague, Dr. Valentine (Valentine and Lawrence, unpub. data). Since dialysable transfer factor is not antigenic in man or rabbits and since the transplantation antigens and other subcellular constituents remain within the dialysis sac, dialysable transfer factor can be cultured with normal lymphocytes without discernible effect on these cells unless the appropriate antigen is added. In the presence of specific antigen as the thymidine uptake curve illustrates in Fig. 18, a small percentage of lymphocytes will transform.

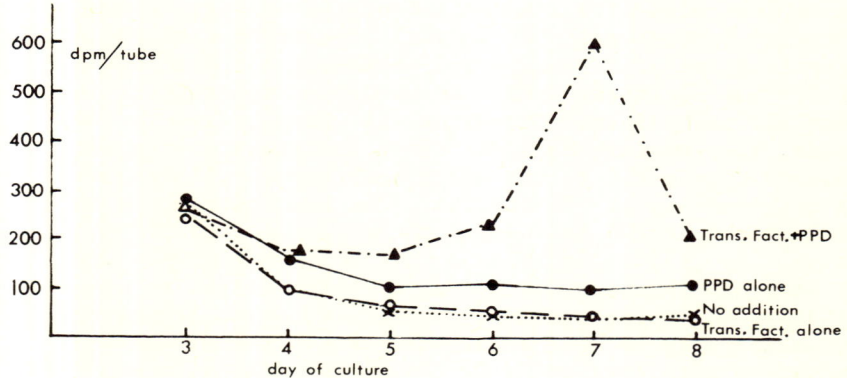

Fig. 18 In vitro sensitization of normal lymphocytes by dialysable transfer factor detected only in the presence of added antigen. Note absence of response (thymidine uptake) of cells incubated with transfer factor alone.

When exquisitely sensitive lymphocyte populations are used, the thymidine uptake affords a discriminating test to detect minute quantities of antigen (e.g. as little as 0.001 microgram PPD/ml is detectable.) In seeking to determine whether transfer factor is an immunogen or antigen-polynucleotide fragment we added dialysate alone to highly sensitive lymphocyte populations and observed no increased thymidine uptake as compared to the same lymphocyte populations incubated without dialysate. However, minute amounts of PPD added to other aliquots of the same cells were effective in causing increased thymidine uptake.

III. TRANSFER FACTOR

We then compared the _in vitro_ effects of dialysable transfer factor with _in vivo_ events in the same recipient. Transfer factor prepared from a tuberculin positive-diphtheria toxoid negative donor was added to lymphocyte cultures obtained from a tuberculin negative-toxoid negative prospective recipient.

As may be seen in Fig. 19, transformation occurred only in those cultures containing tuberculin transfer factor plus tuberculin and no effect was observed in cultures following addition of tuberculin transfer factor plus toxoid; tuberculin alone; toxoid alone or transfer factor alone. An aliquot of the same tuberculin positive-toxoid negative factor was injected into the shoulder of the negative recipient and transferred marked (3+) tuberculin sensitivity but no reaction to toxoid. Blood lymphocytes taken from the same recipient, which were unresponsive to tuberculin alone or toxoid alone before transfer _in vivo_, now responded _in vitro_ to the addition of tuberculin alone with transformation but exhibited no response to the addition of toxoid.†

Although this represents but a single series of combined _in vitro_ - _in vivo_ observations, the approach represents an incisive means of dealing with many of the questions raised. Most importantly it dispenses with the need of testing recipients with antigen prior, during or after transfer. We interpret the result as indicating that the _in vitro_ transfer with dialysate occurs promptly at the level of the circulating, thymus-dependent, small lymphocytes; that this same event occurs _in vivo_; and that dialysable transfer factor is specific when multiple sensitivities are transferred. This type of experiment also suggests that

---

† _Afterthought_: With regard to specificity of dialysable, low molecular weight transfer factor, the donor in addition to being tuberculin positive and toxoid negative, was also SK-SD positive and coccidioidin negative. The _in vivo_ transfer corresponded exactly to these multiple specificities and the recipient became tuberculin positive and SK-SD positive while remaining toxoid negative and coccidioidin negative. The antigens SK-SD and coccidioidin were not evaluated in the _in vitro_ system.

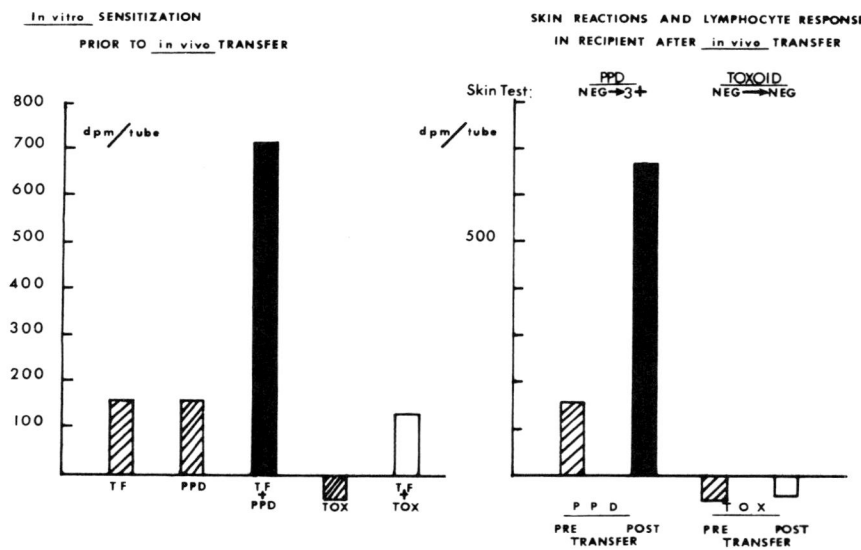

Fig. 19 Specificity of in vitro sensitization of normal blood lymphocytes with dialysable transfer factor (tuberculin positive, toxoid negative) compared to in vivo transfer factor conversion of cutaneous reactivity as well as blood lymphocyte response of recipient to tuberculin but not to toxoid.

the transaction is a peripheral event and transfer factor promptly engages the circulating population of lymphocytes, without obligatory residence in bone-marrow, spleen or lymph nodes to generate its effects. Our results are thus analogous in most particulars to those reported by Fireman et al. (Science, 155, 337, 1967.)

III. TRANSFER FACTOR

Since the magnitude of the in vitro effects of dialysable transfer factor was not as intense as its in vivo effects, (i.e., only 3% of cells transformed when examined on day 7) we recalled an experiment done some years ago which is summarized in Figure 20.

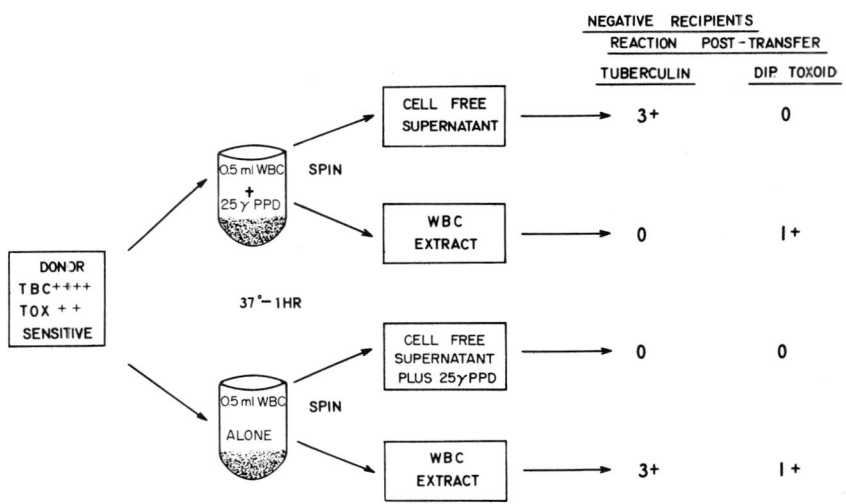

Fig. 20 In vivo activity of transfer factor liberated from sensitive cell population within one hour of incubation with antigen in vitro

(With permission of Journal of Experimental Medicine)

Lawrence and Pappenheimer (J. Exp. Med. 104, 321, 1956; J. Clin. Invest. 36, 908, 1957) had observed that blood leucocyte populations sensitive to tuberculin and to diphtheria toxoid when incubated (37°C - 1 hour) with 25γ PPD resulted in the liberation of only tuberculin transfer factor into the cell-free supernatant as measured by in vivo transfer. The cell pellet had lost the capacity to transfer tuberculin sensitivity but did transfer sensitivity to toxoid. Control leucocyte populations incubated without antigen retained the capacity to transfer sensitivity to both tuberculin and toxoid, whereas neither activity was detected in their supernatant following in vivo transfer.

Valentine and I (J. Clin. Invest. 47, 98a, 1968; Science, in press, 1969) have recently found that supernatants prepared from specifically sensitive lymphocytes incubated with tuberculin when added to non-sensitive lymphocytes, cause them to undergo transformation repeated cell-division and clonal proliferation as illustrated in Fig. 21.

The effect of supernatants containing such activity, as measured by thymidine uptake, is antigen dose-dependent, a property that is illustrated in Fig. 22.

We have found additionally that the material in such supernatants is inactivated at $56^{\circ}C$ for 30 minutes distinguishing it from MIF of either human or guinea pig origin, which is stable at $56^{\circ}C$ (see IV this volume.) The supernatant activity is not sedimented at 100,000 x G, a physical property that sets it apart from the blastogenic transplantation antigens found in mixed leucocyte cultures (Kasakura and Lowenstein, Nature, 208, 794, 1965.) Moreover our material is also non-dialysable.

Thus, earlier experiments demonstrated that supernatants prepared from leucocytes cultured with tuberculin contain antigen-liberated transfer factor within an hour of incubation as shown by in vivo transfer. The supernatant activity which makes non-sensitive lymphocytes antigen-responsive in vitro requires 18-24 hours incubation for its production. Although the latter has not been tested in vivo, it is almost certain that it also contains antigen-liberated transfer factor. The critical question concerning this new supernatant activity produced by antigen-stimulated lymphocytes, is to what extent the effects observed are due to transfer factor alone as opposed to the array of other products now known to result from the interaction of sensitive lymphocytes and antigen. Dr. Valentine and I are

III. TRANSFER FACTOR

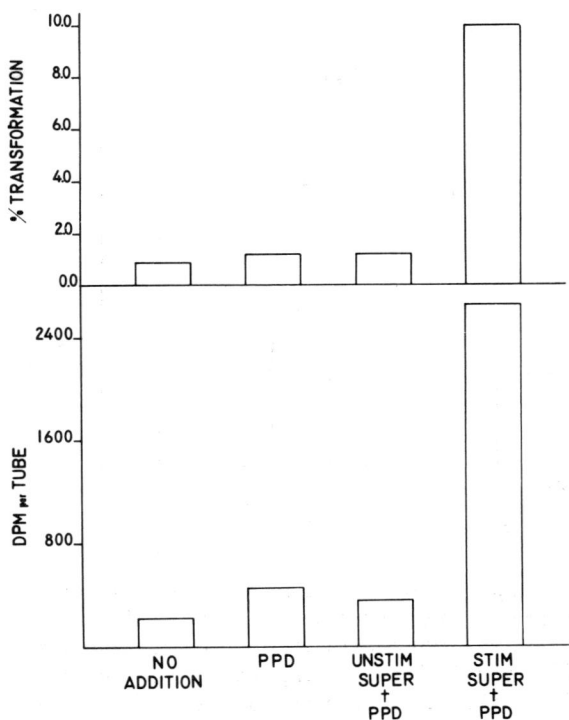

Fig. 21 Response of nonsensitive lymphocytes to cell-free supernatants from sensitive leukocytes. Above, percent blast transformation; below, incorporation per culture of $2\text{-}^{14}C$ thymidine into DNA as assayed by liquid scintillation counting. Each value is mean of three cultures. Final concentration of PPD adjusted to 0.8 µg/ml in all tubes except those marked "no addition." Cultures examined on day 6.

(With permission of Science)

currently engaged in seeking answers to these questions. The <u>in vivo</u> and <u>in vitro</u> relationships of dialysable transfer factor, antigen-liberated transfer factor and the

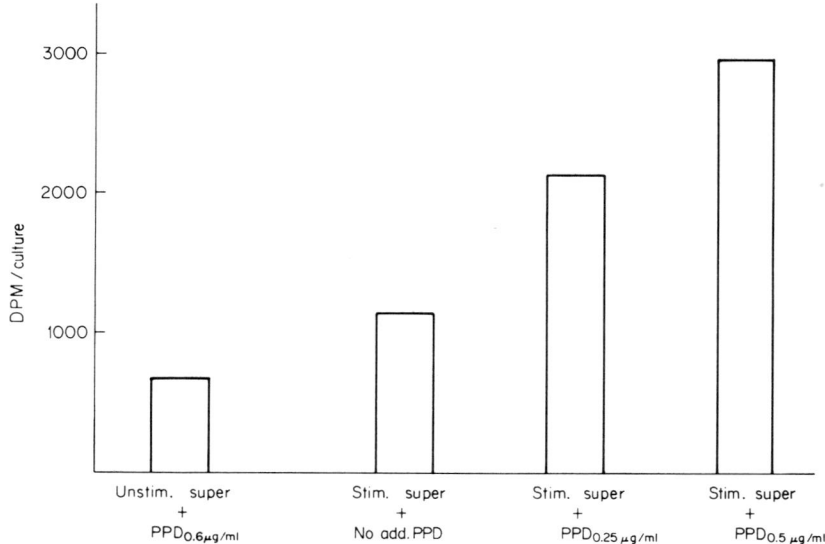

Fig. 22 Response of nonsensitve lymphocytes to 36 hour cell-free supernatants from sensitive leukocytes. Stimulated supernatants were prepared by exposing sensitive cells to PPD (0.25 µg/ml) for 1 hour, washing, and culturing without additional antigen for 36 hours. The amount (0.6 µg/ml) of PPD added as a control to the unstimulated supernatant after separation from the sensitive cells is greater than the maximum possible amount of PPD in any of theother assay cultures even if residual antigen in the stimulated supernatant were assumed to be all of that initially added to the sensitive cells, that is 0.25 µg/ml.

(With permission of Science)

non-dialysable supernatant material insofar as they are currently known is diagrammatically illustrated in Fig. 23.

Thus, we have shown dialysable transfer factor causes a very few (ca 3% by day 7) nonsensitive lymphocytes to become antigen-responsive in vitro and it also results in the immunologic engagement of a similar small number of

III. TRANSFER FACTOR

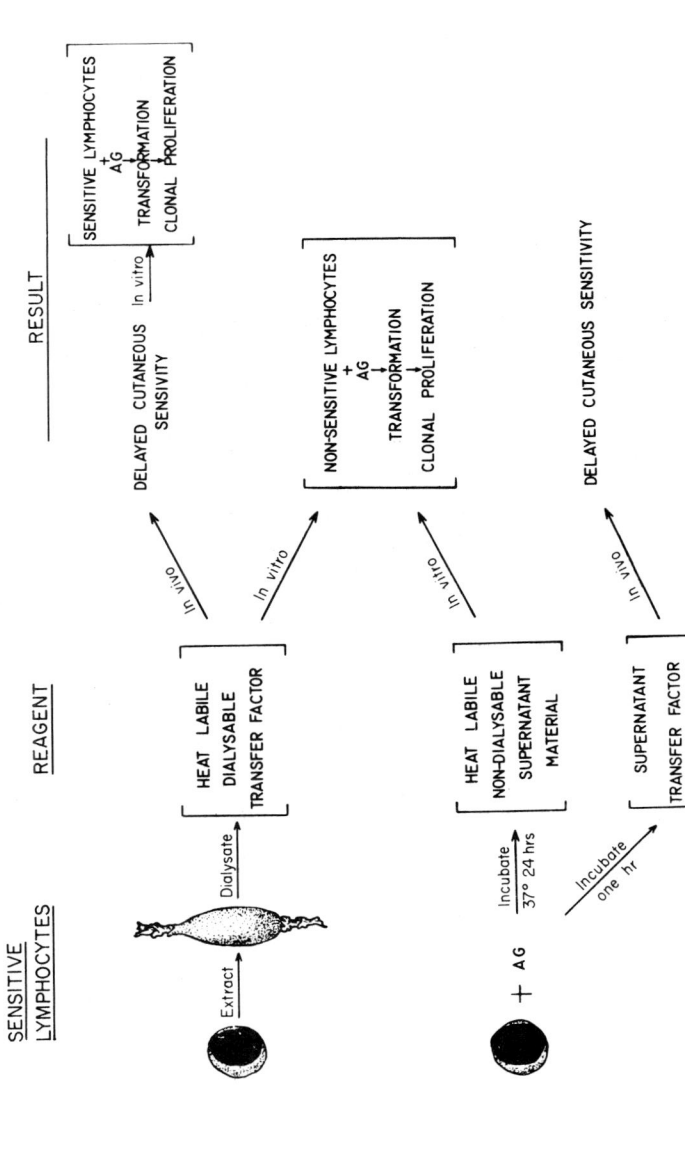

Fig. 23 Diagrammatic comparison of in vivo and in vitro activities of dialysable transfer factor, antigen-liberated transfer factor, and lymphocyte activating material.

(With permission of Advances in Immunology)

circulating lymphocytes of the recipient in vivo, yet it is capable of transferring marked delayed cutaneous sensitivity; whereas, the antigen-produced supernatant material has consistently resulted in a much larger conversion of nonsensitive cells to transformed lymphocytes (15-20%) by the end of seven days culture.

How then are these effects amplified? Does antigen liberate transfer factor from the few sensitive lymphocytes to recruit a large population of nonsensitive cells as originally postulated by Pappenheimer (Harvey Lecture Series, 52, 100, 1956,) or is some other mechanism operative? Drs. Marshall, Valentine and I (J. Exp. Med. 130, 327, 1969) therefore, examined this question with time-lapse cinematography to study populations of blood lymphocytes cultured under continuous observation for seven days. The lymphocytes were held captive under a single microscopic field in a 0.2 - 0.5 mm plastic ring and cells could neither migrate into or out of the field of vision. Initially, tuberculin-sensitive human blood lymphocytes were observed in culture with tuberculin. These studies revealed only an estimated two percent of the total lymphocyte population is antigen-responsive and undergoes transformation, repeated cell-division and clonal proliferation. Thus, at least after an initial 48-72 hours of tube culture, cine studies revealed no evidence of recruitment.

The large number of transformed lymphocytes (20-30%) present at the end of seven days culture thus arose from the very few antigen-responsive cells by a process of repeated cell-division, resulting in the proliferation of a clone of antigen-responsive cells. The important point of these observations is that where it was possible to trace single cells through a series of divisions, large clones were observed to occur. It was usual to see clones of 16 cells develop, common to observe clones of 32 cells and on occasion to follow the development of 64 or more cells from a single cell. A clone of this type arising from a single lymphocyte is diagrammed in Fig. 24 and a representative sequence of still photos illustrating the cine development of two separate clones is shown in Fig. 25.

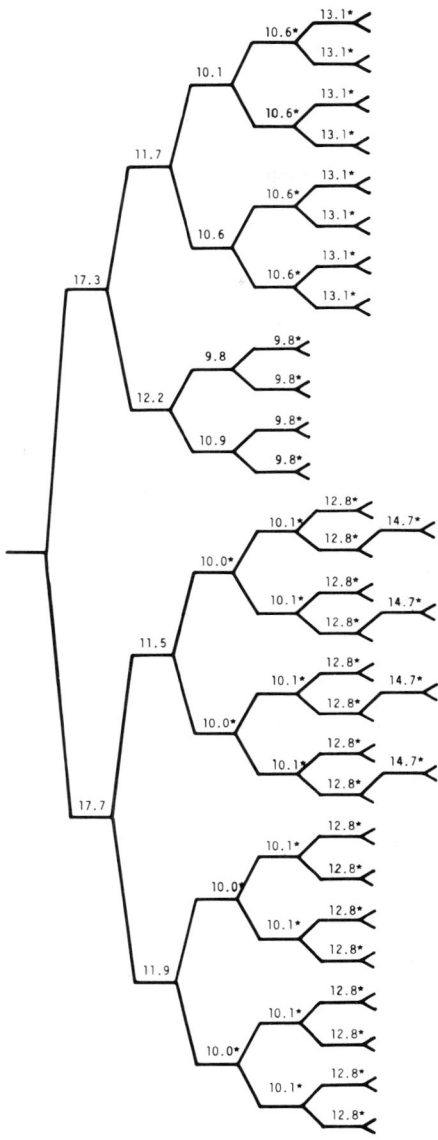

Fig. 24 A diagram to represent the development of a single lymphoblast into a clone that went through to the 7th and in a few cases, the 8th generation after exposure of tuberculin sensitive human lymphocytes to tuberculin. The line at the left represents the initial lymphoblast. Numbers over subsequent lines are generation times in hours. Asterisks indicate that an average generation time as taken for the whole group of cells.
 (With permission of Journal of Experimental Medicine)

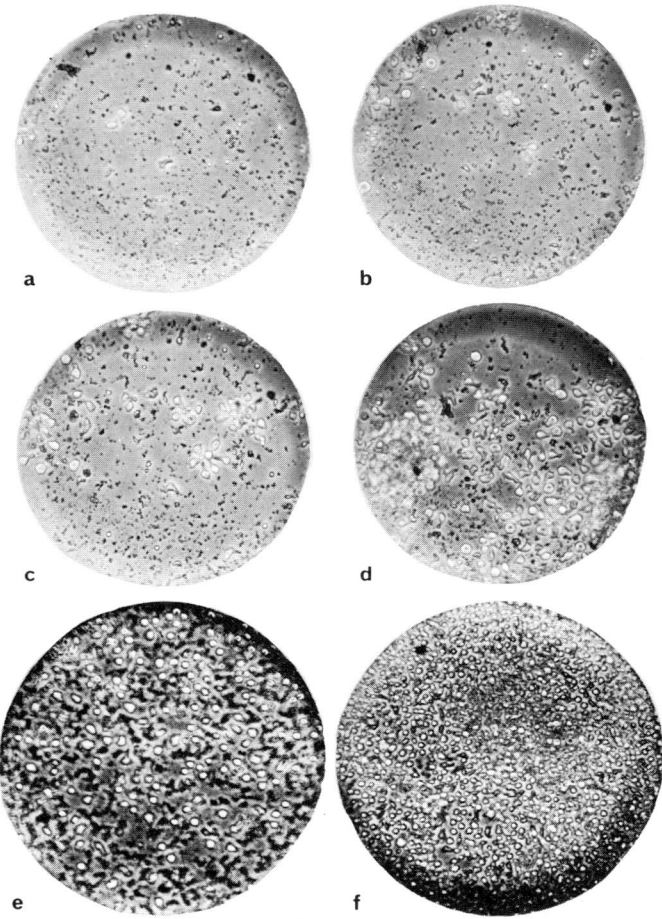

Fig. 25 An individual microchamber demonstrating tuberculin stimulated cell proliferation, photographed on a) day 3; b) day 4; c) day 5 and d) day 6. Photographs e. and f. are two individual microchambers which were not followed by time-lapse but photographed to illustrate the magnitude the proliferating clones may reach by day 7 or 8. The proliferating lymphoblasts are seen as large, light colored, refractile cells often connected in clusters.

(With permission of Journal of Experimental Medicine)

III. TRANSFER FACTOR

It cannot be too strongly emphasized however that the mere observance of clonal proliferation does not exclude other postulated mechanisms of amplification (e.g. recruitment) that may contribute to an increase in the number of lymphoblasts observed in tube cultures. Under the conditions of these experiments there is a gap during the first 48 hours of tube culture; during this critical period recruitment cannot yet be excluded and indeed may actually occur. Our own demonstration that either dialysable transfer factor or antigen-produced supernatant material do confer on nonsensitive lymphocytes the capacity to respond to antigen, is by definition an example of recruitment. Thus, having demonstrated that recruitment does really operate, we are prepared to believe that this mechanism functions under natural circumstances. Nevertheless, the demonstrated ability of lymphoblasts to divide and redivide does argue strongly for clonal proliferation as the major mechanism by which the lymphocyte population is increased <u>after</u> the first two days of culture.

We next applied the cinematography technique to study recruitment in cultures of nonsensitive lymphocytes incubated with tuberculin plus supernatants prepared by incubating tuberculin sensitive lymphocytes with antigen. As had been observed using naturally sensitive cells, here again only an equally small percentage of lymphocytes (ca. two percent) were <u>initially</u> engaged by the supernatant material. This small percentage of cells, in the presence of tuberculin transformed, divided and redivided to form a large clone (15-20%) of lymphoblasts by the 7th day of culture. This entire cinematography sequence was qualitatively, quantitatively and temporally identical to that observed when naturally sensitive lymphocytes were cultured in the presence of tuberculin.

Among the many unanswered questions that remain are the relation of dialysable transfer factor to antigen-liberated transfer factor. Since both have the same <u>in vivo</u> properties, do both share the same <u>in vitro</u> properties? What is the contribution of transfer factor, liberated from sensitive cells after only one hour incubation with antigen, to the non-dialysable, lymphocyte activating material which requires 18-24 hours incubation with antigen for its elaboration into the same supernatant? Do these agents compete for the same few normal lymphocytes that are susceptible to activation or do they act in concert? Is transfer factor in this situation non-dialysable because it has become complexed with antigen during incubation? And finally, is transfer factor a specific recruiter of cells and the supernatant activity a non-specific recruiting agent?

A summary of the more recently elucidated properties of dialysable transfer factor is detailed in Table 19.

TABLE 19

SOME PROPERTIES OF DIALYSABLE TRANSFER FACTOR

BIOLOGICAL	BIOCHEMICAL	IMMUNOLOGICAL
Properties of WBC extract: Prompt Onset (hrs.) Long Duration (>1 yr.) Equal Intensity	Soluble, Dialysable, Lyophilizable	Not Immunoglobulin
	<10,000 mol. wt.	Not Immunogenic
	No Protein, Albumin, α or γ globulin	Immunologically Specific
Dissociable from Transplantation Antigens	Orcinol Positive	Converts Normal Lymphocytes <u>in vitro</u> and <u>in vivo</u> to Antigen-Responsive State
	Polypeptide/Polynucleotide Composition	Transformation and Clonal Proliferation of Converted Lymphocytes Exposed to Antigen
Small Quantities → Magnified Effects	Inactivated 56°C-30 min.	
	Resists Pancreatic RNAse	Informational Molecule/ Derepressor/Receptor Site?
	Retains Potency - 5 yrs.	

(with permission Advances in Immunology)

The nature of the antigen-receptor site residing in or on sensitive lymphocytes and whether it is a cell-associated immunoglobulin of the high affinity type originally postulated by Karush and Eisen or the IgX postulated by Mitchison or yet another type of molecular species with

III. TRANSFER FACTOR

stereospecific configuration, is the focus of much current interest. Since the effect of dialysable transfer factor converting the very few normal lymphocytes to the sensitive state can only be detected following the addition of appropriate antigen, it follows that a specific receptor site must therefore have been conferred on such sensitized cells. These observations raise the question whether transfer factor itself may be the specific receptor site as originally conceived by Pappenheimer, since we had shown antigen to interact with but not neutralize transfer factor, or could transfer factor induce the synthesis of the receptor site? In the conversion of such a select few normal cells to an antigen-responsive state, transfer factor itself is accomplishing a highly specific interaction with a particular lymphocyte receptor site. Since transfer factor is a small, non-antigenic, non-immunoglobulin molecule, this latter event provides at least a handle on the problem of IgX, or whatever receptor sites may be. The _in vitro_ techniques currently available and the separation and characterization of the diverse specific and non-specific immunologic reagents thus far delineated, have brought the problem to the point where an approach to further elucidation of this complicated question finally becomes possible.

Thus, we have reviewed selected _in vivo_ and _in vitro_ properties of transfer factor as an initiator of cellular immune responses at a molecular level. Evidence has been presented that transfer factor is neither antigen nor immunoglobulin and the response transferred is neither passive nor active sensitization, in the usual context of these terms. Transfer factor behaves in some respects like an informational molecule in its endowment of the entire negative recipient or a select portion of his isolated lymphocyte populations _in vivo_ and _in vitro_ with the specific cellular immunological memories of the donor.

Serial transfer from individual A to B to C has also diminished the possibility that transfer factor acts as a super-antigen, as has our inability to make an antibody to transfer factor in man or rabbit. These biological properties of transfer coupled with its _in vitro_ and _in vivo_ effects on nonsensitive lymphocyte populations have demonstrated the repeated cell division and clonal proliferation of lymphocytes bearing transfer factor when exposed to antigen. Thus it is the replication of "activated" lymphocytes bearing transfer factor which yielded results which suggested the notion of replication of transfer factor itself.

Of the materials present in the dialysate, the two main candidates for transfer factor activity are polypeptides and/or polynucleotides. Since transfer factor is unaffected by <u>pancreatic</u> RNAse and is inactivated by heat at 56°C for 30 minutes, <u>if</u> it proves a polynucleotide molecule, it shares two properties unique for double-stranded RNA nucleotides.

Since the polynucleotides present in the dialysate are rather small to code for the amount and specificity of the information required, the interpretation of transfer factor as an informational molecule is difficult to sustain. Our <u>in vitro</u> studies and the concrete visual evidence supplied by time-lapse cinematography, suggest that transfer factor acts as a derepressor of a select population of small lymphocytes which may have been predestined to become antigen-sensitive under other circumstances, such as natural infection with the tubercle bacillus.

In any event, the adaptation of transfer factor to <u>in vitro</u> systems of analysis has led to the beginnings of a molecular basis for cellular immune responses. The principles evolved from the study of transfer factor in normal individuals have found extensive application to the analysis of mechanisms in primary or secondary cellular immune deficiency diseases. Transfer factor has also found practical therapeutic application in the reconstitution of such patients threatened by overwhelming intracellular microbial infections. The increasing validity of Thomas's postulate (in Cellular and Humoral Aspects of Hypersensitive States, p. 529, Ed. Lawrence, Hoeber, 1959) of an immunological surveillance mechanism for disposal of mutant cells, has led to preliminary attempts at immunologic reconstitution of patients suffering from neoplastic disease with an appropriate transfer factor (Lawrence, Adv. Immunol., 1969.)

III. TRANSFER FACTOR

Thus, studies on transfer factor designed to shed light on mechanisms of cellular immune responses and to develop a molecular basis for their further analysis, finds itself central to understanding and effectively managing a much broader area encompassing autoimmune disorders; homograft immunity; tumor surveillance mechanisms; cellular immune deficiency diseases and diverse host-parasite relationships.

CHAIRMAN GOOD: Dr. Lawrence's exposition of our present knowledge of transfer factor is truly a tour de force. To organize our discussion so as to most effectively develop this area of investigation, I propose that we first consider the purely technical factors involved; then move on to focus on the dialysable transfer factor itself; its role in in vitro lymphocyte transformation; the newer evidence for the existence of transfer factor in experimental animal models; and finally to consider its adaptation to the study of clinical immunologic deficiency states.

DR. ROSENAU: I think experiments on enzymatic digestion of transfer factor are very important in elucidating the nature of the material. Has the possible presence of enzyme inhibitors within preparations of transfer factor been considered? Have other proteases besides trypsin been used, such as pronase? Have particular moieties of RNA that may be resistant to pancreatic RNAse been considered, such as certain types of double-stranded RNA? Have you used ribonucleases other than pancreatic RNAse, which have other properties in splitting RNA?

DR. LAWRENCE: To answer your last question first, I indicated that dialysable transfer factor shared two properties which are unique for double-stranded RNA or its polynucleotides, namely inactivation by heat ($56^{\circ}C$ - 30 min.) and resistance to the action of pancreatic ribonuclease. If the biological activity of transfer factor is dependent on the presence of double-stranded RNA polynucleotides, then specific ribonucleases known to cleave double-strands should inactivate transfer factor. Experiments treating dialysable transfer factor with T_1 and T_3 RNAse, as well as phosphodiesterase are in preparation. Should this treatment fail to inactivate transfer factor, we plan to move on to treatment with pronase and attempt sequential peptide digestion, since the main candidates for activity are the polynucleotides and polypeptides in the dialysate. Although our attention and that of others working with dialysable transfer factor has focussed on the polynucleotides present, it would be premature to discount the possible role of a small peptide. Of additional interest in this connection, is our finding that transfer factor is stable in leucocyte extracts prepared by water lysis and held at 25°C or 37°C for 8-10 hours. This result indicates that it is also unaffected by endogenously activated lysosomal hydrolases as well as cell nucleases.

DR. DAVID: My comment is also in reply to Dr. Rosenau's question to Dr. Lawrence concerning enzyme inhibitors present in the dialysate. This is, indeed, a rather important consideration. Our controls for this possibility which showed that in the presence of transfer factor, DNAse and RNAse were perfectly capable of breaking down added authentic RNA or DNA substrate (Lawrence et al. Trans. Assoc. Amer. Phys. 76, 84, 1963.)

As regards the issue of recruitment: in one case, it appeared that the "producing" cells were derived from the sensitized cells, and yet they made a material that affects non-sensitive cells. The question could be resolved if this soluble material were affecting only the cells that could be potentially sensitized to a specific antigen in a normal unsensitized individual. In that event this soluble material would not be recruiting a large number of non-sensitive lymphocytes, but rather affecting the potentially sensitive cells

DR. DUTTON: I wasn't clear whether in any of the experiments the transfer factor represents the only product added to the system. Were there any experiments where transfer factor was injected without any prior tests of the recipient with antigen?

III. TRANSFER FACTOR

DR. LAWRENCE: There are two studies in the literature where leucocyte extracts were used to transfer and the recipients were not tested at any time prior to transfer, nor could they have been exposed to antigen in nature. Maurer's studies (J. Exp. Med. 113, 1029, 1961) on delayed reactivity to ethylene oxide-treated human serum provide the most clearly documented confirmation of the capacity of leucocyte extracts to transfer delayed reactivity. The drastic alteration of human serum proteins by this treatment created new antigenic determinants to which neither donor or recipient had been exposed; consequently the recipient was not skin-tested prior to transfer. Prospective leucocyte donors were actively sensitized to the new antigen and developed marked delayed sensitivity but no serum antibody, even after repeated intradermal immunization over 1-1/2 years. Frozen and thawed leucocyte extracts obtained from these donors transferred strong delayed reactions (20 mm to 35 mm diameter) to five consecutive recipients. Three recipients given viable leucocytes developed degrees of sensitivity comparable to that achieved with leucocyte extracts. The transferred delayed reactivity persisted for at least a year after the initial transfer and skin test, in the absence of repeated exposure to antigen in the environment or via skin test. The latter finding is analogous to our earlier experience with coccidioidin transfer (J. Immunol. 84, 358, 1960) although Maurer's results are the more impressive in view of the additional luxury of transfer without an initial screening skin test.

The other example of transfer without prior skin test is afforded by our earlier studies on the transfer of accelerated skin homograft rejection with DNAse-treated leucocyte extracts (J. Clin. Invest. 30, 185, 1960.) In this study we were aware of the possibility, so frequently raised, that DNAse-treated leucocyte extracts raised in individual B to contain anti-A transfer factor could be contaminated with minute quantities of A's histocompatibility antigens. In protocols deliberately designed to test this possibility, the relevant test graft (A) and control graft (D) were in place for three days in the unrelated recipient and showed all criteria for satisfactory survival on stereomicroscopic examination (pink color, good circulation in graft vessels.) At that time each graft was surrounded by anti-A transfer factor infiltrated into the recipient's skin in a halo fashion about 20 mm away from the graft bed. Within 18 to 24 hours after transfer, the A graft began to show signs of accelerated rejection (i.e., cyanosis, edema, rouleaux formation of RBC followed by thrombosis and hemorrhage microscopically.) In contrast, the similarly treated control graft (D) went through the usual first-set survival time, living through ten days unaffected by transfer factor. If this prompt effect were due to active sensitization, it would be an unparalleled event, in that it would have abolished the latent period usually required for a primary immune response. To control these observations DNAse-treated leucocyte extracts from nonsensitive donors had no effect on graft survival when injected around the target (A) graft nor did serum obtained from the sensitive transfer factor donors. Moreover, when specific transfer factor was injected into the shoulder of a recipient with test and control grafts in residence for three days, only the test graft underwent prompt accelerated rejection in 24-48 hours following transfer while the control graft was accorded a first-set rejection (eight days.) These data appear in Table 20A.

DR. DUTTON: In this situation the graft was placed on the recipient three days before the injection of transfer factor.

DR. LAWRENCE: Yes.

DR. DUTTON: In that case do you have conclusive evidence that the transfer factor preparation itself did not contain antigen as well?

DR. LAWRENCE: No, we can only record that the graft for which transfer factor was specific, was rejected in a period too short to be considered active sensitization and that the transfer factor is highly specific for the one particular individual's transplantation antigens.

III. TRANSFER FACTOR

TABLE 20A

SPECIFICITY OF TRANSFER FACTOR FOR HISTOCOMPATIBILITY ANTIGENS

A. Local Transfer Done 3 Days After Grafts in Residence*:

Donor	Status	Material Transferred	Recipient	Day of Graft Rejection Target "A"	Day of Graft Rejection Control "D"	Score
D4	Sens. vs. "A"	0.2 ml WBC Ext.	R5	4 / 5	8	Positive
		1.0 ml Serum		10	8	Negative
D5	Sens. vs. "A"	0.2 ml WBC Ext.		4	10	Positive
		1.0 ml Serum	R7	10	- -	Negative
Normal	Not Sens.	0.2 ml WBC Ext.		10	- -	Negative
D6	Sens. vs. "A"	0.17 ml WBC Ext.	R8	5 / 6	10	Positive
		0.17 ml WBC Ext.	R9	5 / 6	10	Positive
D6	Sers. vs. "A"	1.0 ml Serum	R10	10	- -	Negative
Normal	Not Sens.	0.2 ml WBC Ext.		10	- -	Negative

* The shorter period of sensitization of the transfer factor donor (e.g. 2 sequential exposures to 11 mm skin grafts) and the lower dosages of transfer factor used to achieve local transfer (e.g. 0.2 ml packed WBC =0=170 x 10^6 cells) were insufficient to cause systemic sensitization of the recipient. Therefore target grafts not in juxtaposition to transfer factor were unaffected.
(with permission Journal of Clinical Investigation)

To answer your objection directly, one would have to repeat the above studies using dialysable transfer factor, since we subsequently showed with Rapaport, Dausset and Converse (Transplantation, 3, 490, 1965) that human histocompatibility antigens are non-dialysable. This was done by showing that materials in the leucocyte extract (mainly endoplasmic reticulum) which remain inside the cellophane sac, actively sensitize recipients to skin grafts from the leucocyte donor. In contrast, the dialysate did not cause sensitization in recipients tested with skin grafts from the same leucocyte donor. Thus, antigenic materials in the histocompatibility system are separable by dialysis from that moiety which transfers sensitivity but cannot

CELLULAR IMMUNITY

TABLE 20B

SPECIFICITY OF TRANSFER FACTOR FOR HISTOCOMPATIBILITY ANTIGENS

B. Systemic Transfer Effective with Sensitized but not Desensitized Transfer Factor Donor[†]

Donor	Status	Material Transferred	Recipient	Transfer in Relation to Skin Grafting	Day of Graft Rejection Target	Day of Graft Rejection Control	Score
D7	Sens. vs. "A"	0.52 ml WBC Ext.[††]	R11	8 days before	4	11	Positive
		0.52 ml WBC Ext.	R12	3 days after	4 / 5	8	Positive
D7	Desens. vs. "A"	0.50 ml WBC Ext.	R13	11 days before	8	8	Negative
		0.50 ml WBC Ext.	R14	" "	9	9	Negative
		0.5 ml WBC Ext.	R15	3 days after	10	14	Negative
		0.5 ml WBC Ext.	R16	" "	8	15	Negative
D9	Sens. vs. "A"	0.7 ml WBC Ext.	R22	8 days before	4	11	Positive
		0.7 ml WBC Ext.	R23	" "	4	8	Positive
D10	Sens. vs. "A"	0.9 ml WBC Ext.	R24	8 days before	4	13	Positive
		0.9 ml WBC Ext.	R25	" "	4	7	Positive

[†] Donor 7 exhibited a "recall flare" at each previous skin graft site coincident with the rejection of 2nd, 3rd and 4th set "A" grafts used to sensitize him. His leucocyte extracts taken at the height of the 4th set rejection transferred accelerated rejection of target but not control grafts to each of 2 recipients. However, leucocyte extracts in the same dosage obtained from Donor 7, (11 days after the above bleeding) failed to transfer accelerated graft rejection to each of 4 additional recipients. Following this unexpected result Donor 7 received a fifth set graft of "A" skin 80 days after his first exposure and now accorded it a first-set reaction with a survival time of 9-10 days (see Rapaport and Converse, Ann. N. Y. Acad. Sci. 1957; Lawrence et al. in Ciba Foundation Symposium on <u>Transplantation</u>, Little, Brown, 1960). It is a pity his serum was not tested at the time his leucocyte extracts failed to transfer since we have shown that incubation of sensitive leucocytes with specific antigen results in the liberation of transfer factor into the supernatant which now can transfer delayed sensitivity while the cells have become desensitized and lose this capacity (Lawrence and Pappenheimer, J. Clin. Invest. 1957).

[††] Transfer factor donors for purposes of systemic transfer were exposed to four sequential applications of 11 mm. skin grafts and larger dosages of transfer factor were used (e.g. 0.5 ml to 0.9 ml packed WBC = 425 to 765 x 10^6 cells).

(with permission Journal of Clinical Investigation)

III. TRANSFER FACTOR

actively induce it. It is worth noting in passing that this result gives some insight into a possible explanation for the prolonged duration (1-2 years) of transferred sensitivity commonly observed in humans. The latter finding has stood in sharp contrast to the short duration (7 days) of transferred sensitivity characteristically observed in outbred experimental animals, where homograft rejection of the transferred cells has been shown to terminate sensitivity (Harris and Harris, Ann. N. Y. Acad. Sci. 87, 156, 1960; Warwick et al., Ann. N. Y. Acad. Sci. 99, 620, 1962.) It has thus become clear in outbred human species, that although the cellular vehicle of transfer factor is rejected via a homograft response, transfer factor itself is not rejected.

Nevertheless, your objection is well taken and we have reported elsewhere many additional control studies directed at answering it among other questions which need not be detailed here (J. Clin. Invest. 39, 185, 1960; Ciba Foundation Symposium on Transplantation, Little, Brown, p. 272, 1962; J. Clin. Invest. 41, 2166, 1962; Ann. N. Y. Acad. Sci. 87, 217, 1960; NAS-NRC Symposium on Histocompatibility Testing, p. 97, 1965; Transplantation, 3, 490, 1965.)

DR. BARAM: I would like briefly to relate some of the work that Dr. Mosko, Mr. Yuan and I did with transfer factor from human peripheral white blood cell lysates (Immunology, 8, 461, 1965; J. Immunol., 97, 407, 1966.) We found in the tuberculin system that there are actually two factors that are capable of transferring tuberculin sensitivity in humans. On Sephadex G-200 chromatography one of these factors was found in the same fraction that contained gamma globulin. There was also a considerable amount of RNA present. This factor has not yet been purified. The second factor, a low molecular weight dialyzable material, could be recycled through one meter columns of Sephadex G-25 and finally yielded activity in a single peak. It was a polynucleotide of less than 10,000 molecular weight, and contained no uridine. Although we could demonstrate only three bases, it was quite capable of transferring tuberculin hypersensitivity to humans.

We attempted to determine by equilibrium dialysis whether the polynucleotide contained antigen; the polynucleotide was placed in one compartment and in the other we placed rabbit antiserum to BCG. It was reasoned that if the polynucleotide transfer factor contained antigen, as the factor equilibrated between the two compartments, the antigen would complex with the antiserum. This would further shift the equilibrium until all of the putative polynucleotide-antigen factor would complex with the antiserum and thus exhaust the compartment originally containing the polynucleotide of transfer capacity. After three days of dialysis the polynucleotide compartment was still capable of transferring tuberculin hypersensitivity to human recipients. Consequently, it seemed that if antigen were present, it would be complexed to the nucleotide in such a way that it could not interact with antibody. The two factors are obviously resistant to degradation by some RNAses. During preparation of the cell lysates the preparations are repeatedly thawed at $37^{o}C$, a situation that allows sufficient time for the cell nucleases to degrade any degradable RNA. Failure to degrade the transfer factors with pancreatic RNAase does not mean the factors are not RNA.

We think there are two transfer factors, both of them insensitive to nucleases, at least those present in the host cell. It may be necessary to use phosphodiesterases to get adequate degradation before one can be sure of the nature of the factors.

DR. OPPENHEIM: Would Dr. Lawrence tell us more about the variables involved in the production of the supernatant. Does more of your material accumulate with time? Are the initial "clone" of cells making this, or are their progeny also involved? Have you been able to reproduce the *in vivo* sequential transfer *in vitro* by taking a supernatant from a culture that had itself been stimulated by an active supernatant?

DR. LAWRENCE: I would like to invite Dr. Valentine to join this discussion inasmuch as he has also been involved in this work.

III. TRANSFER FACTOR

DR. VALENTINE: The supernatants are taken from stimulated sensitive cells at intervals ranging from 18-36 hours, a period preceding cell division. The active supernatants were prepared from stimulated sensitive cells cultured either in media containing autologous plasma or the plasma removed and the cells washed and cultured in non-antibody containing media. Controls which give no stimulation, include supernatants from the sensitive cells cultured with an indifferent antigen or without antigen. Tuberculin (PPD) is added to control supernatants after separation from the unstimulated sensitive cells and also to control supernatants prepared from non-sensitive cells cultured with antigen in the presence of plasma from sensitive individuals. The activity then, presumably comes from the cells.

The media in which active material is produced is unaffected by heating at $56°C$ for 1/2 hour; the media in which it is assayed on the non-sensitive cells can also be similarly heated without diminution of response. The activity itself is destroyed by heating the supernatant at $56°C$ for 30 minutes.

The amount of antigen used is rather small, 0.5 - 1.0 µg/ml. The number of cells employed for production of activity is approximately 10^6/ml. The supernatants are used at a final dilution of 1:4 or more in the media containing the nonsensitive cells. The production of the active material is no greater at four days than at 36 hours; indeed, 36 hour supernatants give a somewhat higher activity than do supernatants taken later.

DR. SMITH: Is the release into supernatant always specific? Will the supernatants which permit uncommitted cells to react to tuberculin also transmit the ability to any other antigen to which the original tuberculin positive individual was sensitive? In other words, was the supernatant transfer factor that had been released specific to tuberculin alone. The derivative question is: does a population of normal cells, which has been treated with transfer factor plus tuberculin (which yields two percent of responsive cells) react to another antigen to which the transfer factor donor was also sensitive? Would this in effect activate an additional two percent of the cells? Or does activation of the original two percent totally exhaust the entire receptive population?

DR. LAWRENCE: In the early studies that Pappenheimer and I did, (J. Exp. Med. 104, 321, 1956; J. Clin. Invest. 36, 908, 1957) incubation of blood leucocytes (425 x 10^6) sensitive to tuberculin and to diphtheria toxoid with PPD (25 µg) for one hour resulted in the liberation into the supernatant of a preformed transfer factor for tuberculin alone but not that for toxoid. The transfer factor for toxoid was only detected in the cell pellet following in vivo transfer. THis result would favor the interpretation that an immunologically specific release of transfer factor from sensitive cells occurred following interaction with antigen. These assays of transfer factor were done entirely in vivo since no in vitro assay systems were then available.

In our more recent approach to this question using both in vitro and in vivo techniques, Dr. Valentine and I (in unpublished experiments) have added dialysable transfer factor prepared from a (tuberculin positive-toxoid negative) donor to (tuberculin negative-toxoid negative) lymphocyte populations obtained from the prospective recipient. The dialyzable transfer factor caused the lymphocytes to respond in vitro following the addition of tuberculin while no response occurred following the addition of toxoid. The subsequent injection of an aliquot of the same dialysate into the recipient resulted in the in vivo transfer of marked cutaneous tuberculin sensitivity (3+) but no toxoid sensitivity. The recipient's lymphocytes, after in vivo transfer, were now found to respond in vitro to tuberculin but not to toxoid.

Thus, the early studies we did with Pappenheimer using antigen-liberated transfer factor were only done in vivo and exhibited specificity. Our more recent approach to this problem with Valentine, employed dialyzable transfer factor which exhibited specificity both in vitro and in vivo.

Our current studies with Valentine (Valentine and Lawrence, J. Clin. Invest. 47, 98a, 1968; Science, in press, 1969), on the lymphocyte-activating material prepared by incubating sensitive lymphocytes with tuberculin has only been studied in vitro. This factor causes nonsensitive lymphocytes to respond to tuberculin by transformation; clonal proliferation as we showed in the film

III. TRANSFER FACTOR

illustrating our time-lapse cinematography studies (cf. Marshall, Valentine, and Lawrence, J. Exp. Med. 130, 1969.)

DR. VALENTINE: Dr. Lawrence has summarized evidence for the specificity of transfer with supernatants as measured by the in vivo transfer in humans. The specificity of release of supernatant activity as assayed by an in vitro system also has been demonstrated. Thus, if you add to sensitive cells an antigen to which they are sensitive then activity is released. Addition of an antigen to which the cells are not sensitive does not release any activity into the supernatant. However, the latter antigen added to cells of different donors sensitive to it is capable of releasing activity. Accordingly, the production of the activity is antigenically specific.

The production of the material is antigenically specific in that it is not released by antigen to which the producing cells are not sensitive. That this failure to release activity is not due to inactivity of the "control" antigen has been checked by showing that this particular antigen involved can stimulate the release of activity by lymphocytes of different donors known to be sensitive to the antigen.

The specificity of the effect of this supernatant activity on nonsensitive lymphocytes is not yet entirely clear. For example, will supernatant activity produced by the tuberculin stimulation of tuberculin sensitive cells also stimulate nonsensitive lymphocytes to respond to other antigens to which they are not sensitive? To test this point one must measure the ability of each of two supernatants prepared with different antigens, to permit doubly nonsensitive cells to respond to either antigen. This sort of experiment is currently being done in our laboratory.

I would like to emphasize a fundamental point which was mentioned but not elaborated on in Dr. Lawrence's introductory remarks. Are the nonsensitive cells responding directly to the material in the active supernatant or has this material rather served to permit the response of nonsensitive cells to antigen? It is obvious that antigen is required for production of the material and that residual antigen inevitably is carried over into the assay system. We have sought to deal with this problem by diminishing the amount of residual antigen in the supernatant. This was done by exposing the sensitive cells producing the activity, to antigen for a very brief period of time, washing them, and then allowing them to continue in culture for an additional 36 hours without added antigen. While this does not remove all antigen from the cells, it certainly decreases the concentration in the medium. Supernatants prepared in this way, when placed on nonsensitive cells, induce a transformation response, but to a lesser extent. Addition of increasing amounts of antigen to these supernatants causes nonsensitive cells to respond to antigen and a dose-response curve is obtained which is comparable to that seen when antigen is added to sensitive cells (see Fig. 22). Therefore, it would seem that the nonsensitive cells are responding to the additional antigen. We have not yet completely removed antigen from such supernatants.

DR. TURK: We know that in experimental animals efforts to transfer sensitivity by extracts *in vivo* have not yet been effected consistently. If you take your transfer factor from human cells and add it to animal cells in culture, do you get the effects you have described using human cells?

DR. LAWRENCE: We have not studied the effects of dialyzable transfer factor from humans on animal cells, but Dr. Smith has done so in the mouse, and dialyzable human transfer factor caused transformation of mouse lymphocytes in the presence of the specific antigen (Adler and Smith, Fed. Proc. $\underline{28}$, 813, 1969). Dr. Baram has also added human transfer factor occurring in blood leucocyte lysates to Rhesus monkey lymphocytes which then undergo transformation in the presence of specific antigen (Baram and Condoulis, Fed. Proc. $\underline{28}$, 629, 1969). I think it more appropriate that they discuss their own work.

DR. TURK: So the *in vitro* transfer experiment does not display the species specificity required of *in vivo* transfers?

III. TRANSFER FACTOR

DR. LAWRENCE: That appears to be a fact that is currently emerging.

DR. TURK: Dr. Lawrence, in those situations where you use fungal or mycobacterial antigens, to what degree were your recipients sensitive to cross reacting mycobacterial or fungal antigens, either above threshhold, or subliminally?

DR. LAWRENCE: You have identified an important point which regrettably is virtually impossible for us to resolve at a practical level. In relation to the question of the specificity of transferred sensitivity to mycobacterial antigens, I refer you to studies of Jensen et al. (Am. Rev. Resp. Dis. 85, 373, 1962). They used leucocyte extracts to transfer sensitivity from donors sensitive to either PPD-S (human), PPD-B (Battey), or PPD-A (Avian), or to all three tuberculins. They achieved simultaneous, multiple transfer of sensitivity to human, Battey and Avian tuberculins and the reactions to Battey and Avian tuberculins were found to be transferred more frequently than reactions to human tuberculin.

DR. TURK: I was more concerned with the reactivity of the recipient prior to transfer. What information is available on your population regarding their sensitivity to these organisms known to be in the environment? I raise this point since such organisms could contain antigens which cross react with the mycobacteria -- or with the mycobacterial or fungal antigens used as test reagents.

DR. LAWRENCE: I have made no specific detailed study of the type that Dr. Turk requests, and cannot answer it for man any more than he can for the guinea pigs used in his work. However, there is a considerable body of experimental evidence dealing with the implications of the question he has raised which has led to the following consensus: 1) with rare exception, donors with negative skin reactions, cannot transfer delayed sensitivity to the antigen involved; 2) there is a direct correlation between the presence and intensity of specific skin reactivity possessed by the donor and the success, frequency and intensity of the delayed reactivity transferred to the recipient; 3) these are quantitative variables which clearly point to the donor's immunological experience, rather than that of the recipient, as the critical determinant of the transferred response. This conclusion has been repeatedly re-emphasized by the exact confirmation of the specificity of the reactions transferred in the recipient to the reactivity expressed by the donor, particularly when multiple sensitivities are transferred in a variety of combinations (cf. Warwick et al. J. Lab. Clin. Med. 56, 139, 1960; Jensen et al. Am. Rev. Resp. Dis. 85, 373, 1962; Kirkpatrick et al. J. Exp. Med. 119, 727, 1964; Salvin and Garvin, Science 145, 52, 1964; Hattler and Amos, J. Nat. Canc. Inst. 35, 927, 1965). The impact of these consistent observations, as well as their meaning, is at direct variance with the conclusion that the entire response following transfer is due to an elevation of a latent or cross reacting sensitivity possessed by the recipient, which I gather is the thrust of Dr. Turk's question.

---

† *Afterthought*: Others have recently published studies of the type Dr. Turk requested which record by state and county the baseline incidence of delayed cutaneous reactivity to mycobacterial antigens. Edwards et al. (Am. REv. Resp. Dis. 99, Part 2, 1, 1969) have compiled a valuable reference Atlas of sensitivity to tuberculin (PPD-S), PPD-B and histoplasmin in the United States. During the years 1958 to 1965, in New York State, the population tested comprised a total of 25,138 white male Navy recruits, 17-21 years of age, who were lifetime residents of one county.

The incidence of positive reactors (10 mm or greater) to PPD-S (0.001 mg) was 4.2% of 25,138 persons tested in New York State compared to 5.4% of 11,662 persons tested in New York City and its suburbs. The incidence of positive reactors (4 mm or greater) to PPD-B (0.001 mg) was 21.5% of 25,138 persons tested in New York State compared to 26.7% of 11,662 persons tested in New York City and its suburbs. The incidence of positive reactors (4 mm or greater) to histoplasmin (H-42, 1:100) was 2.6% of 25,138 persons tested in New York State compared to 1.4% of 11,662 persons tested in New York City and its suburbs.

III. TRANSFER FACTOR

CHAIRMAN GOOD: The most critical population at issue is the coccidioidin negative New York recipients of transfer factor. Is there evidence for cross reacting antigens to coccidioidin in these recipients?

DR. BARAM: I think you may get cross reaction between histoplasmin and coccidioidin skin test reactions, however, neither of these antigens cross react with PPD.

DR. SALVIN: Serologically, antigens from the agents causing blastomycosis, histoplasmosis and coccidioidomycosis, cross react, but animals repeatedly skin tested with coccidioidin do not readily develop hypersensitivity to other fungal antigens. Such animals do not readily respond to cross reacting fungal antigens.

DR. TURK: It would, of course, be important to know the spectrum of reactivity of normal subjects in New York City, to mycobacterial and fungal antigesn that could conceivably cross react with the antigens you are using.

DR. SALVIN: Dr. C. E. Smith, claimed[†] that individuals who had been skin tested repeatedly with coccidioidin did not react nor develop hypersensitivity to coccidioidin. However, the ingredients of potential reaction are present and cannot be entirely excluded. One other point Dr. Lawrence has not commented on involves the passive

---

[†] This was more than a claim. As a prelude to our studies on the transfer of coccidioidin sensitivity, (J. Immunol. $\underline{84}$, 358, 1960), we deliberately studied the effect of repeated skin testing of humans with coccidioidin. We found, as had been known for tuberculin, that although repeated skin tests with coccidioidin may elevate a state of latent sensitivity, this procedure does not actively induce delayed reactions to coccidioidin in negative individuals (J. Immunol. $\underline{84}$, 368, 1960).

transfer of contact hypersensitivity in man. Has such hypersensitivity ever been transferred via transfer factor? If not, what do you think is the basis for the failure? Is it in carrier specificity?

DR. LAWRENCE: I have never studied the transfer of contact sensitivity in man. Among the conferees there are three investigators who have studied contact sensitivity in man using cell preparations containing transfer factor. One, Dr. Good using viable cells; two, Dr. Eisen using leucocyte extracts; and three, Dr. Brandriss, using dialyzable transfer factor. I think it more appropriate that they speak for themselves.

CHAIRMAN GOOD: I think that we have never worked with transfer factor in Minnesota.

DR. LAWRENCE: I would say that whether or not it was his intent, Dr. Good has been working with transfer factor as the active moiety residing in the specifically sensitive viable cell populations he has used in his transfer studies. We apply this term to the equivalent activity liberated from living cells mechanically (lysis, freeze-thawing) or immunologically (interaction of sensitive cells with specific antigen); as well as the more highly purified low-molecular weight preparation separated from sub-cellular constituents by dialysis and concentrated by lyophilization. I think it important that we all appreciate the distinction between the cellular vehicle (i.e. the bus) of transfer factor and the biologically active moiety (the passenger) since transferred cells are rejected via a homograft response but transfer factor is not rejected (cf. Adv. in Immunology, 1969). To cite an analogous operational example, Arthus sensitivity may be transferred by whole serum or by a purified gamma globulin fraction; yet the serum derives its activity only in proportion to its specific globulin content.

III. TRANSFER FACTOR

DR. GOOD: We have not worked with any kind of definable transfer factor, only with transfer using intact cells. We have been able, using intact cells obtained from highly sensitized patients who themselves had shown repeated positive skin test reactions, to transfer contact reactivity to 2, 4 dinitrofluorobenzene. This is not as readily and as easily accomplished, as transferring sensitivity to diphtheria toxoid and it seems to require more cells. If this actually involves transfer factor, it can indeed be accomplished occasionally.

The transfers were most readily achieved in agammaglobulinemic patients, and in unsensitized normal individuals. The initial testing was done at three or four days following the transfer. At the very first test application the reactions were positive, and upon repeated testing over periods of months the reactions remained positive

DR. BRANDRISS: I wonder, Dr. Lawrence, how arbitrary, really, is the definition of tuberculin negativity. The recipients you employed had no reactivity to five micrograms of PPD. However, what is their response to 10 micrograms or a larger dose? Even though skin-test negative, some individuals' lymphocytes are capable of responding to PPD *in vitro*. How many of your recipients were tested by *in vitro* lymphocyte transformation. There could very well be a latent degree of reactivity not revealed by what seems to me, for this purpose, to be a rather arbitrary skin test dose of tuberculin.

DR. LAWRENCE: We have tried to exclude individuals with latent degrees of tuberculin sensitivity by testing with five µg PPD two or three times before transfer. This procedure is known to recall latent sensitivity and yet not sufficient to cause the appearance of *de novo* reactivity in negative individuals. We have been criticized for this precaution. However, the situation in humans is in no way comparable to that in the guinea pig where even a single skin test with PPD may suffice to cause the appearance of a positive tuberculin reaction in control animals. We have only recently turned to *in vitro* lymphocyte transformation to screen potential recipients of transfer factor, as described above in the studies relating *in vitro* to *in vivo* transfer of tuberculin sensitivity.

DR. BRANDRISS: Did those recipients have a minimal degree of baseline lymphocyte transformation?

DR. LAWRENCE: Yes, many of them do. We have only begun to employ this test for routine screening since it obviates completely the issue of introducing antigen into recipients. Furthermore, it is infinitely more sensitive than the skin test for detection of latent sensitivity.

DR. BRANDRISS: That might be one way, I would think, to accomplish these transfers.

DR. LAWRENCE: That is why we are doing it that way now. It so happens that the bulk of our work was done long before the lymphocyte transformation response was an established correlate of cutaneous sensitivity.

DR. BRANDRISS: With regard to Dr. Good's discussion, it would be difficult to know how long the transferred contact sensitivity persists since in this situation the skin doses themselves cause active sensitization.

DR. THOMAS: I would like if we can, to get this matter of contact sensitivity clarified. It never has been at any meeting I have attended thus far. It has been for me surprising that our discussions of delayed hypersensitivity, could have gone on so long and only now reached mention of contact hypersensitivity. How does this matter stand at the present time? Has anyone transferred contact hypersensitivity with transfer factor, and then waited for varying lengths of time before doing any testing at all, in order to see whether persistence of this kind of hypersensitivity can, in fact, be transferred at all. Also, whether it persists for a year or more, a period comparable to those which Dr. Lawrence and his associates have observed with tuberculin.

III. TRANSFER FACTOR

I would also like to reply to the question Dr. Turk raised as to whether, in transferring tuberculin hypersensitivity, one may not be dealing with a population of patients who already have some hypersensitivity which has not come in a specific way. I used to be concerned about this, as was Dr. Lawrence and everyone else; finally, I was convinced that this is indeed not the case. Dr. Lawrence had to go away for a weekend and I was asked to make the observations on a run of patients in a pediatric ward. These were children ranging in age from a year and a half to three or four, all tuberculin negative, and all became violently tuberculin positive as the result of transfer factor.

CHAIRMAN GOOD: I believe we can summarize what is known about contact sensitivity in man by saying this continues to be highly controversial. Positive results have to be accorded more meaning than the negative ones. However, transfer of contact allergy has been achieved only after transfer of very large numbers of cells from patients who have had considerable exposure to the sensitizing agent. In several studies transfer has not been accomplished. I don't suppose we can rigorously rule out the possibility of active sensitization in the successful transfers. Results in the experimental animals seem of course, to be quite different.

DR. BRANDRISS: The idea in attempting to transfer DNCB contact sensitivity with leukocyte dialysate was partly directed to the question previously raised of the possible boost of a minimal underlying degree of sensitivity in the recipient to naturally occurring antigens such as tuberculin and fungal products. This possibility would seem less likely with a simple chemical like DNCB. A simple chemical model would also solve the practical problem of obtaining adequate numbers of suitable recipients. It should also offer real advantages in answering questions on whether antigen or antigen fragments are present in transfer factor. In our work, tuberculin-positive subjects were actively sensitized to DNCB. In this way the positive control of tuberculin was introduced in the attempt to transfer both types of sensitivity from these donors to tuberculin negative normal recipients. Dialysates from these donors did in fact transfer tuberculin sensitivity, but did not transfer DNCB sensitivity. Accordingly, these two modalities appear to behave differently with respect to dialysable transfer factor (J. Clin. Invest., 47, 2152, 1968.)

CHAIRMAN GOOD: Dr. Brandriss, isn't your failure to achieve transfer of contact sensitivity vulnerable to the criticism that you did not take carrier specificity into account. In the in vivo situation, it may not be possible to test with the stimulating antigen. There could occur conjugation of the hapten in both sensitization and skin testing. Furthermore, it is likely that there are antigens in the sensitization that are not revealed by your test system. With the compound you used for sensitization like DNCB, the persons do not express their sensitivity to DNCB but to DNCB-protein. I think the carrier specificity is a crucial issue here.

DR. BRANDRISS: Yes, this is a possibility. I would think it unlikely however in view of the fact that you and others have been able to transfer contact sensitivity with cells or with undialyzed cell lysates.

DR. LAWRENCE: I would point out here that Dr. Good and his associates observed a flare-up of the quiescent leucocyte depots in the recipient at the time of a cutaneous reaction to DNFB applied on the forearm to detect transferred sensitivity. We have observed identical flare-ups of quiescent depots of leucocytes or leucocyte extracts placed in the shoulder coincident with eliciting a positive skin reaction with streptococcal M-substance or with diphtheria tcxoid respectively, in the recipient of transfer (J. Immunol. 68, 159, 1952; J. Exp. Med. 104, 321, 1956). This cccurrence following transfer of DNFB sensitivity suggests, at the very least, that antigen from the skin site percolated up to the shoulder and interacted with the transferred cells or activated host cells to fire a leucocyte site.

III. TRANSFER FACTOR

DR. CHASE: Dr. Brandriss, did you succeed in transferring DNCB sensitivity with living cells from your donors, apart from your attempts to transfer with lysates?

DR. BRANDRISS: I was interested in the dialysate as being more amenable to further analysis and, therefore, did not try living cells.

DR. CHASE: Until transfers with living cells become demonstrable, attempts to transfer with lysates are perhaps premature. The obstacle to exploring the area of transfer factor in contactant hypersensitivity has been an apparent inability to transfer DNCB sensitivity in man by means of cells. If transfer could be done with living cells regularly, the field would be approachable; and I therefore feel that Dr. Brandriss' experiments do not represent the final word.

The difficulties reportedly have been overcome by Dr. E. Klein at Roswell Park, who reports that he has transferred DNCB-sensitivity between human beings with living cells in 12 out of 14 instances. His technique is not yet published, but was mentioned in an article by him (N. Y. State J. Med., 1969). He also reported these experiments at a recent meeting of the American Cancer Society.

If Klein indeed has the technique, then for the first time we can hope to prepare subcellular material such as transfer factor, and pool it until there is a sufficient amount for study as a transfer agent. I think this is the way to approach this particular problem.

Dr. Lawrence, when you prepare dialysate for transfer, what weight of material passes the sac and constitutes an effective transfer dose?

DR. LAWRENCE: It is of course possible to weigh the powdered lyophilized dialysate, but the results are not very informative as the dialysate is comprised largely of extraneous salts.

CELLULAR IMMUNITY

DR. BARAM: As Dr. Lawrence has indicated there are problems in referring to weight because intercellular salts dialyze out; but in terms of optical density material, roughly about 20 percent passes the sac. In the monkey system, much less dialyzes out. We have also transferred <u>in vivo</u> sensitivity in humans with polynucleotide transfer factor (chromatographed on Sephadex G-25) containing 46 μg ribose.

I would also like to comment on the problem of repeated skin testing of recipients which is one that confronted us as well. It is true that we considered tuberculin to be a ubiquitous antigen. There are some reports in the literature claiming that as you test people with increasing concentrations, of tuberculin, up to one mg., eventually all subjects give a positive skin test. Whether these were all specific reactions was not determined. We have also repeatedly skin tested humans, to see how many developed positive skin tests on repeated testing. Using 0.0002 mg of PPD and testing at two week intervals, none of the subjects developed a positive skin test. On the first skin test about five percent were reactors to 0.005 mg of PPD. After the second test about 15 percent reacted. This was probably an anemnestic response. From then on, and some subjects were tested as many as 15 to 20 times, between one and five percent of the group converted with each test.

This is, I think, a pretty low reactor rate considering the frequency with which one can transfer PPD sensitivity using dialyzable transfer factor from donors who are sensitive to tuberculin. It must be emphasized that one cannot convert recipients by means of cell lysates obtained from individuals who are themselves not sensitive to tuberculin. We must be mindful of the fact that only transfer factor prepared from cells of tuberculin sensitive donors specifically causes sensitization of the recipient.

DR. LAWRENCE: I would add the repeatedly documented observations made first by Dr. Chase in guinea pigs and subsequently by ourselves and others in man; namely, that unless an appropriately sensitive donor and an adequate amount of cells are used to transfer, there will be no successful transfer of sensitivity no matter how frequently the recipient is retested. Furthermore, even mixing

III. TRANSFER FACTOR

non-sensitive leucocyte extracts with coccidioidin and testing the recipient repeatedly following transfer with that mixture, does not result in the development of coccidioidin sensitivity by the recipient (J. Immunol., 84, 350, 1960).

DR. FIREMAN: Dr. Chase expressed interest in the quantity of transfer factor preparation obtained per increment of cells. We prepared transfer factor from approximately 1 x 10^9 leucocytes obtained from 500 ml of whole blood. The leucocytes, after they have been frozen and thawed or lysed with distilled water, are dialyzed against approximately 100 volumes of distilled water. Following lyophilization of the dialyzate we obtained between 100 and 400 mg. of crude material which possesses the capacity to transfer delayed hypersensitivity. From the leucocytes in 500 ml of whole blood, we usually obtained sufficient transfer factor to passively sensitize ten individuals. The transfer factor obtained from the leucocytes of the patient with the greatest degree of delayed hypersensitivity to tuberculin thus far encountered, had the potential to passively sensitize approximately 100 adult human subjects.

DR. BACH: I would like to know whether the factor that is released into the supernatant after incubation with antigen can, by itself, stimulate cells *in vitro*? If you wait until later, if you incubate for a longer period of time, of if you incubate with antigen for several hours and then look for the factor days later, is it itself still non-stimulatory? Lastly, have you compared this factor with dialyzable transfer factor, i.e., do they have the same properties?

DR. VALENTINE: I cannot answer the first part of your question. Since we have not removed from the supernatant all antigen necessary for the production of this material, I cannot say categorically that the material itself does not stimulate cells. I can say only that when one decreases the amount of antigen in the supernatant that the amount of stimulation of the nonsensitive cells is less, and that when you add back antigen, the cells respond increasingly, indicating an effect by the additional antigen. Judging by activity per ml of supernatant, we obtained no increase in activity from the sensitive cells upon incubation for periods longer than 36 hours.

Whether this is due to diminished production of activity during the latter part of culture when proliferation and many more blasts are present, or as an alternative explanation, whether activity is being destroyed, I can't say. Late in culture an increased amount of activity is not present even though a much larger number of blasts are present. There does not seem to be any proportionality between activity and number of blasts in the culture. The supernatant material active in vitro is non-dialyzable. This property distinguishes it physically from transfer factor which is dialyzable and is prepared by disruption of sensitive leucocytes in the absence of antigen. I think that one should note here that in the earlier specific release experiments with supernatants, as tested in vivo, by Lawrence and Pappenheimer, (J. Exp. Med. 104, 321, 1956; J. Clin. Invest. 36, 908, 1957) that the material was not subjected to dialysis. This relationship between dialyzable transfer factor, antigen-liberated transfer factor assayed in vivo and the lymphocyte-activating material in the supernatants we have discussed is currently under study in our laboratory.

DR. MÖLLER: The major points that concern me are specificity and the exact number of responsive cells. I think transplantation systems could provide an answer to the issue of specificity. If you have A immunized against B and take the transfer factor from B, you can add it both to the syngeneic B and to A, C, and so on. If this were done quantitatively, I think you could distinguish the effect from a mixed lymphocyte culture response. Furthermore, if B is immunized against A -- has anyone injected B's anti-A transfer factor back into A?

Finally, as regards the number of cells: is the figure based only on a morphological impression from these slides, or have more sophisticated methods been used?

III. TRANSFER FACTOR

DR. LAWRENCE: I don't believe we can answer your first question. When the homograft transfer studies were done, (J. Clin. Invest. <u>39</u>, 185, 1960), reliable *in vitro* assay systems had not yet been perfected.

In reply to your second question, I would ask Dr. Marshall, with whom the cinematography studies were done, to comment on the data and methodology we employed to estimate the figure of two percent antigen-responsive cells (Marshall, Valentine and Lawrence, J. Exp. Med. <u>130</u>, 327, 1969).

In answer to your third question, we did theoretically consider the possible effects of injecting the specific anti-A transfer factor that was raised in individual B, back into the individual (A) who donated the sensitizing skin graft. However, since more than anyone else, I have been impressed with the reality of the potent activity of transfer factor, I did not do the experiment you suggest, which conceivably might have triggered an autoimmune disease in the recipient.

DR. MARSHALL: The controversial figure of two percent which has been repeatedly discussed is an indirect estimate and is based on the following reasoning. From mitosis counts we know that there was no significant mitotic activity before 48 hours (Fig. 26). Suppose that after this time there was only clonal proliferation -- an idea that is quite consistent quantitatively with our findings for single cells recorded by time-lapse cinematography (see Figs. 24 and 25) -- then the number of lymphoblasts present at 48 hours would represent the precursors (Fig. 27). This number by differential cell count is about two percent of the starting population.

DR. WILSON: I would like to know how you determine the number of cells stimulated by transfer factor and antigen?

DR. MARSHALL: Cultures set up with Drs. Valentine and Lawrence where nonsensitive cells were interacted with tuberculin plus supernatant prepared from a culture of tuberculin-sensitive cells were followed by time-lapse

CELLULAR IMMUNITY

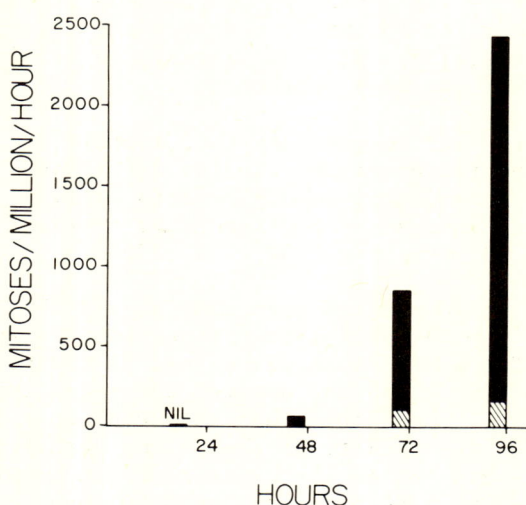

Fig. 26 Histogram to show the number of mitoses found in cultures of sensitive lymphocytes (Subject SIM) incubated with and without tuberculin. The solid parts of the bars represent mitoses in culture with tuberculin, the notched parts of the bars represent mitoses in control cultures without tuberculin.

(With permission of Journal of Experimental Medicine)

cinematography. In these experiments, we saw the same clonal proliferation that we observed with natively sensitive cells. Therefore, using the same argument, the number of cells present at 48 hours can be inferred as the number of precursors that were stimulated. My recollection of those experiments is that the number was not quite as high as two percent. Dr. Valentine may want to comment on this point.

III. TRANSFER FACTOR

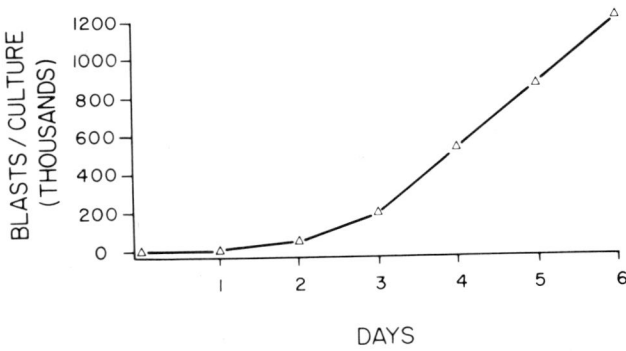

Fig. 27 Absolute count of lymphoblasts in cultures of lymphocytes (Subject CAM) with tuberculin. No lymphoblasts were encountered at the start of the experiment nor after 24 hours incubation.

(With permission of Journal of Experimental Medicine)

DR. VALENTINE: Since the number of blasts present on day six, when nonsensitive cells are incubated with active supernatant, is less than is seen when markedly tuberculin-sensitive donors are used, and since the generation time as measured by cinematography is the same for the "nonsensitive" and sensitive cell proliferation, it is likely that less than two percent of nonsensitive lymphocytes are affected at the beginning of culture period by the supernatant plus PPD. However, because a continuing recruitment of non-sensitive cells may occur during the culture period, actual measurements of the number of nonsensitive lymphocytes activated by the supernatants have not been made.

As Dr. Lawrence has already mentioned, we initially were surprised that only a small percentage of nonsensitive cells were recruited upon incubation with active supernatants or in the presence of dialyzable transfer factor plus antigen. By small percentage, I mean in the order of perhaps one percent or less. We do not have exact figures comparable to those which Dr. Marshall has given for the natively sensitive cell population.

The fact that only a small percentage of cells can be induced to respond by this method is quite meaningful. It is likely that most lymphocytes are already committed to other antigens. The recruitable population could thus be limited to that population of cells which would have become sensitive had the host been natively immunized, as by infection. An alternative hypothesis is that there exists a limited pool of cells from which recruitment can take place, as an initial amplifier for the proliferative immune response to any antigen.

The cinematography studies of nonsensitive cells responding to antigen-containing active supernatants shows that these cells do indeed proliferate. Moreover, the generation times are entirely comparable to those determined for these of sensitive origin.

DR. COHN: If I had a system in which I had induced a dividing clone that had reached the size of 100 cells, I wouldn't discard it; I would continue to grow them and study their properties. Does the clone transfer delayed sensitivity? Does it bind antigen? Does it have all of the properties that you would predict from any simple hypothesis? This seems to me a more direct approach.

DR. BRANDRISS: Dr. Fireman, it was pointed out by Dr. Lawrence that it takes a highly sensitive individual plus an adequate number of cells to get a good transfer. That was certainly my experience also. Did I understand you correctly that the dialysate prepared from cells of a single individual would suffice to effect 100 transfers?

DR. FIREMAN: The yield of transfer factor from the leucocytes in 500 ml of whole blood, from our most highly sensitive donor had the potential to passively sensitize 100 individuals. However, I thought I had pointed out that this represented our most impressive donor and was an unusual example. The average yield is, of course, much less.

III. TRANSFER FACTOR

DR. BRANDRISS: I believe that your estimate is certainly very different from the experience of Lawrence and others in regard to amount required for transfer. I wonder if Dr. Lawrence has ever been able to achieve successful transfers with anything like this small an amount of material.

DR. LAWRENCE: The question of the minimal dosage of cells yielding an effective amount of transfer factor is a complex one and in the absence of a quantitative measure of a defined biochemical moiety, a direct answer is not yet possible. From the outset it has been clear that transfer of delayed hypersensitivity is an all or none response. Cells obtained from a negative donor, with rare exceptions, cannot transfer sensitivity and no amount of repeated testing of the recipient with antigen can make up this deficit. The two most critical quantitative variables which govern the success of transfer are, 1) the degree of specific sensitivity possessed by the donor, and 2) the dosage of cells employed to prepare transfer factor.

The choice of a donor with a minimal or only moderate degree of sensitivity to the test antigen results either in failure to transfer at all or, if sensitivity is transferred, it is feeble in intensity (10x10 mm) and short in duration (weeks). We have examined the role of cell dosage using the same donor-same recipient combinations and found that 0.05 ml (ca. 42×10^6) cells obtained from a single sensitive donor were insufficient to transfer tuberculin sensitivity to each of two negative recipients using the <u>systemic</u> technique of transfer. However, subsequent injection of 0.1 ml (ca. 85×10^6) cells from this same donor into each of the same two recipients resulted in transfer of tuberculin sensitivity to each (cf Table II, Proc. Soc. Exp. Biol. Med. <u>71</u>, 516, 1949).

This finding was confirmed when we subsequently used leucocyte extracts to transfer delayed sensitivity to streptococcal M-substance. Here, 0.08 ml (ca. 68×10^6) lysed cells were found ineffective whereas 0.4 ml (ca. 340×10^6) lysed cells subsequently obtained from the same sensitive donor and injected into the same negative recipient were quite effective in the transfer of sensitivity (cf Table I, J. Clin. Invest. <u>34</u>, 219, 1955).

These results, it must be stressed, were achieved using the <u>systemic</u> technique of transfer and only apply in that situation (i.e., transfer factor injected into the shoulder and antigen injected into the forearm). We have indicated in earlier discussion that the juxtaposition of antigen and transfer factor locally, simultaneously or in sequence, increases the intensity of the result and equivalent degrees of systemic sensitivity can be transferred by this technique using only one tenth the dose of cells required for systemic transfer (e.g., 0.01 ml (8.5 x 10^6) cells vs. 0.1 ml (85 x 10^6 cells).

Further complicating this whole issue are variations in the ease with which each specific delayed hypersensitivity is amenable to transfer. For example, Jensen et al. (Am. Rev. Res. Dis. <u>85</u>, 373, 1962) in an elaborate study evaluating the specificity of multiple transfers using leucocyte extracts, found reactions to Battey and Avian tuberculins were easier to transfer than those to human tuberculin and transfer of histoplasmin sensitivity was more difficult than transfer of other sensitivities. We have also noted that transfer of reactions to tuberculin are more easily achieved and would place in descending order those to streptococcal, diphtherial, coccidioidal and skin homograft antigens.

Our cumulative evidence also suggests the existence of a recipient or "responder" variable. This has been documented deliberately in a controlled fashion by using equal aliquots of cells obtained from each of two tuberculin sensitive donors to transfer the same reactivity to a panel of 16 recipients (cf. Table V, J. Clin. Invest. <u>34</u>, 219, 1955). Nevertheless, despite the admitted role of these variables I would nonetheless conclude the most critical requirement in the whole transaction is the degree of specific cutaneous sensitivity possessed by the donor of transfer factor.

This variable may be expressed in another way; namely, the exact number of circulating lymphocytes bearing the transfer factor for that specific antigen that can be isolated from the donor's blood at that particular moment in time.

III. TRANSFER FACTOR

DR. GRANGER: There are, as I understand, two kinds of transfer factor. One an intracellular material that is rapidly released by freezing and thawing cells, and one that is released in vitro into the supernatant. This in vitro situation could lend itself to careful analysis of the cellular processes necessary for genesis and release of the active material. Have you done any metabolic inhibitor studies or basic release kinetics? It would be interesting to determine the relationship of intra and extra cellular transfer factor and dividing and non-dividing stages of your cultures.

DR. VALENTINE: I can give a brief answer. The material is indeed present in the medium before division. We have not done, but intend to do, metabolic inhibition studies. We cannot find the activity in significant quantities at one hour or four hours. It, therefore, seems reasonable to assume, at least with these small numbers of cells, that the activity is produced rather than released as a preformed substance.

This then would contrast with antigen-liberated transfer factor transferring delayed hypersensitivity in vivo described by Lawrence and Pappenheimer, where using very much larger numbers of cells, (0.5 ml, ca. 425×10^6) activity was detected after one hour incubation with antigen.

DR. BACH: I have a different interpretation regarding the frequency of two percent for the number of blast cells at 48 hours. This frequency at 48 hours may well be different from the frequency of the initially responding unit, which is perhaps best looked at by the limiting dilution experiments, looking for a Poisson distribution. I think the estimates from the literature, and our own estimae for MLC, suggest that the minimum estimate of the frequency of the initially responding unit is between one-half and two percent. On the other hand, while the numbers are similar, the cells involved may be different. I find it much less difficult to interpret that two percent are responding at 48 hours than if two percent were to respond initially to a defined antigen. In our system we are dealing mainly with histocompatibility antigens, known to be complex antigens with multiple determinants.

DR. EISEN: Failure to effectively transfer contact sensitivity to simple chemicals in man deserves further comment. This is a bit worrisome, because we all expect contact skin sensitivity of simple chemicals to be an authentic instance of delayed type hypersensitivity. One could think of three reasons why transfer factor has not been demonstrated with contact sensitivity. 1) First, perhaps the donors are not sufficiently sensitive, and so not enough cells have been used. The experience with intact cells in transfer of contact sensitivity in man is quite variable, implying that relatively more cells are needed than for transfer of tuberculin sensitivity, which can be exquisitely high in many donors. 2) A second possibility is carrier specificity, by which is meant in this situation that the donor who is ostensibly sensitive to a simple chemical, like DNCB is really sensitive to the DNP group plus some neighboring residues, say on a protein carrier; when a transfer is made and the recipient is challenged with DNCB, one is putting the DNP groups back on a protein different from one that functioned in the donor; if the carrier effect were overriding one would expect a negative response in the recipient. I know of no way to rule out this possibility, but I don't find it a very convincing one, because it implies that carrier specificity is so exquisite that we are seeing individual differences, not just protein to protein, but person to person. This does not seem to be the case in animal experiments where one can sensitize a guinea pig to DNCB in an outbred population, take its cells, put them into a recipient allogeneic animal, and get a perfectly good response to dermal DNCB in the recipient. Perhaps one could say that adoptively transferred cells provided the carrier protein for DNP attachment, but I doubt this is either correct or essential. 3) A third possibility, lurking behind some suggestions made earlier is that the transfer factor can function effectively only in systems where there is an underlying low level of sensitivity, perhaps because the corresponding antigens are ubiquitous. In contact sensitivity much ubiquity seems extremely unlikely. I am quite convinced that transfer factor does not function in contact sensitivity to DNP. We tried it because, once in desperation, many years ago, I donated my

III. TRANSFER FACTOR

blood to Dr. Lawrence since I had delayed sensitivity to both tuberculin and to dinitrophenyl. However, the sample was lost and, therefore, we did the experiment ourselves. The experience we had was the same as that of Dr. Brandriss, viz. successful transfer of tuberculin sensitivity, but no transfer of dinitrophenyl contact sensitivity. I suppose the most likely explanation will probably turn out to be that not enough material was used, in view of the low level of sensitivity to simple chemicals.

CHAIRMAN GOOD: Was your attempt to transfer made with cells or with isolated transfer factor?

DR. EISEN: We employed lysed cells, not intact cells.

DR. DIXON: I would like to recall some experiments that Dr. Maurer did some years ago in human subjects, when he was testing blood substitutes for their immunogenicity (J. Exp. Med. 113, 1029, 1961). He induced a delayed hypersensitivity to several synthetic molecules in some medical students. As I recall the experiments, he took buffy coat from about 50 ml of blood, and transferred the killed cells or the supernatant of the killed cells to normal subjects who had never been exposed to the synthetic molecules before. I don't know whether these materials will meet Dr. Eisen's criteria for simple chemicals. However, when the students were challenged with the antigen intradermally the reactions were not merely 70 or 50 millimeters in diameter; they were so large and severe that the students were excused from taking an exam. This synthetic compound at least could induce a sensitivity transferrable by a transfer factor preparation.

DR. BRANDRISS: I think the question of quantitation is worthy of further consideration. It arose naturally in our attempts at transfer with dialysate prepared from cells of a doubly sensitive donor since the transfer of tuberculin sensitivity was successful while, the transfer of DNCB sensitivity was not. In those experiments, the dialysate used was prepared from a large number of cells, $1.4-2.5 \times 10^9$,

the total yield from 500 ml of blood. The donors who were
tested with dilutions of PPD reacted to 0.01 - 0.001 µg
while the recipients were tested with 5 µg a 500 to 5,000
fold difference. I believe that Dr. Lawrence's dcnors are
more highly selected than mine and that in many of his
experiments he may have been working with an even greater
ratio. With DNCB, the donors reacted to 0.5 - 1.C µg while
the recipients could be tested with up to 250 µg, a 250 to
500 fold difference. In most cases then there is a better
chance at transfer with the PPD system. I bring this up
because I think the large ratio between donor and recipient
test doses in the PPD system, with which there is the most
experience, may be important and should be kept in mind
when other antigens are used. For example, we also failed
to transfer delayed intradermal sensitivity to DNP-HSA conjugates with dialysates. Here, large test doses were needed
to elicit reactions in the donors and the degree of donor
sensitivity compared to recipient test dose did not approach
that operative with PPD or DNCB. In this circumstance,
failure to transfer could be attributed to quantitative
considerations alone (Brandriss, J. Clin. Invest. $\underline{47}$, 2152,
1968).

CHAIRMAN GOOD: Yes, I think this is very germane to one
of Dr. Eisen's points. I think contact sensitivity remains
a contentious issue. We have studied contact allergy
intensively and I think factors such as the degree of
sensitivity, the number of cells used, and the route of
administration, are absolutely crucial variables. So far as
I am concerned, the negative reports are not as meaningful
as are the positive ones.

DR. UHR: I think it is clear that the major findings
concerning transfer factor as originally reported by
Dr. Lawrence and his co-workers have now been amply confirmed. Those of us who have watched the "birth" and
development of the studies of transfer factor know what a
long and lonely road Dr. Lawrence has travelled. I am
particularly pleased to see that his findings have been
duplicated now in a number of different laboratories. He
should be congratulated for his perseverance, patience and
prudence in not trying to force a particular interpretation
of these phenomena.

III. TRANSFER FACTOR

In discussing interpretation, I would like to cast a vote for transfer factor being a special and unusual immunogen for the following reasons: the major reason is one of exclusion. I think that the sephadex fractionation experiment shown by Dr. Lawrence and confirmed by Baram and Mosko, Immunology, $\underline{8}$, 461, 1965); Arala-Chaves et al. (Int. Arch. Allergy, $\underline{31}$, 353, 1965) and Fireman et al. (Science, $\underline{155}$, 337, 1967), can be uniquely interpreted. In that experiment each group has found significant transfer factor, indeed the majority of activity in the internal volume of a sephadex G-25 fractionation. This type of gel filtration is in effect a molecular "sieving". Therefore, regardless of whether or not there is activity in the void volume, the presence of considerable activity in the internal volume indicates that the molecule in question has a molecular weight of 10,000 or less. This consideration, to my mind, definitely excludes an informational macromolecule, or an immunoglobulin molecule, for several reasons: first, it is clear that both the repertoire and degree of specificities of delayed hypersensitivity are equivalent to that provided by conventional serum antibody. With conventional immunoglobulin it is known that there are contributions from both light and heavy chains to the antibody combining sites of the molecule. Further, by analogy with enzymes, we can assume that substantial portions of the variable parts of the molecule are concerned with the development of the antibody combining sites.

These considerations exclude both a preformed molecule which would have antibody-type stereo-specificity, and also informational RNA. Thus, a messenger RNA which codes for half the light chain would have a molecular weight of at least 100,000, which is a full order of magnitude higher than that of transfer factor. If we accept the evidence, therefore, that indicates that transfer factor has immunologic specificity, the only possibility left in my opinion is that it is an immunogen of some sort. Moreover, there are several other features concerning transfer factor that suggest that it may be a special type of immunogen. One example is the in vitro study using transfer factor, reported by Valentine and Lawrence. Here, transfer factor appears capable of sensitizing only a very small sub-population of cells which then proliferate.

CELLULAR IMMUNITY

A second point is the prolonged duration of sensitization in vivo when transfer factor is administered to human recipients. A third point is the failure of specific antigen to neutralize transfer factor. A fourth point is the finding of both a dialyzable and a non-dialyzable transfer factor, something consistent with an immunogenic complex that can be broken down. In this connection, I would ask Dr. Lawrence whether he has at any time attempted to block the activity of transfer factor with antibody specific to the antigen in question, such as PPD or toxoid, either in vivo or in vitro?

DR. LAWRENCE: No, we have not done such an experiment, but Dr. Baram has and failed to detect mycobacterial antigens in dialyzable transfer factor by equilibrium dialysis using antisera prepared in rabbits immunized with BCG. This anti-mycobacterial antibody also failed to block transfer factor activity in vivo (Baram and Mosko, Immunology, 8, 461, 1965).

DR. BARAM: Dr. Uhr has suggested that antibodies present may complex with antigen and cause the response observed in lymphocytes. In our work with Rhesus monkeys on the in vitro transfer of KLH hypersensitivity, this did not seem to be the case. Dr. Condoulis and I found that lymphocytes from Rhesus monkeys, sensitized to KLH in complete Freund's adjuvant are stimulated to increased tritiated thymidine incorporation in vitro in the presence of KLH. Peak incorporation rates develop between 3 and 6 days (Fig. 28). If the lymphocytes are incubated with PPD, from animals sensitized to the Mycobacterium antigen in Freund's adjuvant, the peak incorporation of tritiated thymidine in vitro appears later than observed in the KLH system. The time necessary for stimulation of the lymphocytes to appear is related to the antigen used and is not a reflection of concentration of antigen.

Lysates from blood leucocytes of KLH-sensitive Rhesus monkeys incubated with lymphocytes of nonsensitive monkeys cause these cells to incorporate thymidine in the presence of KLH (Fig. 29). Such lysates are also capable of cross species transfers. Nonsensitive human cells incubated with

III. TRANSFER FACTOR

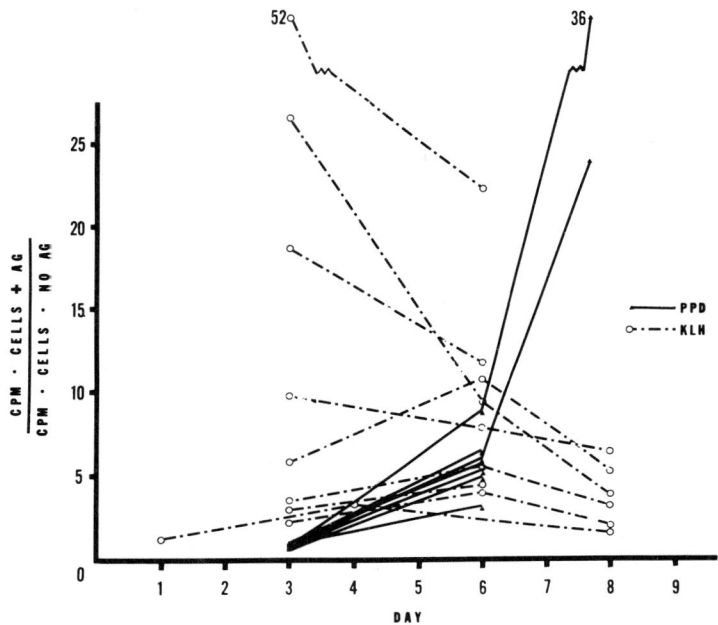

Fig. 28 Thymidine incorporation by hypersensitive cells incubated with antigen. Broken line, KLH sensitive cells; solid line, PPD sensitive cells.

KLH-sensitive cell lysate from monkey plus KLH will also show increased thymidine incorporation. In control experiments, KLH-sensitive cell lysate alone, or lysate of nonsensitive cells with and without KLH added, or anti-KLH antiserum produced in Rhesus monkeys with and without KLH, will not stimulate thymidine incorporation in either nonsensitive human or Rhesus monkey cells

It is also of interest that thymidine incorporation in the lymphocytes incubated with KLH-sensitive cell lysate and KLH, occurs much later than in lymphocytes from KLH-sensitive Rhesus monkeys incubated with KLH. This may be explained by what we have seen in the elegant film shown by Dr. Lawrence. It is possible that only a few cells can

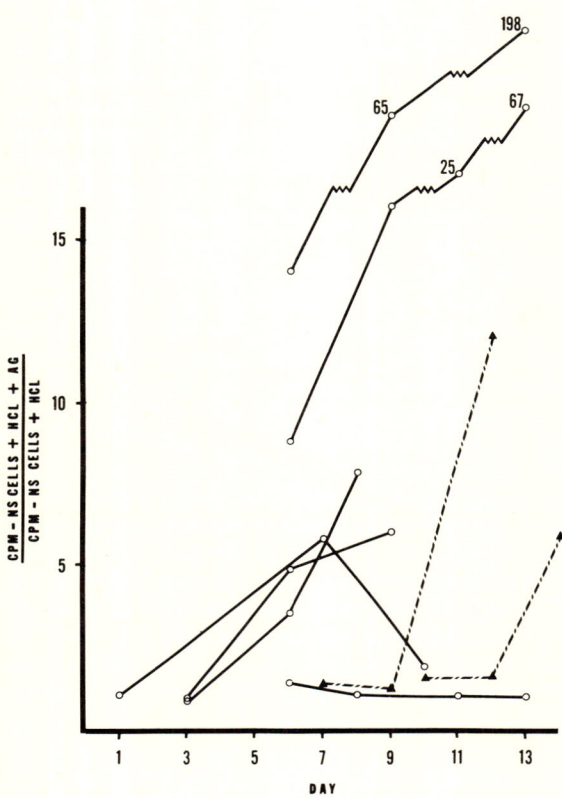

Fig. 29 Transfer of KLH sensitivity to nonsensitive lymphocytes in vitro. Solid lines, thymidine incorporation by nonsensitive Rhesus monkey lymphocytes incubated with KLH-sensitive Rhesus monkey cell lysate and KLH-nonsensitive Rhesus monkey lymphocytes incubated with KLH-sensitive cell lysate. Broken line, thymidine incorporation by nonsensitive human lymphocytes incubated with KLH-sensitive Rhesus monkey cell lysate nonsensitive human lymphocytes incubated with KLH-sensitive cell lysate.

III. TRANSFER FACTOR

be sensitized or recruited from the available cell population by the transfer factor; no increase in tritiated thymidine incorporation would be observed until a sufficient number of progeny of these stimulated dividing cells have accumulated.

Furthermore, attempts to demonstrate processed antigen as a part of transfer factor using equilibrium dialysis, as I mentioned earlier, have been unsuccessful (Immunology, 8, 461, 1965). If antigen is present on transfer factor it is capable only of sensitizing lymphocytes but cannot stimulate these cells to increased thymidine incorporation unless additional antigen is added.

DR. SMITH: The question posed by Dr. Uhr will be very difficult to answer *in vitro* because antibody, in all probability, would result in non-specific activation of cells via an antigen-antibody complex.

DR. UHR: I want to be clear about the blocking experiment with antibody. Of course, antigen-antibody complexes can induce delayed hypersensitivity. Therefore, a negative experiment proves nothing. However, if transfer factor can be specifically blocked with a large amount of antibody of very high binding affinity, that result is interpretable. It would indicate that an antigenic determinant present in the material is playing an obligatory role in the transfer of sensitivity.

DR. VALENTINE: Dr. Uhr is entirely correct in emphasizing that only a positive experiment will provide the needed answer. Nevertheless, I would like to comment that we have found that dialyzable transfer factor prepared from tuberculin sensitive donors does not by itself stimulate tuberculin sensitive lymphocytes in culture.

Tuberculin sensitive cells will detect, by transformation, PPD at a concentration of 0.001 µg per ml. Therefore, one might conclude that if the antigen is in a configuration which is capable of stimulating cells, a function quite suitable as a test for immunogenicity, then any antigen present in the dialysate must be a very small amount indeed.

DR. SILVERSTEIN: I want to comment on Dr. Uhr's pertinent and cogent review of the four possibilities for the nature of transfer factor. He has dealt reasonably with the possibility of transfer factor as the sole recognition factor, or as an informational intermediate in the recognition process. He cites the evidence to suggest that it is a super-antigen or some kind of derepressor. But it seems to me that these alternative raise the problem of the rapidity with which one can elicit a response in the transferred recipients. As I understand the situation, the response can be elicited within hours. To have any appreciable proliferation in order to build up that level of cells necessary to mediate the reaction, and further, to have those cells synthesize the recognition factors required for the elicitation event during that short interval would, I think, present formidable problems.

DR. UHR: I don't think that is inconsistent, Dr. Silverstein, because the contributions of specific and nonspecific events to the red spot in the skin are not known. For example, it could be argued that transfer factor is a special immunogen which sensitizes a very small number of cells, which however are particularly effective in disseminating non-specific factors for recruitment of nonsensitive cells. In other words, the red spot that appears in the skin so quickly after antigenic challenge of an individual who received transfer factor, might represent a predominance (beyond the usual) of non-specific to specific cells. We don't know enough about these *in vivo* events to exclude this possibility.

I want to make clear, however, that the concept that transfer factor is an immunogen, is not an entirely comfortable position in the face of several excellent experiments which suggest an absence of immunogen. I emphasize, however, that there is no critical experiment that presently excludes this possibility.

III. TRANSFER FACTOR

CHAIRMAN GOOD: I wonder if we could consider the possibility that derepression need not involve a super-antigen, but rather a molecule that has conformational characteristics, perhaps somewhat similar to antigen, but still a molecule of a different class. I think small molecules could achieve this effect.

DR. UHR: I think that the concept of a stimulator that has specificity for a very small population of cells sounds suspiciously like a description of antigen. In fact, from the informational point of view I think this is a virtual impossibility. The concept that you are suggesting is that a small molecule other than antigen can recognize and recruit a clone of immunologically reactive cells. I contend that from the informational point of view, this simply is not possible. It took nature a long time to evolve an immunoglobulin system which has an enormous amount of information expressed by the production of antibody specific to any injected antigen. The system you suggest ends up being operationally similar to antigen-antibody specificity, but with molecules other than antigen and antibody interacting on a cell surface. There are not other mammalian systems except for the central nervous system that in any way approach this repertoire of specificities.

CHAIRMAN GOOD: I would suggest that long before the immunoglobulins had evolved there had already occurred specificities in nature; this is what I have called the third biological language, the surface language.

DR. UHR: Right, but that language has a much smaller vocabulary. We are looking for vocabularies equivalent to the specificity of antibodies.

CHAIRMAN GOOD: That may very well be, but we can't yet be sure.

DR. SCHLOSSMAN: We spent considerablt time previously discussing the specificity of delayed reactions and the specificity of antibody. One of the major difficulties with Dr. Uhr's postulate is in terms of the specificity of antibody. An accumulating body of evidence suggests that much of the antibody made is to conformational aspects of the immunogenic molecule. These determinants defined by the conformation of native molecule will not be retained following degradation to a small molecular weight fragment. So now we have a process which has to degrade the antigen and yet after this antigen is markedly degraded, give information to a cell that will recognize the native antigen. This is really very difficult to support because dialyzable transfer factor is assuredly less than 10,000 molecular weight. Consequently, the retained antigenic fragment must be extraordinarily small. The exquisite specificity of delayed hypersensitivity reactions involve not only the hapten but the area adjacent to the hapten. How can the immunogen retain all these specificities and be of low molecular weight. On that basis alone, I find it personally difficult to visualize a markedly degraded macromolecule still retaining a determinant that can induce a sensitized cell specific for the original highly organized molecule.

DR. MÖLLER: I think that basically Dr. Uhr must be correct. Transfer factor is either an antigen or else acts as a super adjuvant of some kind.

DR. BRAUN: Why not both?

DR. MÖLLER: Yes, it could be both. The concept of super antigen could involve an adjuvant action as well. But in both cases specificity studies become important. I think that with the in vitro techniques available it should be possible to study and resolve this issue. If antibody of high affinity is added in large amounts to the cells exposed to transfer factor and antigen, one should get at least a quantitative decrease if an antigenic determinant is involved. Another possibility is to induce tolerance, because as Dr. Smith reported, you can now work with the

III. TRANSFER FACTOR

human transfer factor in mice. If tolerance is induced in mice to the antigen involved no effect would be obtained if the material were a super adjuvant or an antigen; if, however, it were entirely non-specific, one would then still get a response.

DR. CHESSIN: Dr. Möller, I don't see how you are going to discriminate between transfer factor and antigen using high-affinity antibody. The antigen-antibody complex itself would act as a trigger thus making the model untenable.

DR. MÖLLER: Few antigen-antibody complexes are very strong stimulators. Furthermore, you could remove a complex by centrifugation or precipitation of the antibody by ammonium sulphage.

DR. SMITH: The suggestion of Dr. Uhr regarding transfer factor as a super-antigen is logically derived, cogent and cannot as such be denied. However, transfer factor by itself has no discernible effect and requires addition of antigen to activate the cells in the various _in vitro_ systems. We must in some way get around this issue before we can label transfer factor a super-antigen. In addition, there is no evidence for stereochemical affinity between PPD and transfer factor, nor between transfer factor and antibody to tuberculin.

DR. CHASE: The fact that Dr. Lawrence has hit upon an effector molecule contained in somewhat crude material is certainly well established, and that the dialyzate does indeed transfer, is also well established. However, my review of the literature suggests that we have insufficient evidence to prove that we are dealing with a molecule bearing the attribute of specificity. I would suggest, then, that those who do transfer work in human beings should make it a practice to test both donor and recipients with a battery of allergens, just as Dr. Good did in studying patients with Hodgkin's disease. In this way, data can be built up to affirm the principle of specificity in a molecule of <10,000 molecular weight. It is my opinion that one should test by intradermal injection, and build up one's evidence, rather than that one should lean upon findings with MIF, for which specificity has not been demonstrated. I do not myself believe that Dr. Lawrence is working with a non-specific material; but I do seek documentation.

DR. LAWRENCE: I agree that extensive documentation of specificity for dialyzable transfer factor is desirable, particularly in view of its low molecular weight. Nevertheless, our own studies (cf Lawrence, Adv. Immunology, 1969) and those of many other laboratories (Warwick et al. J. Lab. Clin. Med., 56, 139, 1960; Jensen et al. Am. Rev. Resp. Dis. 85, 373, 1962; Kirkpatrick et al. J. Exp. Med. 119, 727, 1964; Hattler and Amos J. Nat'l. Cancer Inst., 35, 927, 1965) working with viable cells or leucocyte extracts have demonstrated specificity over and over again. Especially convincing in this regard is the repetitive demonstration, where multiple sensitivities have been transferred, of the exact correlation between the specificity and intensity of the delayed reactions in the donor and the specificity and intensity of delayed reactivity transferred to the recipient. If, as seems very likely, dialyzable transfer factor is the active moiety present in the viable leucocytes and the leucocyte extracts effective in achieving the transfer of sensitivity in such experiments, it is also likely that extensive documentation of its specificity will be forthcoming. In the experiments that Valentine and I did, dialyzable transfer factor prepared from tuberculin-positive, toxoid-negative, SK-SD-positive, coccidioidin-negative donor transferred cutaneous sensitivities to tuberculin and to SK-SD but not to toxoid or to coccidioidin into the negative recipient in vivo. The in vitro transfer was also specific, but we tested only for tuberculin and toxoid and not for SK-SD or coccidioidin.

DR. BARAM: I would like to add some information from in vitro experiments with human transfer factor done jointly with Drs. Pakque, Dray and Knishem. As an indicator system, we used MIF released from human peripheral lymphocytes to inhibit guinea pig macrophage migration. Transfer factor (whole cell lysate) from

III. TRANSFER FACTOR

humans sensitive to histoplasmin, incubated with non-sensitve human cells alone, or with unrelated antigen (PPD, coccidioidin) did not result in the production of MIF by the cells. On the other hand cell lysates from histoplasmin sensitive donors incubated with nonsensitive cells plus added histoplasmin does result in the production of MIF, i.e., the reaction is quite specific. This kind of experiment has also been done using coccidioidin sensitive cell lysates, incubated with nonsensitive cells. Here too, only addition of coccidioidin will cause production of MIF. Moreover, a few experiments of this type have also been done with tuberculin. Therefore, I think these findings argue for the transfer of sensitivity being specific rather than simply a matter of an adjuvant action.

DR. UHR: In reply to the comment of Dr. Baram. It is possible that when non-dialysates are used other immunologic ingredients in addition to transfer factor are likely to be present. For example, in your lysates, there may be a small amount of antibody in addition to transfer factor. Thus, antigen-antibody complexes may be formed which cause release of MIF. We cannot assume that in each different experimental situation using whole leucocyte lysates, whether _in vivo_ transfer or MIF production, that we are dealing with transfer factor only.

DR. LANDY: Dr. Uhr has been persuasive in marshalling arguments in favor of transfer factor being an immunogen. He has properly emphasized that in our interpretations we have to favor experiments that yield positive results. I wonder how Dr. Uhr would square his view of transfer factor as an immunogen with the experiments on serial transfer that Dr. Lawrence did some years ago. In that work he effected sequential transfer of specific sensitivity starting in the first instance with a leucocyte extract obtained from a natively sensitive donor. This product conferred sensitivity to a primary recipient whose cells could then be extracted to yield a product capable once again of transferring sensitivity, to still another recipient. This seems to me to imply a generating or replicating function that I do not associate with antigen.

DR. UHR: As regards Dr. Landy's point concerning serial transfer, I think this experiment could be interpreted as support for the immunogenic idea. The only other possibility for serial transfer is an informational macromolecule which has been excluded.

DR. LANDY: In that event, how would you account for the amount of transfer activity being generated. If one is successfully effecting transfer serially from A to B to C, as I recall the report; by any standard applied, the dilution factor would be prodigious. If transfer factor were an immunogenic component how could this activity be so greatly expanded in vivo?

DR. UHR: One of the best magnifiers known is the immune response. A small amount of immunogen results in a large amount of stereo-specific reactants. I am assuming that the transfer is immunologically specific.

DR. BLOOM: I would like to develop some evidence that relates to the observation in guinea pigs that, under appropriate conditions, a single skin test can lead to prolonged sensitization. Accordingly, it would seem to me that one has to withhold skin tests and in the work in humans this has not been done.

CHAIRMAN GOOD: I believe that was Dr. Thomas' point also; it is clear this aspect of the work has not been done properly.

DR. BLOOM: In the serial transfer case, I would postulate after transfer and the initial test plus the reaction it elicits, the individual has become sensitized so that when a secondary cell transfer is performed, the primary recipient may be already actively sensitized.

III. TRANSFER FACTOR

DR. LAWRENCE: The suggestion that tests with antigen before and after transfer prepares or conditions the recipient of transfer factor to develop a specific delayed reaction has also been raised repeatedly in the literature. We have deliberately examined this possibility and have provided critical experimental answers to this question in at least two publications -- data which somehow continues to escape notice.

In transferring delayed sensitivity to diphtheria toxoid, donors were deliberately chosen with sensitivity to tuberculin as well as toxoid (Lawrence and Pappenheimer, J. Exp. Med., 104, 321, 1956). The test with tuberculin was used as an indicator that transfer had occurred and allowed the test with toxoid to be withheld at will. It was demonstrated that withholding the first test with toxoid post-transfer for as long as 19 days had no effect on the quality or intensity of the transferred sensitivity to toxoid. This response was comparable to the reactions elicited 19 days after transfer in other recipients who had responded to previous tests with toxoid at four and again at 11 days after transfer. We also documented that the screening test with toxoid to determine the recipients negative state before transfer, also had no effect on the quality of transferred sensitivity. This was clearly the case whether the recipient had been tested as long as two years before or as recently as three days before transfer.

An entirely similar result was obtained when we transferred accelerated skin homograft rejection (Lawrence et al. J. Clin. Invest. 39, 185, 1960). These studies provided additional critical data insofar as no prior testing of the recipient was necessary and the placement of the target homograft following transfer was withheld for varying periods of time. The tempo and intensity of the accelerated rejection of the specific graft against which transfer factor was directed, was identical whether transfer factor had been injected eight days before or three days after the homograft was applied. Negative results were obtained in control recipients of leucocyte extracts obtained from nonsensitive donors as well as recipients of serum obtained from sensitive donors.[†]

CELLULAR IMMUNITY

DR. CHASE: I wish to make some remarks about cellular transfer of hypersensitivity in the guinea pig, not for the purpose of contrasting the species with man, but to recognize the working model which is represented by the guinea pig. For what are we to regard and accept as an "in vitro correlate of delayed type hypersensitivity?"

Following intravenous transfer of cells the recipient animal is usually able to make a maximal response within 16 hours or so, but only to the specific allergen to which the donors have been sensitized. Cellular transfer isolates the events and dissociates any response from circulating antibody which the donor may possess. If "trained" cells are injected intravenously at D_0 (Day 'zero') and a contact test T_0 is made close to the time of transfer -- say three hours before, up to three hours following transfer -- the reaction to test is strong and can be fully expressed by 24 hours, as is shown in Fig. 30, curve "i.v." I have seen maximal sensitivity to be present before sixteen hours; Metaxas also reported the same early responses which we have noted likewise in cellular transfer of tuberculin hypersensitivity. If the cells are injected intraperitoneally, recipient animals exhibit sensitivity more slowly; indeed, withholding the first test for 48 hours is usually optimal in terms of the 24 hour response (Fig. 30, curve "i.p.").

---

†Afterthought: This is the situation in man. However, I would agree with Dr. Bloom that in the guinea pig a single test with tuberculin is frequently sufficient to induce feeble yet rather long-lived, cutaneous sensitivity, while two sequential tests increase the incidence of conversion. This has also been our experience over the years in extensive, unpublished and almost uniformly negative in vivo attempts to transfer tuberculin sensitivity from guinea pig to guinea pig or from man to guinea pig, using leucocytes or leucocyte extracts. Because of this experience with the guinea pig, I can understand the origin of Dr. Bloom's concern about the possible contribution of screening skin tests performed in humans. Earlier discussions by Baram and by myself have cited evidence that man differs from the guinea pig in failing to acquire sensitivity by means of a skin test alone, particularly when tuberculin and coccidioidin are used as antigens.

III. TRANSFER FACTOR

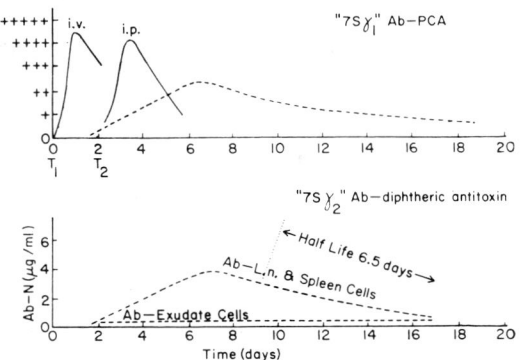

Fig. 30 Cell transfer of contact sensitivity and antibody synthesis. The upper part of the figure is a schematic representation of the temporal differences, following cellular transfer, between the appearance of contactant reactivity (solid lines) and the appearance of antibody (dashed line) having the specificity of the hapten employed for sensitizing the donors, as determined in randomly bred guinea pigs. The antibody was evaluated by the method of passive cutaenous anaphylaxis (PCA).

The lower part of the figure shows a similar temporal course of appearance and decay of another type of immunoglobulin, diphtheric antitoxin, following similar cellular transfer, in the absence of delayed-type sensitivity.

(With permission Harvey Lecture Series)

Transfers between non-inbred guinea pigs and practical relevant details are given in Table 22, including examples of the speed of acquired sensitivity with use of the intravenous route of transfer. Nearly always, the 24 hour reading of test T_0 (presented in the column bearing this heading) is seen to be fully expressed. One rare exception is listed; one recipient injected with an aliquot of a pool of lymph node cells was slow to respond: the maximal

CELLULAR IMMUNITY

TABLE 21

Cellular Transfer, Living Cells [a, b]

Cell Source	Vol. (ml)	Count $\underline{n}$ x 10^8 ($\underline{n}$)	Donors per Recipient	Contact tests, 1% PCl			
				T_0	T_1	T_2	T_3
A. Intravenous route							
Peritoneal exudate	0.28	8.3	2:1	++++±	++++		
"	0.15	2.6	1.5:1	+++++	+++		
Lymph Nodes	---	{5.7[c] "	1.5:1 "	+++++ +±	$(++)$ [d]	$(++++)$	
" "	---	{7.2[c] 3.6	2:1 1:1	++++ ++			
Spleen	---	3.9	3:1	+++++			
"	---	{6.0[c] 3.0	2:1 1:1	++++ ++++±			
B. Intraperitoneal route							
Peritoneal exudate	0.15	---	1.5:1		+(++++)	++++	
Lymph Nodes	{0.50[c] 0.25 0.13 0.25	--- --- --- ---	4:1 2:1 1:1 2:1	(i.v.)	++(+++±) 0 (++++) +±(++++) +++++	++++ ++++ +++++ +++++	+++++ +++++ +++++ +++++

[a] Data from Appendix Tables in Bloom, B.R., 1963, Dissertation, "Studies on delayed hypersensitivity .....," The Rockefeller University. Available from University Microfilms, Inc., Ann Arbor, Michigan.
[b] Donors were sensitized by the "Combination method" (loc. cit. and Chase, M.W., Intern. Arch. Allergy, 5, 163, 1954), sacrificed between 33 and 60 days after initial intramuscular injection.
[c] Brackets indicate injection of recipients from the same pool of cells.
[d] Figures within parentheses show 48 hour readings of tests made at the indicated time.

response of this individual occurred on day four, the 48 hour reading of Test T_2.

Some typical experience with the intraperitoneal route are shown in Fig. 30. It is evident that such recipients should not be tested until at least 24 hours have elapsed; when initial testing is then practiced (T_1) about 48 hours are necessary to attain the maximal response at this test

III. TRANSFER FACTOR

site; the response is duplicated -- or even exceeded -- when initial testing T_2 is employed, for both T_1 and T_2 reach their maximal reactions simultaneously.

Following injection by either route, the newly acquired sensitivity is to be discovered only by making a contact test within four or five days. Sequential contact tests on the same animal, or spaced primary tests on parallel recipients, show a decline in the sensitiveness within the week, probably a reflection of homograft-type rejection of the transferred cells. When no test is made within the first days following transfer, the potential capacity to respond to the specific allergen is lost and no information is passed to the cells of the recipient animal. The data in Fig. 30, apart from the two curves showing cellular transfer of contact-type hypersensitivity, bear on the transfer of cells from selected donors which possess both contact-type sensitiveness and circulating anti-hapten immunoglobulin. Antibody has never been detected following transfer of paraffin oil-induced peritoneal exudate cells; it is synthesized by cells of lymph nodes and spleens after transfer from these selected donors, but only at a rate which shows that the contact reactivity is maximally established very early. There is considerable evidence that guinea pig cells must continue to metabolize after transfer to secure expression of contact-type sensitivity by the recipient animal. Dr. Bloom has secured excellent evidence of this point by treating cells with mitomycin C as metabolic inhibitor. This evidence is consonant with the demonstrated inability to strip off a transfer factor from cells that suffice to transfer sensitivity and even from many multiples of the required amount; methods used have included sonication, freezing and thawing, and steeping in media containing PPD, cells which are capable of transferring tuberculin hypersensitivity. Antigen has not been detectable in cells highly effective in transferring hypersensitivity when concentrated cells were incorporated in a type of complete Freund's adjuvant and injected into nuchal muscles intramuscularly or into the footpad. The injected animals neither become sensitive to contact nor do they synthesize PCA-type antibody. One question for which there is no present answer concerns the requirement for transferring fewer and fewer cells as the hypersensitivity of the cell donors ascends. Does the exquisitely sensitive animal simply possess more cells having competency to transfer, or does the competency per cell ascend? The question may be irritating to some, but we need solid information. Having mentioned the early allergic conversion after cellular transfer in which maximal sensitivity is attained in relatively few hours, I will now briefly identify additional events that occur later on. In the actively sensitized animal (I have not investigated the matter by passive transfer between inbred animals) there accumulates around the site of an apparently purely delayed contact test, as repair occurs, cells which make antibody of the same anti-hapten specificity. We know also from the work of Inderbitzen that within and around prior test sites there accumulates a high local concentration of histamine, probably a consequence of higher than normal concentration of mast cells.

In cellular transfer of contact sensitivity to allergenic chemicals, a special phenomenon is seen: the placing of a contact test <u>in conjunction with an injection of</u> "<u>sensitized</u> <u>cells</u> results in an active and permanent sensitization to that allergen. Viable cells are required, and they must convey the sensitivity that is specific for the particular allergen employed. Active sensitization takes place around day seven to ten, as a new event which follows the initial sensitivity attributable to the transferred cells and their metabolic products. Evidently the "trained" living cells provide a processing step for active sensitization, yet a step which is allergen-dependent. Accordingly, some process occurs in a reacting test site which appears to be curiously effective in "training" the cells of the recipient to recognize the fixed hapten-tissue conjugate (Macher and Chase, J. Exp. Med., <u>129</u>, 81, 1969). A labile factor could be involved. These various points bear on what may be expected of "an <u>in vitro</u> correlate of delayed type hypersensitivity" as hypersensitivity is presented by an animal model. Certain events must occur within 16 hours, events for which cellular changes taking place over six to eight days could not be viewed as appropriate. Perhaps our chief concern should be directed at the early metabolism of the cells. Later events, about which we must learn every detail, could represent "<u>in vitro</u> parallelisms" more than "<u>in vitro</u> correlates," and yet yield highly useful information.

III. TRANSFER FACTOR

CHAIRMAN GOOD: Dr. Lawrence, do you wish to respond to Dr. Chase's remarks?

DR. LAWRENCE: The major difference between guinea pig and man in respect of cell transfer rests on the fact that cell-free preparations of transfer factor are effective for in vivo transfer in man and not in the guinea pig. When viable cells are used for transfer, both man and guinea pig display similarities with regard to 1) the indispensible requirement for a donor with specific sensitivity; and 2) the dependence of successful transfer on quantitative variables such as the degree of the donor's sensitivity and the dosage of cells employed.

The phenomenon in humans, however, is of a different order of magnitude in respect of the small numbers of blood leucocytes required for transfer per surface area of recipient (e.g., as few as 8×10^6 WBC or 85×10^6 WBC using "local" or "systemic" technique of transfer respectively). Moreover, our ability to transfer delayed sensitivity from one donor to several recipients simultaneously or to many recipients over a period of years, differs from the general, and perhaps obligatory, use of several donors to yield a pool of cells sufficient to sensitize one guinea pig.

The prolonged duration of transferred sensitivity observed in humans (mos. to 2 years), stands in contrast to the short duration (seven days) seen in outbred guinea pigs where sensitivity is terminated when the transferred cells are rejected via a homograft response (Harris and Harris, Ann. N. Y. Acad. Sci., 87, 156, 1960; Warwick et al., Ann. N. Y. Acad. Sci. 99, 620, 1962). Why the latter event does not occur in man may find explanation in our recent finding that dialyzable transfer factor is readily separated from human histocompatibility antigens of blood leucocytes which are non-dialyzable (Transplantation, 3, 490, 1965). Therefore, although the cellular vehicle of transfer factor may be rejected via a homograft response in man, transfer factor is not rejected.

It is also noteworthy in man, that blood leucocytes are capable only of transferring delayed hypersensitivity and not capable of transferring the capacity for serum antibody synthesis (Lawrence and Pappenheimer, J. Exp. Med., 104, 321, 1956; Good et al., Ann. N. Y. Acad. Sci. 64, 882, 1957). However, transplantation of lymph node slices to an adult agammaglobulinemic patient has resulted in the transfer of both tuberculin sensitivity and a serum antibody response. Here again the synthesis of antibody comes to an end at 100 days coincident with the rejection of the lymph node slices whereas the transferred tuberculin sensitivity still persisted a year later, (Martin et al., J. Clin. Invest., 36, 405, 1957). We conclude from these findings in humans: 1) that recipients of transfer factor, unlike the donors, are expressing delayed hypersensitivity without concomitant circulating antibody; 2) leucocytes in the circulation have either few or no functional precursor cells for antibody synthesis; and 3) the function of transferred antibody producing cells of lymph node populations, unlike delayed hypersensitivity cells, seems to depend upon viable cells and is brought to an end by their rejection. This last fact may serve to clarify my earlier insistence that Dr. Good, as well as others who have used viable cells for transfer of delayed sensitivity in man, are only able to do so by virtue of the presence of transfer factor in the cellular vehicles destined for rejection that they elect to employ.

DR. BILLINGHAM: Dr. Chase, how many cells have you transferred from sensitized guinea pigs to each normal host? What is the minimal number that will transfer a detectable level of sensitivity.

DR. CHASE: The cells that Dr. Bloom and I transferred from the order of 2.6 to 8.3 x 10^6. These cells represented the yield from a single source, such as lymph nodes or peritoneal exudate cells of one to three, usually one and a half to two donors. If one transfers cells of all three sources, pooled, it is possible to reduce the donor:recipient ratio to 0.5 - 0.3. The cell number can be further reduced, but one then enters the range of "dose-dependent" responses, and also individual donor differences.

III. TRANSFER FACTOR

DR. MITCHISON: Dr. Lawrence, do you think that there is any comparison to be made between transfer factor and scrapie? I hate to compare the unknown with the unknown, yet the history of that disease has been that it too was argued whether it is, in fact, a virus or an immunogen? On the whole, and in spite of cogent arguments to the contrary, hasn't the evidence grown in favor of an immunogenic causation of scrapie?

DR. LAWRENCE: Yes, I think so -- and I too have considered scrapie as having certain resemblances to transfer factor. However, it has been established that the scrapie agent resists boiling, whereas dialyzable transfer factor is inactivated at $56°C$ or $100°C$ for 30 minutes.

DR. GOOD: I would point out that there can nonetheless be information contained in molecules that tolerate boiling. Mucopolysaccharides and mucoproteins are such examples.

DR. BRAUN: First, a very brief comment on the exchange between Uhr and Landy. It seems to me that even without an informational molecule, one may trigger, with the help of a non-specific derepressor, events that can be self-replicating and can result in the formation of another material like the one that initiated the replication. Now, in regard to the extensive discussion about the in vivo and in vitro results, I think it might be useful to recall that in a related area, namely, in antibody formation, it has been demonstrated that one antigen-dependent event that includes nucleic acid material of unknown function can activate a clone. It has also been shown that there is a second set of events (again dependent on the presence of antigen and again involving polynucleotides) which is required to support and to stimulate the subsequent multiplication of antibody forming cells. To reiterate, the first event seems to be concerned with the initial activation of a clone, and the second with a stimulation of the further propagation of a clone.

I am wondering whether in the debate on transfer factor produced in vivo and in vitro, two distinctly different phenomena have been placed into one pot. I am wondering whether what we have been discussing may also represent two separate and distinct phenomena; one a possible true activation of a clone from a stem cell, and the other a stimulus to further multiplication of an already existing clone.

DR. WAKSMAN: Dr. Braun has in part said what I wanted to comment on. There are really two difficulties about the proposal Dr. Uhr has made. One is the fact that dialyzable transfer factor has at no time been found to stimulate either sensitive or nonsensitive lymphocytes in an in vitro system as though it were antigen. That is a real difficulty that requires explanation. The other is a quantitative one implied by serial transfer in the absence of testing with antigen. In other words, successive transfers that ought to lead to dilution of the material with no increments of antigen.

It seems to me that the Fishman-Adler type of RNA experiment with regard to antibody forming systems should be thought about in this connection. Work in that sphere has led us more and more to the suggestion that the substance extracted from macrophages after incubation with antigen cannot be an informational type of RNA. People began, therefore, to view it as a super antigen with the demonstration that it was actually an antigen-RNA complex Recent work has led to a shift of emphasis about what the RNA may mean. There is no question of entry of the complex into the cell, since it appears that immunogenicity is a surface phenomenon. Antigen apparently acts at the surface, perhaps with an antibody type of receptor, to trigger the immune response. I don't think we have a clue at this point as to what the RNA is doing. One possibility is that it is merely a highly efficient carrier. Dr. Zanvil Cohn has shown that macrophages in culture are activated by certain acidic molecules. The most active are nucleic acids, for which there must be some type of specific receptor at the macrophage surface. Whatever the RNA may actually do, it is a tenable hypothesis that transfer factor is a super-antigen.

III. TRANSFER FACTOR

Now, what about the two problems in regard to this viewpoint? First of all, with regard to the quantitative problem, the Nossal group have shown that fantastically small amounts of certain specific antigens, like the Salmonella adelaide flagellin, are immunogenic in rats. I don't remember the latest lower limit; it seems to me that 10^{-13} mole is still active in the intact animal. Certainly smaller amounts of antigen in super-antigen form might be effective in immunizing the whole individual.

As to the second point, in spite of the work showing that one needs an immunogenic molecule to elicit an in vitro phenomenon of the delayed type, we don't know that that immunogenicity has exactly the same molecular attributes as those required for in vivo immunization. This discrepancy should not stand in the way of giving very serious consideration to the interpretation suggested by Uhr.

DR. LAWRENCE: In this context it is of interest that most of the RNA-antigen complexes reported on in the literature are inactivated by treatment with pancreatic ribonuclease, while transfer factor is not.

DR. BRAUN: No, they are not.

DR. LAWRENCE: The Mannick and Egdahl and the Fishman and Adler type RNA complexes that have been described, have their activity abolished following treatment with ribonuclease. It may be that the ribonucleic acid in such preparations is presenting the antigen fragment to cells in an appropriate stereospecific configuration, and following treatment with RNAse this configuration is lost.

DR. DUTTON: I want to come back to the interpretation of the serial transfer work and the question of dilution. It seems to me that if one assumes that the antigen is more or less universally distributed in the environment, dilution ceases to be a problem. At the first transfer one would sensitize the recipient who is then able to collect enough antigen so that more of the transfer factor, containing antigen, can be made for the next time around. Thus, it would not be necessary to propose the specificity part of the complete factor replicated by the individual.

DR. LAWRENCE: I would ask Dr. Dutton to cite a replicating antigen, other than a virus or bacterium where more antigen is made following injection of non-living material.

DR. DUTTON: That is beside the point. What I am saying is that there is no problem in the recipient making a non-specific factor. If, however, the factor is specific, then we are faced with the problem of how it was that there was replication of the antigen portion. What I am saying is that if one collects the antigen ready made from the environment, then it is not necessary to replicate the specificity.

DR. LAWRENCE: Your argument would be an attractive one provided transfer factor were non-specific. The fact of the matter is, however, that rigid criteria for specificity have clearly been met, by our own results and those of others, successively with viable cells; leucocyte extracts, cell-free supernatant preparations and most recently with dialyzable transfer factor.

DR. COHN: A point of clarification. Didn't you inject PPD in the serial transfer experiment to determine whether you had successfully transferred sensitivity?

DR. LAWRENCE: Yes.

DR. COHN: Therefore, you did provide some antigen to the individual.

III. TRANSFER FACTOR

DR. LAWRENCE: Yes, five μg PPD was injected into the primary and the secondary recipient of transfer factor. Since the capacity to transfer in any case will depend upon the degree of sensitivity of the donor as well as the dose of cells used for transfer, I had to know the primary recipient's reactivity to determine whether he could be expected to transfer any reactivity at all. Otherwise, if the primary recipients possessed only moderate or lesser degrees of cutaneous sensitivity following transfer, they would not be capable of transferring sensitivity to the secondary recipients. In that case a negative result would have been recorded and it would have been meaningless. However, I find it difficult to conceive that this amount of antigen would provide the necessary requirements to fulfill your postulate.

DR. HIRSCHHORN: In our first description of PPD activation of lymphocytes in vitro, we had the opportunity to test the cells of an infant which did not respond to the antigen. Following a single skin test with PPD, there was a transient but definite response to the antigen in vitro. I think this indicates that a single skin test dose can give some kind of sensitization.

I would like to get back to what I referred to previously as numerology. One must differentiate between activation of cells on one hand and their division on the other. I believe that we can look at this in the in vitro system by means of autoradiography with tritiated uridine to determine how many cells at the beginning are activated in regard to new RNA synthesis, as compared with those which divide. We know that only a minority of lymphocytes that respond to PHA go to division.

I would like to suggest a method which may be adapted to studying the kinetics of the production of transfer factor. I previously mentioned our recent success in establishing essentially permanent long-term lymphoid cell lines from a great variety of donors. We are now trying, by means of agents like measles vaccine, to induce a cell population in vivo that will perform like stem cells, i.e., that will go into permanent culture in vitro. Perhaps this could also be done with specific transfer factor, if this component could induce such stem cells.

An additional approach which suggests itself is to take the already established cell line induced by means of a variety of the stimuli I described previously and search for transfer factor in such cell populations, notably those that had been derived from tuberculin positive individuals.

DR. WILSON: Dr. Lawrence, I wonder if it might be possible to approach some of these distinctions in the following way.

Suppose you were to use cells from sensitized individuals or animals, and add transfer factor and antigen. In the presence of transfer factor would you get a greater amount of stimulation than could be accounted for on the basis of cooperative events?

DR. LAWRENCE: This was an inescapable result of the *in vivo* studies with addition of dialysable transfer factor alone, to either sensitive or nonsensitive lymphocytes did not result in any detectable change. Transformation only occurred in those tubes to which the appropriate antigen had been added.

DR. WILSON: You will get some response with sensitized cells plus antigen. My question is, if you add the appropriate transfer factor, how is this situation altered?

DR. LAWRENCE: Fireman *et al.* (Science, 155, 337, 1967), have reported results where addition of transfer factor to natively sensitive lymphocytes plus PPD resulted in an additional increment of six percent transformed cells above the figure obtained with PPD + cells alone. Moreover, transfer factor plus PPD placed on lymphocytes from recipients of an *in vivo* transfer of tuberculin sensitivity, resulted in an additional increment of four percent transformed cells above that obtained with cells + PPD alone. These observations suggest recruitment of non-reactive lymphocytes by dialyzable transfer factor *in vitro* over and

III. TRANSFER FACTOR

and above the pool of committed cells available in nature or after transfer factor's original recruitment in vivo.

DR. BARAM: Dr. Hirschhorn has emphasized the numerous events occurring in stimulated lymphocyte cultures and particularly the likelihood that no single one of them need reflect all that is going on. I believe, Dr. Valentine said that if you add dialysate to nonsensitive cells plus antigen, you begin to see the thymidine incorporation in about three or four days.

DR. VALENTINE: With dialysates plus specific antigen we see thymidine incorporation comparable in timing to that seen in natively sensitive cells.

DR. BARAM: On the other hand, the experiments we did with MIF, as pointed out earlier, showed that a considerable release of MIF had already occurred at 36 hours. I think this bears out that there is more than one event, and the probability that more than one group of cells is involved.

DR. BRANDRISS: I would ask Dr. Lawrence if the fact that in some circumstances, such as the sarcoid patients, a good local transfer is obtained but little or no systemic transfer, influences his interpretation of the mode of action of transfer factor. I was thinking that one might expect these results if transfer factor were an effector substance. How would this observation fit with the idea that it is an instructional molecule or an immunogen?

DR. LAWRENCE: The only conclusion we have drawn is that the response of sarcoid patients to transfer factor is another proof of the requirement of a host contribution to the transaction and that the event is decidedly not a "passive" transfer nor is transfer factor an effector molecule. I think transfer factor in this instance endows the patient with local sensitivity by engaging the few uncommitted lymphocytes that are still available for cell-mediated immunity. This is a situation where the preponderance of such cells may be committed to and responding to the Kveim antigen and are thus difficult to deflect from this exclusive antigenic preoccupation (Lawrence and Zweiman, Trans. Assoc. Amer. Phys., 81, 240, 1968).

My colleagues and I (Solowey, Rapaport and Lawrence, In, Histocompatibility Testing, S. Karger, Basel, p. 75, 1967) have also studied the response of 10 patients with systemic cancers, anergic to a battery of antigens (SK-SD, PPD, Toxoid, Histoplasmin, Coccidioidin, Mumps) to dialyzable transfer factor. We found that such patients respond by acquiring both local and systemic delayed sensitivity to SK-SD. Such patients differ from normals, however, in that the systemic reactions transferred were all feeble in intensity (10x10 mm) and short in duration.

This experience differs of course from the situation disclosed in Hodgkins disease. In the latter, the deficit seems absolute and there appear to be no immunocompetent host lymphocytes either capable of or available to provide the initial interaction between cells and transfer factor necessary for even a local transfer to be expressed (Good et al., Progr. Allergy, 6, 187, 1962; Fazio and Calciati, Panminerva Medica, 4, 158, 1967).

As regards clues to the nature of transfer factor, I can only say that if it were an effector substance, like MIF, one should be able merely to utilize any Hodgkins patient's skin and in the presence of antigen elicit a passive reaction, as Dr. Bloom has done using MIF in the guinea pig. This is, in fact, not possible with transfer factor.

The studies on sarcoidosis, unhappily, do not allow a choice between an informational molecule or an immunogen. However, if transfer factor turns out to be an immunogen, as Dr. Uhr has proposed, it would have to be unique indeed in view of the inability of the majority of these patients to develop tuberculin sensitivity following living BCG vaccination, despite having recognized and responded to bacillary antigens as evidenced by the production of specific serum antibody (Carnes et al., Am. J. Path., 27, 743, 1951). This result would suggest that transfer factor is an "immunogen" for delayed reactivity exclusively in this situation, whereas replicating bacilli can only function as immunogens for serum antibody production.

III. TRANSFER FACTOR

CHAIRMAN GOOD: This was a point that was of great concern to us in our attempts to transfer delayed sensitivity to Hodgkins patients by means of cells. We used as many as ten times the number of cells known to transfer sensitivity to immunologically competent individuals. We were nonetheless unable to transfer sensitivity to Hodgkins patients (Good et al. Progr. Allergy, 6, 187, 1962).

My belief in transfer factor has recently been enhanced by Dr. David's observation on another group of patients who were immunologically unresponsive despite the presence of excessive quantities of antigen in their tissues. With transfer factor he converted at least one of these patients to a fine, if temporary, state of reactivity. These are patients who have a mucocutaneous form of candidiasis and are unreactive to Candida antigens or to other antigens to which sensitivity occurs on high frequency in normal individuals.

DR. DAVID: I referred to this result earlier, but it may be more appropriate in this context. Dr. Good refers to three patients we studied with chronic candidiasis who did not make any MIF, and were skin test negative to Candida.

What was remarkable was that one of these anergic patients who was incapable of making MIF on three prior occasions, following transfer with dialyzable transfer factor became skin test positive within a week. Moreover, following development of skin reactivity the patient made MIF when examined for it, on two subsequent occasions, and then again became skin test negative. I would point out that this was accomplished in someone whose tissues are loaded with antigen.

CHAIRMAN GOOD: Yes, that is true but it may not be antigen in the proper form or delivered to the proper site.

DR. BACH: I want to make a comment about the specificity of the cells involved in the various reactions we are discussing. Dr. Wilson brought up the issue of adding transfer factor to already sensitized cells, and inquired whether the amount of transformation increased; and whether a different population of cells were now making transfer factor because factor production preceded cell division. With respect to the first approach, the *in vitro* systems discussed are very difficult to use for these questions and several points must be considered.

First of all, there is a dose response curve for all stimulants. The addition of more antigen initially increases the response and eventually with addition of still more antigen the response is diminished. Thus one has to be sure one is working in the range of peak response and thereby gets a true summation with the addition of two stimulants rather than a dose response. Even if such criteria are met, there are substances which themselves stimulate an individual cell very little or not at all, and yet when added to an MLC reaction, enhance that reaction a great deal.

We have previously published data showing that within a family, stimulating cells differing from a responder by two alleles at HLA (the major histocompatibility locus in man), stimulate the responding cells more than cells differing by one allele and, in fact, stimulate approximately as much as the sum of the two cells each differing by one allele. I think such evidence also cannot be interpreted critically to indicate that different cell populations are responding to the antigens associated with the two different alleles -- although that is clearly one possible interpretation. This is not at all understood, and therefore interpreting the "specificity of the responding cells" with reactions such as these, is I think rather difficult.

I would be inclined to question the interpretation that there are two different populations of cells -- those that engage in division and those that make the supernatant lymphocyte activating factor of Valentine and Lawrence referred to earlier, because the factor is present before cell division is detectable. First, we do not know whether there has not in fact been some division; secondly, we do not know whether there is a responding cell that disseminates information to a much larger percentage of cells, which are then seen at 48 hours. Thirdly, it may well be that the cells do not divide until 48 hours, but that the same cells go through the G-1 phase of the cycle

III. TRANSFER FACTOR

when they are making this factor and this is actually the same population of cells.

CHAIRMAN GOOD: We are all very much indebted to Dr. Lawrence for his persistence in the face of the difficulties involved in the studies of transfer factor. I think one of the real problems with working on transfer factor is that it is really a difficult model to study since it requires the use of human volunteers. We will now move on to a consideration of other assay systems for transfer factor.

DR. SMITH: It has already been referred to earlier that Adler and I (Fed. Proc. 28, 813, 1969) have observed that mouse lymphocytes treated with human transfer factor dialysate react to PPD. This result is exactly as Dr. Lawrence described for the human system *in vitro*. The kinetics involved suggest that there is a threshold level to achieve activation with transfer factor, but after the addition of the transfer factor, the response is as dose dependent and the dose response curve exhibits exactly the same pattern I described for the primarily reacting, tuberculin sensitive mouse lymphocytes.

DR. BACH: If I understood you correctly Dr. Smith, this is an extremely important finding with respect to Dr. Uhr's earlier argument that transfer factor is an immunogen. For every lymphocyte reaction known, (including PHA, antigen to which an individual is sensitized, allogeneic cells, ALS, etc) as more stimulant is added, there eventually occurs less and less response and even total inhibition.

If the addition of transfer factor does not induce such inhibition, it would seem to me that there has been realized a very important distinction. It would, however, be important to make such tests at a concentration of transfer factor at least five or ten fold greater than the amount needed to attain peak stimulation.

CELLULAR IMMUNITY

DR. SMITH: That is why I made this distinction.

DR. BACH: To what extent did you increase the dose of transfer factor over and above that which was maximally stimulatory?

DR. SMITH: With increasing dose levels the response plateaued, but we may not have gone far enough. Experiments are still in progress and we will have to await a more definite answer.

DR. BRAUN: In the context of Dr. Uhr's earlier discussion on the possibility that transfer factor may function as an immunogen, I would like to show some provocative but preliminary data which I think raise still another possible interpretation. I have been for some time preoccupied with the possibility that the initiation of immune responses may involve the antigen-guided entrance of a non-specific activator into pre-existing stem cells with specific capacities.

Accordingly, Dr. Lawrence and I had a discussion last fall about the possibility that transfer factor could also represent a complex of antigenic determinants and non-specific activators (a complex in which it may be difficult to detect the antigenic determinant) the antigenic moiety serving as the pilot to bring the non-specific activator into appropriate responsive cells.

On the remote chance that such an activator, obtained from human sources, might operate in a murine system, we decided to test human transfer factor in mice, i.e., the dialyzed material given to us by Dr. Lawrence, the test conditions selected were those that, on the basis of our prior data, support the entrance of stimulators or activators into lymphocytes. As I indicated in my earlier remarks, the presence of ALS or epinephrine appears to provide us with such conditions.

III. TRANSFER FACTOR

Table 22, shows that, in test with mice, the combination of transfer factor and epinephrine and also, to a lesser extent, the combination of transfer factor and ALS, elicited an increase in the number of splenic PFC specific for sRBC and also elevated to some extent the PFC specific for hRBC. Transfer factor alone, or epinepherine alone or ALS alone, had no effect on the number of PFC.

These preliminary data are shown to focus attention on the possibility that transfer factor may indeed represent a complex of non-specific activator or stimulator and a difficult-to-detect antigenic determinant providing a "homing instinct" for the non-specific activator material.

TABLE 22

Effect of Dialysable Human Transfer Factor on Development of PFC in Mice

Treatment of spleen donors	Average number ($\pm$ S.E.) of antibody-forming cells per 10^8 spleen cells, assayed 48 hours after immunization or treatment, on:	
	sRBC	hRBC
	56.9 $\pm$ 16.1	
Transfer Factor	57.6 $\pm$ 8.5	21.2 $\pm$ 4.2
" " + epinephrine	239.5 $\pm$ 68.5	44.7 $\pm$ 8.0
" " + ALS #2	97.3 $\pm$ 20.5	45.3 $\pm$ 15.1
Epinephrine	58.7 $\pm$ 7.8	16.0 $\pm$ 5.2
ALS #2	42.6 $\pm$ 6.9	
sRBC (10^8)	440.7 $\pm$ 71.2	19.6 $\pm$ 10.0

CF1 females; 5 animals/group
Transfer factor (Josephson 4-21-61, WBC 0.32 in 3 ml saline), 0.1 ml per mouse i.v.
Epinephrine, 250 x dil., 1.0 ml per mouse i.p. (at 0, 6, 12, 18, 24 hrs.)
ALS #2, rabbit anti-mouse lymphocyte serum, 2 x dil., 0.1 ml per mouse i.p.

CELLULAR IMMUNITY

DR. HIRSCHHORN: It may be conceptually important to realize that overdoses of antigen and PHA, may decrease the response of lymphocytes because they are cytotoxic. I think it would be important to know whether transfer factor is cytotoxic and whether there are effects from overdosage with this material.†

DR. BARAM: We have done experiments with blood leucocytes lysates in the Rhesus monkey system (Fed. Proc. $\underline{28}$, 629, 1969). As I pointed out earlier we found that we could transfer KLH sensitivity in vitro with KLH sensitive cell lysates containing 25 micrograms of ribose; ribose being used to determine the RNA concentration. We have done transfers using lysates containing up to 200 micrograms of ribose. Increasing the concentration of the lysates added does seem to cause a slight inhibition of the transfer reaction.

Using KLH-sensitive lysate concentrations containing 3, 25, 50, 70, 100 and 200 µg of ribose we found that once the concentration of lysate was reached (25 µg of ribose) necessary to transfer KLH sensitivity to nonsensitive cells, then further increase in concentration did not, either increase the response of the cells or change the time of thymidine incorporation. Further increases in amounts of the KLH-sensitive cell lysate alone did not effect a stimulation of thymidine incorporation. For this to occur it was always necessary to add KLH.

---

† Large increments of transfer factor are not discernibly toxic either to sensitive or nonsensitive lymphocytes in culture during a 7 day period. In the absence of appropriate antigen transfer factor has no discernible effect.

III. TRANSFER FACTOR

DR. THOR: We have been evaluating the capacity to transfer in vitro reactivity using a human RNA material and a guinea pig RNA extract. Since much of this work has been published with Dray or Jureziz, I will only summarize those data that are germane to this discussion. Two animal species of RNA extracts have been studied -- human and guinea pig. Our human material may differ from Lawrence's transfer factor in that it is obtained from lymph nodes rather than peripheral blood leucocytes. The RNA in the human system was ribonuclease sensitive (0.1 μ/500 μ RNA).

In the guinea pig, Dr. Schlossman and I have studied this system using alpha DNP-L-(lys) 8.4 and epsilon DNP-L-(lys) 14 as immunogen. These DNP-oligolysines have been found by Benacerraf et al. and others to be immunogenic in strain 2 guinea pigs, but not immunogenic in strain 13 guinea pigs, who are uniformly found to be non-responders. Using RNA extracts obtained from sensitized strain 2 guinea pig lymph nodes, we have been able to transfer to lymphoid cells of both nonsensitive strain 2 and, non-responder strain 13 the ability to: 1) produce MIF, and 2) undergo radioactive incorporation of H_3 thymidine and blast transformation. In two recent experiments we have passively transferred cutaneous sensitivity in vivo with specificity to each of these antigens -- using either the strain 2 or strain 13's own lymph node cells after incubation with RNA and injection back into the same inbred animal.

If you challenge the guinea pig after injection of the RNA-incubated cells whether it be the non-responder strain 13 or the non-immunized (responder) strain 2, these recipients will develop a classical delayed hypersensitivity skin test within 24 hours. However, if they are not challenged within three days, this ability to recognize either the alpha DNP (lys) antigen or the epsilon DNP (lys) antigen diminishes and is not recalled on subsequent testing after two weeks have elapsed. This phenomenon is inexplicable at present, because if sensitive inbred strain 2 cells are transferred within strain 2 animals, the duration of transfer is much longer than this period of time.

Finally, I would take issue with the concept of transfer factor as a possible super antigen effect and the notion of widespread sensitization resulting from prior and subsequent skin testing. It may be a super immunogen not behaving as antigen, but I rather think there are striking differences. A super antigen would be expected to show stimulation of cells or MIF production when we concentrated the RNA extract greatly and used up to 500 micrograms of RNA purified as a 5 to 12 S RNA. In fact we do not see stimulation. I think it is feasible to hypothesize that if we had super antigen in this extract that we should have seen some stimulation, especially since we do obtain stimulation with antigen at a concentration of 0.1 µg provided the cells have been incubated with specific RNA.

DR. FIREMAN: I wonder if we can get a consensus among those who have been studying transfer factor in terms of species specificity. I am very perplexed by some of the data presented earlier, because we have been unable to transfer tuberculin hypersensitivity to the rabbit or the guinea pig *in vivo* or *in vitro* by the lymphocyte transformation methodology using human transfer factor. I present this negative data because Dr. Smith had earlier mentioned the effect of human transfer factor on mouse lymphocytes *in vitro*. Additionally, Dr. Baram has described the effect of monkey transfer factor on human leucocytes *in vitro*.

Is there any other experience along this line?

DR. CHASE: There is one such observation: rabbits rendered sensitive to tuberculin yield living cells which effect transfer between rabbits, not guinea pigs; conversely, guinea pigs made sensitive to tuberculin transfer only within their own species. One example worth rethinking was described by Bacon and Wallace some years ago; rat cells were injected into guinea pig skin in the belief that the latter represented a good reaction tissue; a short time later they injected into the cell depot the antigen which, in their case, was, I think, tuberculin. They described obtaining a specific reaction which would not have been got if the rat cells had been dispersed by intravenous or intraperitoneal injection. Perhaps with extract of

III. TRANSFER FACTOR

foreign cells, this technique could represent a possible approach, if some of the extract can be fixed locally. In this way, a subsequent injection of antigen, locally, might minimize species differences and allow use of guinea pig skin as an effector tissue.

DR. GOOD: I think transferring with cells across the species barrier is associated with several hazards, among these I would emphasize that natural antibodies are almost certainly present which could provide a pathway for elimination of the transferred cells.

IV
ELABORATION OF EFFECTOR MOLECULES
BY ACTIVATED LYMPHOCYTES

Spectrum of effector molecules released by antigen-stimulated lymphocytes — Adjuvant effects of delayed-type hypersensitivity reaction — Separation and physicochemical properties of MIF — Inhibition versus activation of macrophages by lymphocyte products — Macrophage activation correlated with adherence to surfaces — RNA transfer of MIF production does not involve an informational RNA — Blastogenic factor is not a transplantation antigen — "Immune Macrophages" ⇌ cells carrying antigen to stimulate responsive lymphocytes — Variables that determine potency and expression of mediators influence their individual detection —Supernatants of activated lymphocytes evoke characteristic cutaneous histology — Prior cellular accumulation in cutaneous test site intensifies and accentuates response to antigen — Transfer of tuberculin sensitivity and homograft immunity via plasma factor released by X-irradiation.

IV. BIOLOGICAL ACTIVITIES OF LYMPHOCYTE PRODUCTS

DR. BLOOM: As biologists we are concerned with the reason why there are two major kinds of immunologic responses. At this conference particularly we should seek to determine what evolutionary selective value, and hence function, the delayed type hypersensitivity response offers that would help account for the persistance of a system that surely has been operative for many millions of years. It is now ten years since Dr. Lewis Thomas first suggested that cell-mediated immunity evolved as a defence against mutant cells and neoplasia, (In: Cellular and Humoral Aspects of the Hypersensitive States, Ed. H. S. Lawrence, p. 529, Hoeber, N. Y. 1959)an idea which has since been termed "immunologic surveillance" (Burnet, Lancet, $\underline{1}$, 1171, 1967) and focused our attention on such a fundamental function of the immunologic apparatus. We all accept on faith that the cell-mediated immune response is to some extent involved in the elimination of cells altered by somatic mutation, by viral infection or perhaps by certain bacterial infections. In our discussions of possible effector substances, I would urge that we try to relate these agents to events that occur _in vivo_. It seems to me that the evidence is overwhelmingly convincing that there is indeed immunological 'surveillance' operative in the normal individual all the time. It is not my intent to review all the evidence here, but rather to mention as examples the markedly increased incidence of tumors in animals that have been thymectomized and in humans who have been on immunosuppressive therapy. We seek to determine the possible mediators of this surveillance mechanism.

A second aspect of the biological role of delayed-type hypersensitivity _in vivo_ that we propose to consider, is what is termed 'cellular immunity', an increased resistance of certain cells, particularly macrophages, to the destructive effects of certain bacterial infections, an immunity brought about under the influence of delayed-type hypersensitivity. The mechanisms by which sensitized cells are able to inflict damage on various target cells, and their relation to immunological surveillance, will be taken up by

CELLULAR IMMUNITY

Dr. Granger later on and I will therefore omit consideration of the cell destructive aspects of lymphocytes at this time.

The first point I would make about the delayed-type hypersensitivity reaction in vivo, and to a degree in vitro, is that it is at least a two-cell reaction. The evidence for this is abundant, but on the simplest level one need only look at the histologic picture of a classical tuberculin reaction. Clearly two cell types are present. Previously pathologists tended to hedge and call the picture a round-cell infiltrate. By more modern methods, it has been possible to define one of the components involved as a small lymphocyte, most likely thymus-dependent. The second cell has been shown to arise in the bone-marrow, to pass through the blood stream, and upon appearing at the site of a delayed-type reaction become recognizable as a macrophage or histiocyte. There are clearly variations in the histology of various type of delayed-type hypersensitivity reactions, depending on the nature of the antigen and where in the body it is localized, yet I believe a strong case can be made that both lymphocytes and macrophages are involved. It seems clear from the elegant work of Dr. Mackaness and his collaborators on cellular immunity that in a functional sense there occurs an immunologically specific event which is followed by a rather non-specific effect on macrophages which activates them to deal effectively with a variety of bacteria. I would like to think that the specific event is initiated by the small lymphocyte, which in turn influences the macrophages. Thus, in the context of Dr. Mitchison's schema presented at the previous session, I would suggest that:

a) small lymphocyte + specific antigen $\longrightarrow$ macrophage. Later in my argument, I will suggest that this can also work in a reverse fashion, to complete a circle.

b) macrophages + antigen $\longrightarrow$ small lymphocytes

I would bring to an end my cursory comments on the salient features of the delayed-type reactions in vivo with a consideration of the cell transfer technique, since that was the means by which it was established that lymphocytes from hypersensitive individuals have the information to effectuate the specific delayed-type reaction within a normal individual. The difficulty with the cell transfer

IV. BIOLOGICAL ACTIVITIES OF LYMPHOCYTE PRODUCTS

experiment is simply that once the cells are transferred, even with the most careful observation and highest degrees of labelling, it is impossible to ascertain where the cells mediating the reaction go, let alone to analyze the metabolic and biochemical processes they undergo that eventuates in the cutaneous reaction detected. It is for this reason, that a number of the conferees have devoted considerable time and effort trying to unravel the phenomenon of cell-mediated immunity utilizing *in vitro* models. There are now about eight kinds of biologic activities demonstrable in the culture supernatants of sensitive lymphocytes that have been challenged with specific antigen or have been activated by a mitogenic agent. My preference is not to discuss my own work with Boyce Bennett here in any detail but rather to mention briefly each of the systems studied and later on have the current experimental data dealt with in the general discussion.

It seems to me that some justification is in order regarding the use of any of the *in vitro* systems for the study of delayed-type hypersensitivity. In the case of the migration inhibitory reaction, with which I am most familiar, the basic correlations are as follows:

1) To effect reactions *in vivo* or *in vitro*, sensitized lymphocytes must be capable of synthesizing new RNA and protein. Treatment of sensitized lymphocytes with mitomycin C irreversibly blocks their ability to effect passive transfer or to produce the migration inhibitory factor *in vitro*. Interestingly enough, mild treatment with mitomycin C, under conditions where small amounts of DNA are crosslinked and where cell division would not be possible, does not inhibit passive transfer reactions *in vivo*. This indicates that it is the transferred cells that can mediate the reaction.

2) In the cell migration system, the migration inhibitory factor has been found to be produced only by lymphocytes from animals with delayed-type hypersensitivity. In this case, involving guinea pigs infected for six days with viable BCG, no circulating antibodies are detectable. Conversely, immunization with alumina as adjuvant produces high levels of circulating antibodies even to PPD and under these circumstances it is not possible to find MIF produced, as judged by migration inhibition experiments.

3) The effector molecule, MIF, is not produced continuously but only following contact of the sensitized lymphocytes with specific antigen. Hence, in contrast to antibody which would be present all the time in an immunized individual, this factor would be expected to be produced after antigenic challenge and then only locally.

The kinetics of production of the various biologic activities or factors has been studied for some but by no means all. In our experiments it is worth emphasizing that MIF is released quickly from the cells; it can be detected in culture supernatants within six hours after addition of antigen, long before DNA synthesis, cell division or blast cell transformation. Moreover, MIF continues to be produced long after the cells are initially "triggered" by antigen. In experiments involving daily change of medium for five successive days, MIF was found in all the supernatants. Consequently, under these conditions it is likely that MIF is being synthesized continuously rather than merely released from some preformed state.

The various activities associated with cell mediated immunity *in vitro* are assembled in Table 23. This represents an attempt to select from the literature those salient physico-chemical features which might enable us to distinguish the mediators of these reactions, one from another. The first of these, MIF, can be released by sensitized lymphocytes cultured in the presence of specific antigen. This factor, the first to be studied, has the property of inhibiting the migration of normal macrophages. In fact, it appears that human MIF will inhibit the migration of guinea pig macrophages, although the relative effectiveness across species lines has not yet been ascertained.

A second putative effector molecule is lymphotoxin, liberated under generally similar conditions. Most interestingly, it is also liberated from normal lymphocytes by PHA. This factor, now designated LT, has the ability to kill a variety of target cells from many species, and Dr. Granger will shortly discuss it in detail. Probably related to LT is a cloning inhibitory factor which, without killing the seeded cells, e.g. HeLa cells, inhibits their capacity to divide more than once or twice, thereby blocking the formation of detectable clones.

IV. BIOLOGICAL ACTIVITIES OF LYMPHOCYTE PRODUCTS

TABLE 23

POSSIBLE EFFECTOR SUBSTANCES RELEASED BY LYMPHOCYTES

Putative Effector	M.W.	$\Delta 56°$	$\Delta 80°$	Phenol	Protease	Urea	+Red. Alk.	Electrophoresis R_f	Species Specificity
Migration Inhibitory Factor	70,000	+	−		±	+	+	> alb	±
Lymphotoxic Factor	80,000	+*, −**	+*	−					−
Skin-reactive Factor	70,000	+			±			< alb	±
Chemotactic Factor	60,000	+			−			< alb	−
Mitogenic Factor	25,000		±						
Interferon	25,000	+			−	+	−		+
Antibody	140,000	+			+		−	<< alb	±[‡]

+ stable   − destroyed or none   ± partial or variable   * mouse   ** human

[‡] although antibodies function across species, the ability to fix to cells and tissues varies.

The skin-reactive factor, which Bennett and I found to be present in purified preparations of MIF, upon inoculation into the skin of normal guinea pigs, produces an indurated and erythematous lesion apparent in three hours, maximal at 6-10 hours, which has disappeared by 30 hours. Our interest in this factor relates to the distinctive lesion characterized by a predominantly mononuclear infiltrate, produced early after its intradermal injection. Later on there occurs an infiltration of polymorphonuclear cells with focal epidermal necrosis. The histological picture is remarkably similar to that seen in an active delayed-type cutaneous lesion, with the main and understandable exception of an accelerated time course.

Recently a factor that is chemotactic for macrophages has been described, released from sensitized lymphocytes under the same conditions as MIF. This factor rather than causing inhibition, causes macrophages to migrate through a millipore filter in a Boyden chamber in the direction of the chemotactic factor gradient.

Another activity, that of causing blast cell transformation in normal lymphocytes, has been found in relevant circumstances such as: the stimulation of human or of guinea pig sensitized lymphocytes by specific antigen, and in MLC supernatants. These could represent more than a single mitogenic factor.

Next on this list is interferon, produced by stimulation of human lymphocytes either by mitogens or by PPD, an agent known to cause human tissue culture cells to become resistant to viral infection.

Lastly, I have included antibodies themselves, since they too have been found to be released and synthesized by sensitized lymphocytes stimulated with specific antigen. The "cytophilic" varieties are especially appropriate for our consideration, since their role in delayed-type hypersensitivity has by no means been completely excluded.

My construction of Table 23 makes it evident that the available data are rather incomplete. This is understandable, since the field of in vitro mediators is a rather recent development. I have sought to assemble whatever data

IV. BIOLOGICAL ACTIVITIES OF LYMPHOCYTE PRODUCTS

were available on these activities associated with sensitized lymphocytes in the hope that similarities and differences would become apparent, and thus enable us easily to merge or to distinguish various factors. Unfortunately, this is not yet possible. The estimates of molecular weights for the first five factors, as determined by gel filtration, are so similar as to be indistinguishable. The heat-inactivation data seem to offer more possibilities but it should be noted that species differences and differences in the contaminating proteins in the mixtures are important considerations;hence, it is not possible to accept the data as proof of real differences in factors. The most hopeful avenue for dealing with the five factors is the most tedious; namely, separation of activities by acrylamide gel electrophoresis. Preliminary findings suggest that MIF activity can be separated from chemotactic activity and skin reactive activity, although the precise results from different laboratories are not yet in agreement. Clearly, the only factors that can be presently distinguished are antibody immunoglobulin and classical interferon. However, I hasten to point out that there are many interferon-like substances which are less well characterized than the viral-induced interferon given in this table. Accordingly, it may be that at this moment even the possibility that one of the other factors may have interferon-like activity is not to be completely excluded. We have reached the point where we simply must have more data to unravel the various activities and factors.

The problem can be approached from another vantage point. It is pertinent to ask whether any of these putative factors could be excluded on intuitive grounds as being unrelated or irrelevant to delayed-type reactions. Again, regretably, I believe this cannot be managed presently. Indeed, if I may be permitted a teleological kind of argument, I believe that I can weave all these activities into a rather attractive, albeit fanciful, model for delayed-type hypersensitivity reactions.

Upon introduction of antigen into a local area in a sensitized individual, the first event would be for sensitized lymphocytes to appear in the site, either on an entirely random basis or by attraction of an antigen gradient which is chemotactic. The next step would be the interaction of the sensitized lymphocytes with the specific antigen leading to the elaboration of some or all of the various factors previously mentioned. First, the chemotactic factor would cause the accumulation of cells, especially macrophages, to help the reaction. Once there, it would be reasonable to keep them there with MIF to do the effector job, and possibly to activate them in the sense of producing rather drastic changes in their lysosomal hydrolases and respiration, and even division; changes such as are found in macrophages surrounding a tubercle focus. Obviously, to fulfill the function of surveillance a cytotoxic factor would be perfectly suited to preserve the natural state of affairs by wiping out altered cells. To handle such a large job, it would probably be valuable to have a mitogenic factor produced, which would amplify the reaction by triggering non-sensitized lymphocytes that traverse the affected area and thus cause them to release still more of all the factors. Additionally, it is a curious fact that the great majority of viral infections produce a delayed-type hypersensitivity in vivo. The one exception which comes to mind is that of the picornaviruses, small RNA viruses like polio. But the point here is that the tumor viruses and other viruses which either denature or alter antigens at the plasma membrane, give rise to delayed-type hypersensitivity. Once inside cells, these viruses are mostly immune to the effects of antibodies, so that a substance like interferon which confers upon unaffected cells resistance to virus infection, would be most appropriate. And lastly, it is not proposed to ignore the potential usefulness of antibodies locally, and especially cytophilic antibodies, which might be distinctly valuable in guiding activated macrophages, or perhaps lymphocytes, quite specifically to the cells which they are to destroy, thereby imparting a bit of control on the specificity of some effector cytotoxic processes.

The last consequence of a delayed-type hypersensitivity reaction which I would tentatively submit as possibly having some significance, would be an adjuvant effect. Initially, I argued for a sequence in which lymphocytes interacted with antigen and affected macrophages, and now I propose that, for the second stage of the reaction, macrophages interact with antigen and feed information back to lymphocytes. Dr. Chase described earlier an experiment in which some

IV. BIOLOGICAL ACTIVITIES OF LYMPHOCYTE PRODUCTS

normal animals were given sensitized cells in a passive transfer. All animals received one skin test at various times, and three months later were all tested for only the second time. It was found that those animals that had received sensitized cells and reacted within the first week to an initial test were positive to a second test three months later. Those animals receiving sensitized cells and were not tested until after the first week, i.e. after the transferred cells had been rejected, reacted neither to the first test, nor to the second test, behaving as did normal controls that had simply been tested twice. The only reasonable explanation for the fact that the first group became and remained positive for a long time is the presence of a positive delayed-type reaction coincident with application of the first test site. This ongoing event enabled the test antigen to be used efficiently for a phase of active senzitization. Other animals receiving the same amount of test antigen, in the absence of an accompanying delayed-type reaction at the test site, could not use it as efficiently; consequently, no active sensitization took place. Consistent with this association is the well established observation of Turk and Humphrey, that when a new antigen is introduced into a tuberculin sensitive guinea pig together with PPD, there occurs unusually high levels of antibody production to the new antigen (e.g. diphtheria toxoid). Dr. Halpern in my laboratory, has repeated this type of experiment with bovine gammaglobulin (BGG) as the irrelevant antigen, and we have looked for delayed-type sensitization. The experiment was performed in the following manner: guinea pigs were sensitized to tuberculin with Freund's adjuvant, and after four months, were skin tested either with 25 μg PPD, 25 μg PPD + 100 μg BGG or BGG alone. Two to four weeks later the animals were skin tested for delayed-type hypersensitivity to BGG. As shown in Table 24, a little over 50% of the animals that had BGG at the site of an irrelevant delayed-type reaction, became sensitized.

Pursuing this line of reasoning it is possible to visualize the delayed-type hypersensitivity response as being a basic immune response of great economy. One needs perhaps, as in Dr. Mitchison's model, a separate line of antigen-reactive cells, with the capability of initiating specific delayed-type reactions. By "triggering" the cells

TABLE 24

POSSIBLE ADJUVANT EFFECT OF DELAYED-TYPE HYPERSENSITIVITY REACTIONS

Sensitized to	Challenged with	Positive to BGG
Tuberculin	BGG alone	0/9
Tuberculin	BGG +PPD	6/9
Nothing	BGG + PPD	0/5

with antigens, the reaction would be started and macrophages would be involved. In my view, the macrophages would serve both as effector cells in a sense, and also with the capacity of amplifying the reaction. They might, perhaps, also carry antigen to other lymphocytes both locally and in the nodes, i.e. they could involve more lymphocytes, thereby still further amplify the reaction. One could thus visualize a kind of continuing cycle of escalation or resonance. The condequences of such a proposal are anything but inconsequential.

I am intrigued with Dr. Good's observations on the effects of injecting Freund's adjuvant in primitive species such as the lamprey and the guitar fish, leading to the development of granulomatous lesions which progress to such an extent that they overwhelm and eventually kill the host. A corollary of this idea might be the rather chronic and progressive nature of those diseases in man regarded as having delayed-type hypersensitivity involvement. I am also intrigued with the possibility of explaining ways in which a delayed-type hypersensitivity reaction can be initiated to one antigen, which then somehow involves other antigens. This is a situation entirely conceivable in some viral or post-vaccinial encephalomyelitides, where a specific reaction to the virus could bring in macrophages capable of carrying brain antigen back into the immune system, thereby

IV. BIOLOGICAL ACTIVITIES OF LYMPHOCYTE PRODUCTS

leading to a vicious overkill reaction which could lead to destruction of the organ. If one accepts any of these speculations or this line of reasoning, the next logical issue is the problem of what control mechanisms for this type of response exists in higher animals. Clearly not all delayed-type reactions are lethal, yet the basis for control has not been brought up for discussion and it is certainly not readily apparent.

As a last major issue, I would like to turn from the possible usefulness or hazards of the effector molecules in a clinical sense, to what I regard as their possible importance to the molecular biologist. The possibility exists that these molecules, which can be 'induced' at will by adding antigen to sensitized lymphocytes, provide a basis to probe mechanisms for macromolecular control and regulation in mammalian cells, a subject which has thus far been extremely difficult to approach experimentally. There is a vast gap in our knowledge on control of gene function; in the bacterial cell this information is considerable because life in the bacterial cell is so much simpler; in contrast to the paucity of analogous information on mammalian cells. For example, in E. coli the DNA is naked, a polymerase transcribes a gene and puts an RNA next to the gene, a few polysomes cluster and protein synthesis proceeds right there. In the mammalian cells, gene transcription takes place in the nucleus, but protein synthesis occurs at a geographically distant site in the cytoplasm. The DNA in mammalian cells is not naked, but buried in chromatin and coated with nuclear proteins and RNA. Thus it has not been easy to find mammalian models for studying how genes are activated, or how coordinated synthesis of batteries of proteins in development are controlled. One of the best models in my opinion, is that of Tomkins, in which tyrosine aminotransferase levels in a cultured line of hepatoma cells can be greatly increased by steroid hormones. The system is facinating and the results are really quite exciting. Nevertheless, this system presents certain problems: first the cell studied is neoplastic and aneuploid; secondly, the enzyme is already present in all the cells and the 'inducer' merely increases an already existent function rather than unmasking a new gene; and lastly, the functional relationship between the inducer, the steroid, and the product, tyrosine aminotransferase, is not at all clear.

It occurs to me that a detailed study of the production of the various putative effector molecules we have been discussing here might well provide important insights into the problem of cell control. Clearly, lymphocytes, while they have the information for making these factors, require 'triggering' by antigen or mitogens in order to elaborate them. If any of the factors are already present, prior to stimulation, they are in amounts too small for us to measure with any of the existing methodology. Inasmuch as the inducers are antigens, and the producers elaborate products with properties consistent with those expected of effector molecules, the process clearly has biological meaning. However, for the system to be relevant to the study of gene control, it is necessary to demonstrate that the factors are, in fact, gene products, not merely precursor-derived products released without gene activation. The evidence that the production of most of the factors is inhibited by mitomycin C, actinomycin D and puromycin suggests that indeed they may be genuine gene products, requiring mRNA and protein synthesis. However, at present, the evidence is suggestive rather than conclusive. If this indication can be fully validated I believe that study of these systems, in a molecular sense, would surely provide a good deal of insight into a fundamental biological problem, in addition to the important immunological information entailed.

In closing, I would like to identify those issues that seem to me to be of immediate importance in understanding the relation of the putative effector molecules to cell-mediated immunity. Hopefully we will deal with many of these issues in the course of our discussions.

1) Which of the factors produced by lymphocytes _in vitro_ can be demonstrated at the sites of active delayed-type hypersensitivity reactions _in vivo_?

2) Which factors are identical chemically and which are separable and distinct? It seems obvious that some of these activities may be attributable to the same molecule, and to me it seems equally clear that at least two will not. For those activities, produced by the same substance, we must determine which assay is the more sensitive, and which is the more relevant to the complex _in vivo_ situation.

IV. BIOLOGICAL ACTIVITIES OF LYMPHOCYTE PRODUCTS

3) Which factors are species-specific and which are not, and what is the importance of species specificity in principle and in practice? Dr. Chase raised the question of effecting passive transfer with living cells across unrelated species. I for one am not aware that this has, in fact, been accomplished. Yet some of the putative effectors themselves, i.e. in the isolated state, are effective across different species barriers, at least in vitro. In practice, this becomes a most urgent question, because one wants to measure human effector molecules, and at present it is frequently much more convenient to do this in vitro or using animal cells as targets.

4) Which factors are induced only by antigens; which can be produced by so called non-specific agents that activate lymphocytes? From the point of view of cell biology, this question asks whether, when a lymphocyte is activated, it is in effect 'turned on' for everything it is capable of making, or whether there are circumstances where this is selective and only certain activities are released.

5) Are two cell types required for release of these putative effector molecules? I raised this question previously and I believe it is an important one for us to consider. There seems to be a good deal of evidence that specific antigens do not act directly on the lymphocyte so as to induce it to become activated. In fact, many believe that the direct pathway is the means by which immunological tolerance is produced. The question then develops whether macrophages have to be present before lymphocytes can be stiumulated to release these factors?

6) A number of paradoxical situations have emerged. Thus, lymphocyte culture preparations effect both macrophage migration inhibition and chemotaxis for macrophages. Then too, LT preparations are cytotoxic for fibroblast target cells and macrophages and yet lymphocytes elaborating these factors seem to be refractory. How are these seeming conflicts to be resolved?

7) At the most basic level we must eventually deal with the question of whether all cells produce all the known factors, or whether some effectors are produced only by some cells, etc? Which are the cells that produce the effector

molecules, are they thymus-dependent or bone-marrow derived? What is their origin and the basis for their specificity?

DR. DAVID: I would like particularly to discuss three of the issues identified by Dr. Bloom. One concerns recent studies we have done in an effort to characterize the migration inhibitory factor (MIF). The second will describe the chemotactic factor produced by sensitized lymphocytes challenged *in vitro* with specific antigen. And the last will deal with the question whether MIF acts directly on macrophages itself to inhibit migration, or whether it forms a specific complex with antigen to do so.

With Drs. Remold and Haber, we have been attempting to isolate and purify MIF. The system I shall discuss is the production of MIF by lymphocytes from guinea pigs sensitized to the soluble protein antigen, O-chlorobenzoylated bovine gammaglobulin (OCB-BGG). Lymph node lymphocytes were incubated in tissue culture overnight in serum-free medium, under the conditions shown by Bloom and Bennett to permit elaboration of MIF in medium not contaminated with large amounts of extraneous serum proteins. One aliquot of the sensitized cells was incubated without antigen, while the other was incubated with the specific antigen. MIF is produced only when sensitized cells are cultured with antigen, the other aliquot thus serving as a control. Supernatants and fractions derived from them were tested for their ability to inhibit the migration of normal guinea pig peritoneal exudate cells. The supernatants were concentrated and fractionated on Sephadex G-100 columns, and we have shown that there is an indication of some protein in the void volume, but very little in the region where albumin would elute. Since Bloom and Bennett and we have shown that MIF is found in the albumin region, I_{125}-labelled rabbit albumin was added to our samples to delineate this region. When material eluting with the albumin marker was concentrated and subjected to acrylamide gel disc electrophoresis, one sees a number of protein bands. The patterns are shown in Fig. 31. The first tube shows the electrophoretic pattern of serum. The second is concentrated migration inhibitory supernatant purified on Sephadex. Obviously, some of the bands correspond to serum components while others are

IV. BIOLOGICAL ACTIVITIES OF LYMPHOCYTE PRODUCTS

different. I must note here that the patterns obtained from control and migration inhibitory supernatants are not distinguishable.

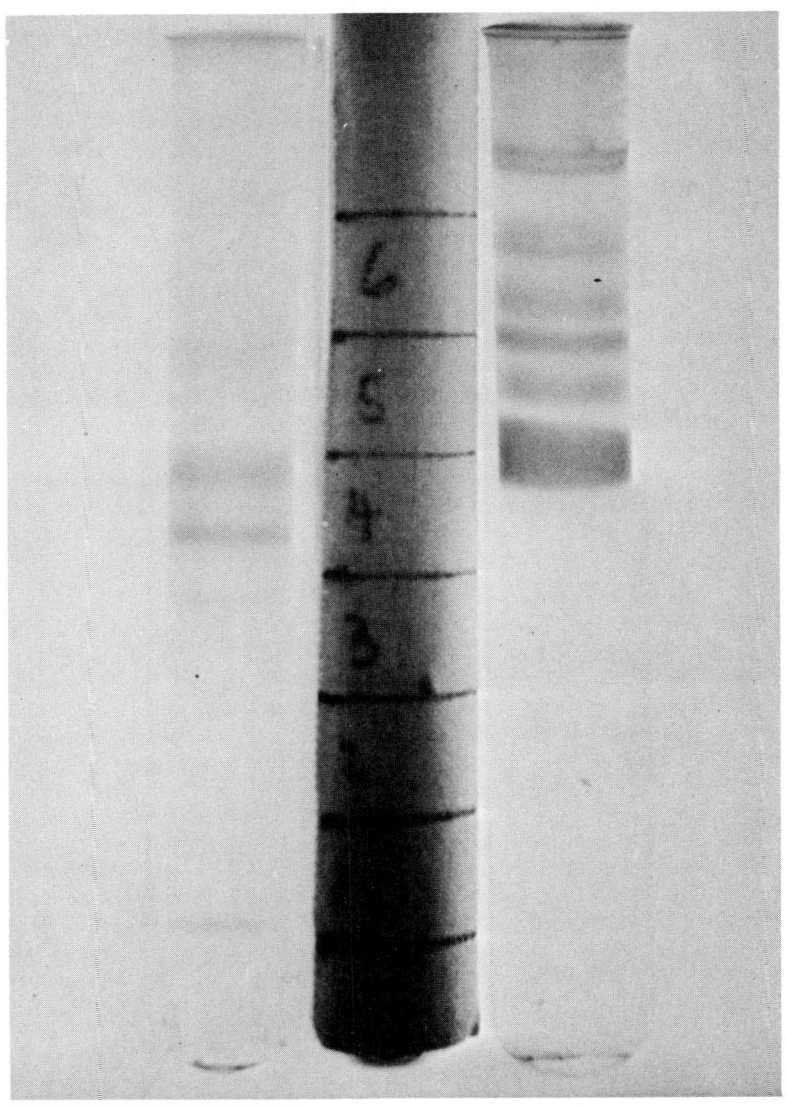

CELLULAR IMMUNITY

Fig. 31 Disc acrylamide gels stained with Coomasie blue. The tube on the left shows the staining pattern of MIF containing supernatant pre-purified on Sephadex G100; the tube on the right shows the staining pattern of normal guinea pig serum. The middle tube indicates the manner in which the gels were cut and labelled. The area above fraction 6 was pooled with fraction 6. Note that MIF activity is found in fraction 3 and that no albumin is contained in that fraction. The staining pattern of control (not antigen stimulated) supernatants is the same as the pattern of supernatants from antigen stimulated cells. (From H. Remold, E. Haber and J. David).

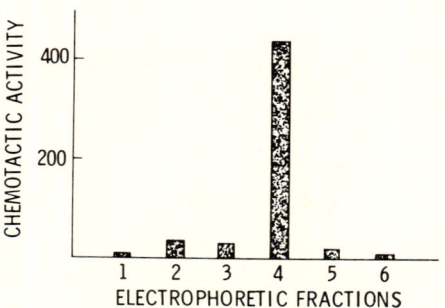

Fig. 32 Representation of chemotactic activity for macrophages of fractions eluted from acrylamide gels following electrophoresis of prepurified MIF-containing supernatants. Chemotactic activity assayed by Dr. Peter Ward, is measured by the number of cells which have crossed a millipore filter. Note that chemotactic activity is in fraction 4 and not in fraction 3.

(From P. Ward, H. Remold and J. David).

IV. BIOLOGICAL ACTIVITIES OF LYMPHOCYTE PRODUCTS

When unstained gels were cut into four mm slices starting from the buffer front, and the material in each eluted by further electrophoresis, MIF activity was consistently found in fraction 3, (Table 25) that migrating anodally to the albumin. Albumin is found in fraction 4. This active fraction 3, contained one clear band and two faint ones. Since no new bands could be seen in the MIF-containing fraction, not present in the control fraction, some people have suggested that instead of being called MIF, it should be known as ENCF, or the Emperor's New Clothes Factor.

TABLE 25

DETECTION OF MIF ACTIVITY IN FRACTIONS ELUTED FROM DISC ACRYLAMIDE GELS

Disc Fraction	% Migration				
	Exp. 1	2	3	4	Average
6	102	77	99	97	94
5	88	98	93	92	93
4	109	91	100	96	99
3	62	58	44	--	55
2	102	81	98	104	96
1	96	94	90	100	99

While I was working on this system at N.Y.U. with Drs. Al-Askari, Lawrence and Thomas, Dr. Thomas raised the possibility that chemotaxis might play a role in this reaction. Bennett and Bloom showed that MIF-containing Sephadex purified material produced a skin reaction resembling delayed-type hypersensitivity lesions, which raised the question of how the mononuclear cells got to the injection site of the MIF. In collaboration with Dr. Ward, supernatants rich in MIF have been assayed for chemotactic activity *in vitro* using Boyden chambers. In this system, two small chambers are separated by a millipore filter and mononuclear cells from normal peritoneal exudates are placed in the top chamber. If a chemotactic agent is added into the lower chamber, the cells will migrate through the millipore filter and can be counted on the undersurface. We found that MIF-containing supernatants were consistently chemotactic both for rabbit and guinea pig macrophages, whereas supernatants from sensitized cells is not stimulated with antigen, were not. Thus, the chemotactic factor is similar to MIF in that its production is antigen specific, it is heat stable at $56^\circ C$ for 30 minutes, and it is eluted from G-100 Sephadex with the albumin marker. When fractions of activated lymphocyte supernatants prepared by acrylamide gel electrophoresis, were tested simultaneously for migration inhibitory and chemotactic activity, the latter was found only in fraction 4, while fraction 3 still contained the MIF activity but was not at all chemotactic. Thus MIF and the chemotactic factor seem to be separable from one another by acrylamide gel electrophoresis (Fig. 32).

While it is clear that MIF can inhibit the migration of macrophages, there has been much speculation as to the possibility that MIF might somehow activate the macrophages as manifested by a heightened reactivity to microorganisms may be detectable. We have hints that this may be the case, but it has been very difficult to obtain consistent proof. Clearly, however, MIF does not kill macrophages at least in the concentrations available to us. If one takes monolayers of macrophages and incubates them with migration inhibitory or control supernatants, there are times when one cannot see any difference, while at other times the macrophages seem to spread more in the culture containing MIF. Dr. Hawrylko in our laboratory has measured C_{14}-leucine incorporation into protein of macrophages exposed to control or MIF-containing supernatants. Incorporation of leucine appeared to be greater in both control and MIF-containing supernatants than in normal media. At the moment, though, we do not have definite proof that the macrophages are activated.

IV. BIOLOGICAL ACTIVITIES OF LYMPHOCYTE PRODUCTS

The last matter I would like to consider is whether antigen is necessary for MIF activity. At the outset, let me say that it is very difficult to remove every molecule of antigen in the supernatants of antigen-triggered cells. There are certain experiments, however, which suggest rather strongly that antigen is not necessary for MIF to act. In the first set of experiments, carried out with Drs. Meyers and Shoji, BGG sensitive lymphocytes were incubated with BGG for 24 hours, washed three times and incubated for an additional 24 hours without antigen. The resulting supernatant had considerable MIF activity. This supernatant was divided into two aliquots; one was tested directly while the other had 100 µg of BGG added to it. Both aliquots inhibited migration equally well, and the ability of the supernatant to inhibit migration was not augmented by further addition of antigen. One may still question just how much antigen was present in the first aliquot. When the experiment was repeated using I_{125}-labelled antigen only about 0.15 µg of antigen was detected. Thus the migration inhibitory activity of supernatants was identical whether antigen was present in amounts as small as 0.15 µg or as large as 100 µg. This argues against MIF having to combine with antigen in order to inhibit migration. If this 0.15 µg were added directly to sensitized exudates, one would get negligible inhibition, even less than seen here with the supernatants tested on normal macrophages. In the case of the inhibitory acrylamide gel fraction 3, we can detect no I_{125}-labelled antigen above background for the gel.

In pursuing this question further with Dr. Schlossman, using the dialysable low molecular weight antigen, alpha DNP-lys_{11}, which was radioactively labelled, we found that supernatants of sensitized cells triggered by antigen were active even after exhaustive dialysis. In this case, the amount of antigen remaining was only about 0.02 µg and here too, further addition of antigen did not increase the migration inhibitory activity.

All of these experiments indicate that MIF activity is not dependent on the presence of antigen. While there always remains a trace of antigen, it seems most unlikely that this trace is involved in the activity. We would therefore conclude that MIF is a molecule which acts directly and non-specifically on macrophages to inhibit their migration.

DR. BLOOM: I should like to interject a personal note, if I may, to confess a bias or prejudice that all of us working on effector mechanisms in hypersensitivity were unwittingly captive of. As the elaborate gyrations of Dr. David's experiments on the presence of antigen in the MIF fractions indicate, we had all started out conditioned to look for an antibody as the mediator of delayed-type reactions, but we never found one. In retrospect, it seems to me that the preconception that there had to be an antibody to mediate this response proved to be the major impediment to progress in this field for the last 25 years. We all know that for some immunologists it is almost unthinkable to consider reactions in terms other than involving antibodies. Thus, when Bennett and I were trying to demonstrate some in vivo biological activity for MIF, we obviously started by injecting a few ml intraperitoneally into normal guinea pigs, and challenging in the skin with tuberculin at various times. When that didn't work we persisted in injecting more and still more and we wasted liters of active supernatants before we finally gave up. We then turned to injecting the concentrated supernatants intradermally into normal guinea pigs and followed that by injecting PPD and OT intravenously. We were disturbed by two observations -- first, a rather high degree of non-specific toxicity resulting from culture supernatants, made in the presence of 10-15% serum and concentrated tenfold before injection into normal guinea pig skin, and second, the fact that injection of antigen intravenously had no effect. We then devised simple culture conditions for the production of MIF, by triggering lymphocytes with antigen in completely serum-free medium. When that was accomplished, we found that upon injection of the control supernatants into normal guinea pig skin, no toxicity or reactions of any consequence could be seen. In contrast, injection of migration inhibitory supernatants alone, in the absence of antigenic challenge of the animal, resulted in reactions of induration and erythema, detectable as early as three hours, maximal at six to ten hours, and markedly diminished at 24 hours. Upon histological sectioning of these reaction sites we found that, at the early intervals (4-6 hours), the lesions were predominantly mononuclear, and looked very much like typical active delayed-type hypersensitivity reactions; later on, there was clear focal epidermal necrosis with an infiltrate consisting of half neutrophils and half mononuclear cells. Using inbred

IV. BIOLOGICAL ACTIVITIES OF LYMPHOCYTE PRODUCTS

guinea pigs to eliminate any histoincompatibilities, the same reactivity was found in Sephadex purified MIF preparations injected in amounts as small as 1 µg protein containing only 1% residual PPD.

While it seems that MIF does not require antigen for its activity, one must recognize that in unfractionated supernatants of cultures of sensitized lymphocytes, some antibody is also invariably present. By adding C_{14}-leucine to the medium and doing co-precipitation studies, a very slight amount of newly formed specific antibody is detectable in these cultures. It is noteworthy that antibody is found both in the non-stimulated and in antigen-stimulated cultures, although there is probably more present in the stimulated cultures. In cultures of lymph nodes taken two weeks after immunization, such demonstration of antibody should occasion no surprise. It does, however, point up the hazard of working with unfractionated supernatants if one wants to prove an effect attributable to MIF.

DR. GRANGER: Have you tested your MIF fraction to determine whether, in appropriate dilutions, it would have any chemotactic effect?

DR. DAVID: The chemotactic fraction loses its chemotactic activity with increasing dilution. However, the MIF preparations do likewise.

DR. GRANGER: What I really was trying to get at is whether it is possible to dilute the MIF fraction down to the level where instead of inhibiting macrophages it would be chemotactic.

DR. DAVID: When the preparations are diluted, they are less and less inhibitory; at no time have we seen stimulation.

DR. WAXSMAN: Dr. Johanovsky has published data which seem to show stimulatory effects of antigen on sensitized cells. How is one to account for these findings. Have you an explanation?

DR. DAVID: We have tried to do some of the things that Dr. Johanovsky reported. For instance, he has incubated cells with small amounts of antigen, and one gets to a point where they make no MIF, even after the addition of more antigen, or alter natively, they are making MIF which is not increased by additional antigen. Our experiments utilized BGG as antigen whereas Johanovsky used PPD in the experiments you cite. There may be still other differences that I don't know about.

It should also be noted that in this experimental situation, antibodies are also present. Consequently, antigen-antibody complexes can be formed and their possible effect should be reckoned with. In our system, however, they don't seem to make any difference since controls in which antigen is added to the supernatant evokes no further effects.

DR. BLOOM: In answer to Dr. Waksman's query, I think that both his question, and Dr. David's careful elucidation of one component of the reaction system are important. If one removes antigen after stimulating cells the supernatants are slightly inhibitory, however, upon restoration of antigen, the degree of inhibition doubled. The question has been repeatedly raised whether the 0.15 µg BGG, or 0.02 µg of DNP-$(lys)_{11}$ in Dr. David's experiments, or 0.03 µg PPD in ours, are amounts of antigen really sufficient to bind to the very small amounts of MIF present in these fractions. I believe this issue, at least for now, is best relegated to the Talmudic scholars.

Dr. David has shown, and we have subsequently confirmed that if one deals with the Sephadex purified material from the second peak, the addition of antigen to that fraction is without effect. More recently Dr. Weiser has reported that in the first peak of G-100 sephadex, using similar supernatants, there is a molecule which comes out in the first peak which has the characteristics of a cytophilic antibody, and an immunoglobulin, specific for antigen. In the presence of antigen this molecule will inhibit migration.

We are all in agreement that under appropriate conditions, antigen-antibody complexes inhibit migration, but then again, there is nothing mystical about the antigen dependent inhibitor of migration. The point to be made is that from now on if one is to do meaningful experiments with the effector known as MIF, it is mandatory to go beyond whole culture supernatants and employ instead the more purified

IV. BIOLOGICAL ACTIVITIES OF LYMPHOCYTE PRODUCTS

sephadex second fraction.

DR. WILSON: I wonder if it would be possible to get a little more directly at the problem of whether antigen is participating in MIF activity by using antigen coupled to an immuno-adsorbent. Have you tried this, or do you know if anyone has?

DR. DAVID: Amos and Lachman have used an antigen attached to solid particles. With PPD they could remove the antigen by centrifugation and decrease the amount of inhibition. However, when PPD was restored the degree of inhibition was increased.

DR. DIXON: How can you distinguish a chemotactic effect from MIF not only in vivo, but also in the *in vitro* systems? If chemotaxis occurred at a given anatomical site there would be an accumulation of cells if cells wandering at random through a similar site were immobilized there would also be an accumulation of arrested cells. Whatever you are liberating in the capillary tubes, whether it is inhibitory of chemotactic, the end point also would be the same.

DR. DAVID: We were surprised to find that you could separate the effects, but the fact is that they do appear to separate by gel electrophoresis. For chemotaxis, one needs a gradient. If the chemotactic agent is put in Boyden chambers on the same side as the mononuclear cells, they do not move through the millipore filter. It is of interest that the material in fraction 4, which did not inhibit macrophage migration *in vitro* was chemotactic, whereas the fraction which did inhibit macrophage migration was not. As a result, the familiar situation involving sensitized peritoneal cells in capillary tubes represents either an absence of sufficient gradient of the chemotactic factor or else that the inhibitory effect of MIF dominates the reaction.

DR. DIXON: But the only way you can measure chemotaxis is by putting the factor far away from the cell to establish a gradient; by definition you can't do that either *in vivo* or in the capillary tube, can you?

DR. DAVID: I would think you could establish a chemotactic gradient in vivo, whereas it would be exceedingly difficult to do so in a migration chamber.

DR. DIXON: I would like to speak to two of Dr. Bloom's comments at this point. First, I think it is difficult to use the histological character of the lesions in various hypersensitivity diseases as evidence for more than one cell type being specifically involved. In some delayed type reactions such as experimental allergic encephalomyelitis (EAE) in the rat, the great majority of the cells found about blood vessels in the central nervous system (CNS) are small lymphocytes; in some more granulomatous lesions associated with bacterial hypersensitivity most of the cells are larger mononuclear cells and macrophages. This spectrum of histologic lesions may not reflect the cell types specifically sensitized but rather depend upon secondary events related to the tissues involved etc. The second point I would like to touch on is the idea that Dr. Bloom mentioned in relation to the viral encephalitides. He suggested that viral infections of the CNS might liberate or spill central nervous system antigens as a result of injury and that the host might then develop a hypersensitivity to these antigens. While this is a possibility, it is also possible to develop perivascular mononuclear infiltrates in the CNS with circulating antibodies to virus residing there. In mice with chronic lymphocytic choriomeningitis (LCM) infections there is readily demonstrable viral antigen in the CNS, choroid and meninges with little or no apparent histologic reaction. If one injects intrathecally into such an LCM carrier mouse, homologous or heterologous anti LCM antibody there will be focal perivascular exudates of polymorphonuclear cells within an hour or two and within one or two days there will be sizeable perivascular exudates of mononuclear cells. In this situation only serum antibody has been added to a chronically infected animal and perivascular mononuclear infiltrates result, suggesting that the specific immunologic message was carried by circulating antibody even if the final lesion involved a mononuclear infiltration.

DR. SMITH: I have a question to pose on behalf of the uninitiated. Is MIF produced only by the reacting cells? Do the other cells in the population produce it in

IV. BIOLOGICAL ACTIVITIES OF LYMPHOCYTE PRODUCTS

sympathy or reactively? Does the same two percent of the population which transforms, produce MIF?

DR. DAVID: The initiation of the reaction requires interaction of specific antigen with specifically sensitized cells as shown by many studies, with various antigens. We do know that only a few sensitized lymphocytes suffice to produce enough MIF to effect many macrophages, however, we do not know whether in this process other lymphocytes capable of synthesizing additional MIF are recruited. Until such time as it is possible to label these cells elaborating MIF, it will not be possible to provide any quantitative data on the number of responding cells.

DR. MOLLER: What is the evidence that a factor is produced and not that an inhibitor is used up.

DR. DAVID: First, inhibitors of protein synthesis prevents MIF production. Secondly, fractions are either dialyzed against normal tissue culture media and then serum added before assay on macrophages, or are reconstituted in normal media so that inhibitors would not result from the lack of a nutrient factor.

DR. MOLLER: I do, of course, believe that a factor is produced but my alternative is a theoretical possibility. As long as you can't positively identify it as a factor actually present in the challenged cultures and lacking in control cultures, there is still a possibility that you have instead removed something.

DR. UHR: In regard to Dr. Dixon's comment, what happens if a known chemotactic factor is placed in the capillary tube with peritoneal exudate cells; is migration inhibited?

DR. DAVID: We have not done that.

DR. UHR: The puromycin experiment clearly shows that protein synthesis is necessary, but it does not show that the protein that is produced is necessarily MIF. The protein could also be concerned with the transport or secretion of MIF, or its conversion from an inactive to an active form.

DR. BLOOM: It seems to me that we already have convincing data for synthesis. I have already pointed out that we can change the medium daily, and find that about the same levels of MIF are produced again and again until the culture dies. We have made as many as five daily changes of media. It is hard for me to believe that this represents other than net-synthesis -- can you visualize these cells continucusly releasing pre-existent materials; I think not.

DR. DUTTON: To come back to Dr. Smith's question, am I right to think that there is no evidence as to how many of the cells are actually making MIF? But is there any evidence to decide between the opposing alternates whether it is all the cells or an extremely small number?

DR. DAVID: No, I know of no evidence on what proportion of the lymphocytes are making MIF.

DR. SALVIN: I would like to introduce the thought that the process of macrophage inhibition is more than merely migration inhibition. We have been looking at the reaction of individual cells rather than the mass migration of cells. To this end, we have devised a technique whereby we can observe the activity of individual cells on an agar surface. We use peritoneal exudate cells, lymph node cells, purified cell fractions from these sources, and a filtrate from sensitized lymph node cells after exposure to specific antigen. Such cells are washed, then placed on the surface of the agar and incubated in a moist chamber at $37^{\circ}C$. We have found that there is a very striking correlation between the morphologic appearance of the cells and the inhibition of migration. This is shown clearly in the photographs of these migrating cells taken under phase microscopy (Fig. 33).

When normal peritoneal exudate cells are migrating in the presence or absence of antigen, or when purified macrophages are migrating in the absence of specific MIF, the cells have extensive cytoplasmic processes extending from the cell and appear to be actively motile. Large quantities of granules and vacuoles are consistently absent (Fig. 33A).

IV. BIOLOGICAL ACTIVITIES OF LYMPHOCYTE PRODUCTS

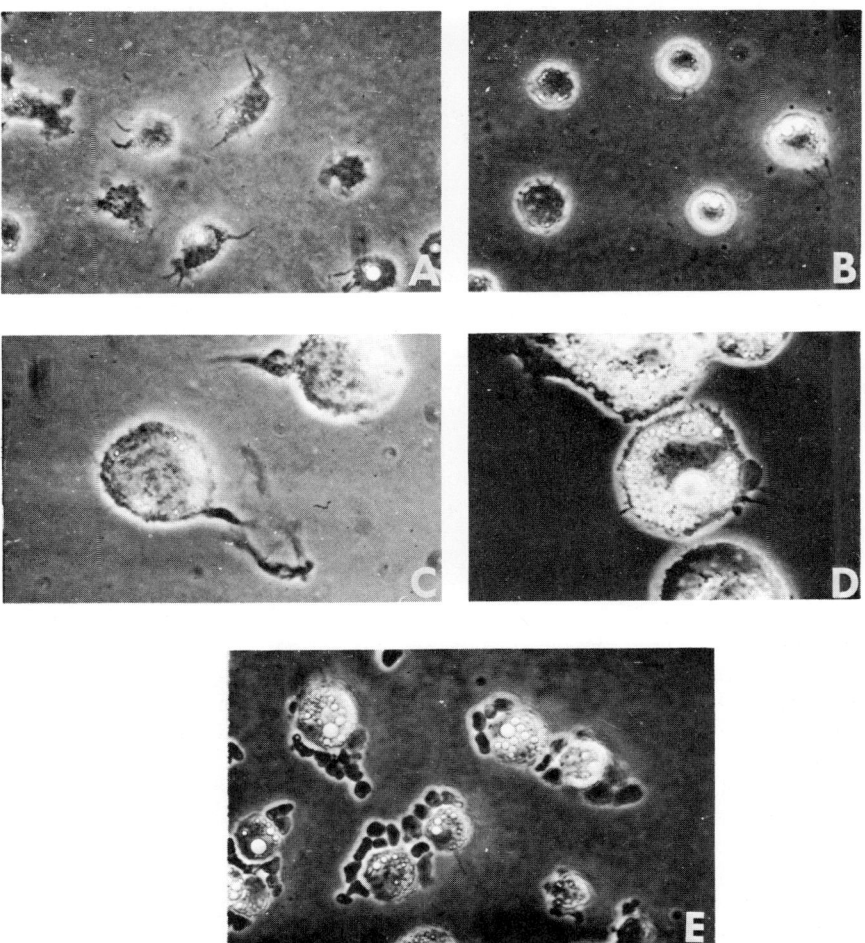

Fig. 33 Lymphoid cells maintained on agar for 48 hours at 37^8C.

    A. Living peritoneal macrophages from guinea pigs sensitized to the tubercle bacillus. No PPD in agar. X350

B. Living peritoneal macrophages from guinea pigs sensitized to the tubercle bacillus. 30 µg/ml PPD in agar. X350

C. Sensitized peritoneal macrophage fixed in vapors of 1% osmium tetroxide for 30 minutes. No PPD in agar. X750

D. Sensitized peritoneal macrophages fixed in vapors of 1% osmium tetroxide for 30 minutes. 30 µg/ml PPD in agar. X750

E. Sensitized lymphocytes with normal macrophages. 30 µg/ml PPD in agar. X350

When we induce migration inhibition of macrophages, the morphology of the cells undergo profound changes. When there is extensive inhibition, the cells are rounded up, have a more refractive cell wall, and are highly granular or vacuolar. In neither the migrating nor the inhibited cells is there an indication of active mitosis. Yet, at least at this point, the cells are still alive (Fig. 33B). In further attempts to differentiate between migrating and inhibited cells, the macrophages have been fixed "in situ" with osmic acid vapor. Under higher power magnification, a normal macrophage that has been killed with osmic acid and examined under phase microscopy, possesses few visible cytoplasmic inclusions (Fig. 33C). However, on exposure to sensitized lymphocytes with antigen, or on exposure to MIF itself, such macrophages develop large quantities of yellowish cytoplasmic granules (Fig. 33D).

We have noted that when normal macrophages from strain 13 guinea pigs are mixed with sensitized lymphocytes from strain 13 guinea pigs in the presence of antigen, or when sensitized peritoneal exudate cells are incubated with antigen, there is a tendency for the sensitized lymphocytes to adhere to the macrophages (Fig. 33E). This adherence indicates more than cells merely sticking to each other. The lymphocytes look as if they are trying to embrace the macrophages. What is actually happening cytologically is under study and still remains to be determined.

IV. BIOLOGICAL ACTIVITIES OF LYMPHOCYTE PRODUCTS

Another quite separate point I would like to make is with regard to the induction of hypersensitivity with soluble vs. insoluble antigens, and with the detection of this hypersensitivity by in vitro procedures. When whole tubercle bacilli are injected into the footpads of guinea pigs to induce delayed hypersensitivity and the lymphoid cells are examined from about one week to about nine months after sensitization, there is a gradual increase in the ability of lymphocytes to inhibit the activity of macrophages in the presence of specific antigen. In other words, if in vitro macrophage inhibition is plotted against time after sensitization, there is a gradual increase with time in the amount of inhibition - at least for the nine months during which our studies were conducted.

This behavior is strikingly different from that associated with a soluble antigen, such as BGG or diphtheria toxoid injected in footpads for sensitization of the guinea pig. When peritoneal exudate cells from such animals were examined in vitro, macrophage inhibition appeared at about day five after sensitization; the time sensitivity could be detected by skin testing. By day eight, this ability of the lymphocytes in the presence of antigen to inhibit macrophages in vitro rapidly declined. Such diminished response corresponded in time with the appearance of circulating antibodies. Thus, the decline of in vitro delayed hypersensitivity coincides with the development of conventional antibody. Does antibody therefore directly regulate the development of in vitro delayed hypersensitivity or does it combine and thereby inactivate the antigen that may still be in the tissues? Lymphocyte-macrophage interaction may therefore involve a good deal more than migration inhibition.

DR. GOOD: I believe Dr. Salvin has raised what continues to be a crucial issue in this work and was the focus of the previous session. Are we dealing with inhibition or is this really activation? The cells that Dr. Salvin has shown us with the processes extruded, look to me rather like my children ready for Sunday dinner, whereas the cells after treatment with MIF remind me of the way my children look later on after the big Sunday meal. Have these macrophages been phagocytizing and then settle down to digest their meal? I still believe the crucial issue is whether these factors, such as MIF, etc. are stimulating in appropriate dilution or whether in higher concentrations they are somehow damaging the cells. The question raised by Dr. Granger concerning Dr. David's experiment seems to me especially relevant; can you dilute out the acrylamide fraction 4 so that the migration-inhibiting factor then produces a chemotactic effect?

DR. DAVID: I do not know how far Dr. Ward has managed to dilute fraction 4; this will have to be determined. Dr. Good, you have asked previously whether inhibition of migration was analogous to immune adherence. I would like, finally, to answer this question. With Dr. Cochrane we have treated our inhibitory culture supernatants with cobra venom factor, which is known to destroy $C'3$. Since this produced no loss in MIF activity it is assumed that this phenomenon does not require a functional complement system and would therefore be distinguished from immune adherence.

DR. WAKSMAN: I would like to address myself to a question that several conferees have raised. Are we talking about something that is really inhibition, i.e. something negative about the target cell, or are we really dealing with stimulation. We published a study of this question ten years ago with Mrs. Matoltsy, using monolayers of guinea pig peritoneal exudate cells that contained an unknown number of sensitized lymphocytes. The principal finding was a clearcut stimulation of glass-adherent macrophages in the presence of specific antigen. This could be measured in two ways. First we estimated the actual number of surviving mononuclear cells in the culture; counts were made of remaining viable (trypsin-resistant) cells at various times. By this technique, in cultures exposed to specific antigen, the number of cells was sustained over 24 or 48 hours or even increased above the starting level. This finding clearly implied an actual cell multiplication in macrophages of the target monolayer. In addition, there was a rapid morphologic change in the macrophages over 24 to 48 hours from small monocytic cells, that were hard to distinguish from lymphocytes, to large active macrophages, full of vacuoles which took up neutral-red.

In all discussions of in vitro tuberculin sensitivity, since the original Rich and Lewis reports, the emphasis has always been on inhibition, or cell killing. Yet among

IV. BIOLOGICAL ACTIVITIES OF LYMPHOCYTE PRODUCTS

the better recent studies, which, for example, quantitate cells that migrate out of spleen fragments, there are several that suggest under some conditions, <u>stimulation</u> of the cells rather than killing can be obtained. There are some reports which show stimulation first, followed by killing and others which suggest that there is stimulation when the culture conditions are favorable and killing when the culture conditions are poor.

Thus the migration inhibition studied by Drs. David and Bloom is semantically misleading, not that they have ever sought to mislead their colleagues. However, the fact of inhibition has somehow suggested damage, yet it does not really imply anything of the kind. It is well recognized by people who study macrophages that an activated macrophage is more sticky than the non-activated monocyte. Migration inhibition could be therefore accounted for simply as cell stickiness.

I want to tell you about two experiments which demonstrate that macrophages are activated in the presence of supernatants of the type which contain MIF, presumably they also contain all the other factors that Dr. Bloom has listed. I would like to demonstrate some of the findings in the original Matoltsy work. The difference between monocytes as they appeared on the day the culture was started and the macrophages remaining in culture at 48 hours when they have been exposed to the specific antigen are shown in Fig. 34. The control cultures, meaning those to which no antigen was added, or those of unsensitized peritoneal cells exposed to the antigen, did not develop cells of the type seen on the right for a long period of time in culture. They tended to remain in the original inactive form. Here then we have clear evidence of activation.

In current experiments in our laboratory, Dr. Mooney uses rabbits sensitized by footpad injection of Freund's adjuvant. The draining lymph node cells are removed from these rabbits at either ten or fourteen days, washed, and then cultured for 24 hours with PPD, at concentrations of 10 or 20 µg/ml. The supernatant is either used immediately or kept at $-70°C$ and used several days later.

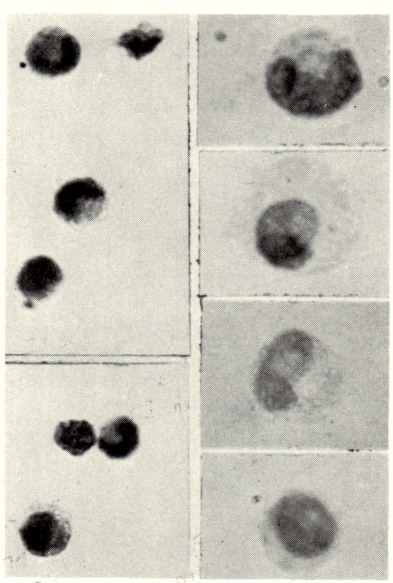

Fig. 34 Change in size and character of peritoneal exudate monocytes from tuberculin-sensitized guinea pig when cultured in presence of control medium (left) or OT 1:300 (right) for 48 hours. Sensitized lymphocytes in original suspension remained present in culture (Reproduced with permission of Journal of Immunology).

The data summarized in Table 26 consist of results from two experiments in which such a supernatant was added to a fresh culture of normal rabbit peritoneal exudate macrophages. These cells had been allowed to settle on the plastic of a Falcon flask and then washed very vigorously, to remove non-adherent cells. The overwhelming majority are macrophages. Counts were made of fully extended cells, partially extended cells, and round cells.

These data show two things. First of all, with the supernatant from sensitized lymph node cells and PPD, that is in the actual test culture, a considerably higher proportion of the total cells remained adherent after 24 hours. That represents stickiness. At 48 hours the difference is even more marked; the stimulated macrophages continue to adhere to the plastic.

IV. BIOLOGICAL ACTIVITIES OF LYMPHOCYTE PRODUCTS

TABLE 26

Macrophage Activation by Supernatant Factors

Experiment	No. of flasks	Adherent Cells x 10^5 24 hrs.	48 hrs.	Percentage Activated 24 hrs.	48 hrs.
Sensitized LNC + PPD					
I	4	48	35	44	32
II	3	36	33	47	37
Sensitized LNC only					
II	3	31	18	30	16
Normal LNC + PPD					
II	3	33	24	40	28
Normal LNC only					
II	2	30	17	29	12
PPD + medium					
I	4	24	16	22	11
II	2	27	17	36	26
Medium					
I	3	18	12	17	20
II	2	21	13	21	15

Supernatants harvested from 24 hour cultures of sensitized or unsensitized lymph node cells exposed to PPD 20 µg/ml.

The last two columns show the percentage of cells on the plastic which are partially or fully extended at 24 and 48 hours and can be regarded as active, vigorous cells. Again, the proportion is much higher in the flask containing the test culture. Similar results were obtained in three additional experiments under slightly different conditions. There can be no question that these macrophages are activated in the presence of the supernatant from sensitized lymph node cells incubated with antigen.

The standard error of the mean in the various numbers in Table 26 was less than five percent of the actual numerical values given, so that the overwhelming majority of differences shown are quite significant. With the new data obtained in the subsequent experiments, I expect they will be still more so.

These cultures were carried out in medium containing 20 percent serum, which is a culture condition that favors activation of macrophages; so the control levels are high. I expect that when we repeat this experiment in lower concentrations of serum, control values will be substantially lower.

Shown in Fig. 35 is a summary of unpublished data from experiments of Nomoto, Gershon and myself, working with a hamster tumor in our laboratory. We also showed that when sensitized lymph node cells were incubated with tumor cells, that is to say with the antigen, and the supernatant was then added to normal macrophages, up to 50 percent of the macrophages after 6 to 12 hours in culture showed a similar activation. Dr. Nomoto called them motile cells, but this represents cells that are spread out and, i.e. activated in the same sense as indicated previously. The supernatant obtained from normal lymph node cells incubated with tumor did not produce this effect, nor the supernatant from sensitized lymph node cells incubated without antigen.

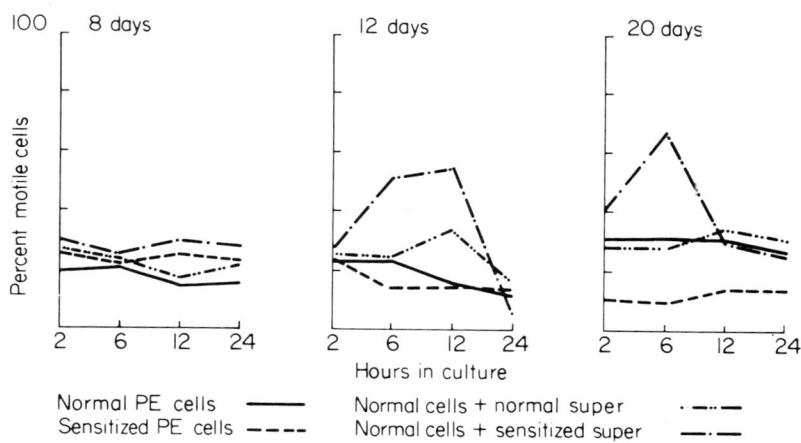

Fig. 35 Rapid increase in percentage of macrophages showing spreading on plastic, in cultures of normal macrophages exposed to supernatants from incubation of

IV. BIOLOGICAL ACTIVITIES OF LYMPHOCYTE PRODUCTS

specifically immune lymphocytes with hamster lymphoma. Control supernatants were obtained by incubating normal cells with tumor.

Here then, in a different animal species with a quite different system, one sees what appears to be numerically almost an identical result. These experiments provide strong evidence that macrophages under favorable culture conditions are indeed activated by the factors released from sensitized lymph node cells when they have reacted with antigen. Inhibition in the David system may be simply a manifestation of stickiness as shown in Table 26.

DR. SALVIN: I don't believe our present knowledge enables us to determine whether migration inhibition means stimulation or degeneration. Much more to the point would be to determine whether a macrophage under the influence of sensitized lymphocytes and antigen has altered metabolism and phagocytic activity. We are therefore now seeking to relate migration inhibition to skin reactivity as well as cell respiration, phagocytosis and enzyme changes in macrophages from guinea pigs sensitized with various antigens.

DR. TURK: Dr. Diengdoh and I did some experiments a few years back, looking at enzyme activity in macrophages. The system we used was an *in vivo* variant of the system of macrophage inhibition of migration, the system of Nelson and Boyden with the injection of antigen intraperitoneally in the sensitized animals, whereby the cells stick onto the walls of the peritoneal cavity. If you look at the cells before they stick you can see certain changes in the macrophages. Briefly, what we found was that they had decreased cell membrane permeability, and that molecules of around 800 molecular weight using DNP and TPN in the enzyme studies, could not get through the macrophage membrane. We followed this by showing that the macrophages also had a decreased electrophoretic mobility and thus a decreased electrostatic charge on their surface. We could reverse both of these phenomena by the use of either insulin or potassium ions. This is consistent with the effects on the macrophage cell surface being a charge effect and in some way this could be related to the decreased cell permeability and a decreased ion flow across the cell membrane.

DR. COHN: I want to know if the following statement is correct: In order to elicit the delayed hypersensitivity reaction, you require a substance which can also sensitize the animal. You can't elicit with a substance that cannot sensitize. In other words sensitization and elicitation require an immunogen. Is it also correct that in order to induce the migratory inhibitory factor in vitro that you also require an immunogen?

CHAIRMAN BILLINGHAM: You have achieved concurrence on these points. The answer is yes.

DR. GOOD· I am interested in hearing from Dr. Salvin whether those macrophages he showed us were full of agar, since if they are, it would do no good to give them something else to eat.

DR. SALVIN: We obviously have not determined this directly. We are currently studying macrophages for the presence of digestive enzymes.

DR. HIRSCHHORN: Dr. Conover when in Dr. Kuschner's laboratory at N.Y.U. utilized purified rat alveolar macrophages on glass to study the effect of industrial toxins, he was able to demonstrate that within short time that the macrophages resembled those shown by Dr. Salvin. This change did not occur if the cells were killed prior to the exposure to toxins, and eventually these cells died more rapidly than cells not exposed to toxin. I can't help wondering whether the phenomenon we observe, then, is endocytosis of a detrimental substance. I believe we have activation expressed as phagocytosis, then inhibition, resulting in some cases in cell death.

DR. SALVIN: Regarding the question of increased metabolism or respiration, it is known that phagocytizing macrophages do show increased respiration but it is not established whether macrophages under the influence of MIF show any of the same respiratory changes.

DR. BLOOM: There are at present at least two published reports and much unpublished data that I know if, consistent

IV. BIOLOGICAL ACTIVITIES OF LYMPHOCYTE PRODUCTS

with Dr. Salvin's finding that in the presence of a migration inhibitory supernatant, macrophages don't stick well to glass and they round up and look unhealthy. In Dr. Salvin's case on an agar substrate, he gets the same effect. In Waksman's experience on the other hand, and in some of David's experiments, it seems clear that the cells appear stimulated. It seems to me that further discussion of this point, will not resolve the issue in the absence of concrete metabolic data.

DR. THOR: There have been a number of questions raised about the cell migration system, and perhaps a discussion of some of our own work would serve to clarify a few of the problems. The first point I would make concerns our adaptation of the cell migration assay for use with human cells. In what I shall refer to as the "direct assay", we used human lymph node cell suspensions obtained from tuberculin hypersensitive patients cultured _in vitro_ for 72 hours to allow development of a migrating cell population. These cultured cells were collected, packed in capillary tubes and allowed to migrate in the presence or absence of specific antigen. Under these conditions we found that their migration was inhibited only by specific antigen.

Drs. David and Bloom reviewed primarily what I refer to as the "indirect" assay, i.e. one in which sensitized lymphocytes are cultured in the presence of specific antigen. Cells cultured with antigen elaborate MIF into the medium. Provided a highly sensitive donor is used, such culture supernatants can be used directly as a source of MIF without further concentration. When prepared in the absence of serum, other MIF preparations can be concentrated by pressure dialysis; fractionated on sephadex columns; and lyophilized without any diminution of activity. In the case of supernatants from human cells, we can easily test their MIF activity using guinea pig peritoneal exudate cells as the target or migrating cells. Thus MIF prepared from human lymphocytes is capable of inhibiting the migration of guinea pig macrophages.

In the indirect assay, normal macrophages are cultured in MIF containing supernatants. However, we have also looked at these normal macrophages, examined as cultured monolayers in control and MIF containing supernatants. The macrophages in culture for seven to nine days with serum

CELLULAR IMMUNITY

and MIF remain viable. When MIF is present and there is real inhibition of migration at 24 hours, the inhibited cells subsequently begin to escape and after 72 hours again migrate; i.e. they are affected but not killed.

We have also conducted some experiments in the cell migration system using both responder and non-responder guinea pigs to DNP-oligolysine antigens. The data in Table 27 were derived from an indirect assay in which guinea pig lymph node cell suspensions of strains 2 and 13 were incubated with specific antigen to which the donors had been sensitized. The culture supernatants were harvested, concentrated and added to normal guinea pig peritoneal exudate cells of the same strain.

TABLE 27

Direct Assay for Migration Inhibition. Capillary Tube Migration Indexes Using Peritoneal Exudate Cells from Sensitive Strain 2 or Non-Responder Strain 13 Guinea Pigs

Strain of Guinea Pigs	Immunogen[1]	Test Antigen[2]	Migration Indexes[3]					Mean M.I.[4]
2	α-DNP (lys)$_{8.4}$	α-DNP	35	43	27	39	46	38.0
		ε-DNP	108	96	99	111	95	101.8
2	ε-DNP (lys)$_{14}$	ε-DNP	48	29	32	21	36	33.2
		α-DNP	94	103	109	97	92	99.0
13	α-DNP (lys)$_{8.4}$	α-DNP	93	95	97	101	102	97.6
		ε-DNP	99	112	96	95	108	102.0
13	ε-DNP (lys)$_{14}$	ε-DNP	104	102	113	107	111	107.4
		α-DNP	109	106	102	104	105	105.2

1 - Immunizing material given in Complete Freund's Adjuvant.

2 - Respective antigen placed in tissue culture media inside the Sykes-Moore closed tissue culture chambers.

3 - Migration Indexes (M.I.) given here represent duplicate values for 3 chambers or 6 individual measurements calculated as
$$\frac{\text{Average Area of Migration with Antigen}}{\text{Average Area of Migration without Antigen}} \times 100 = \text{M.I.}$$

4 - Mean M.I. is the mean of the 5 preceding different animals.

IV. BIOLOGICAL ACTIVITIES OF LYMPHOCYTE PRODUCTS

The first immunogen used in the responder strain 2 guinea pigs, was α-DNP-(lys)$_{8.4}$. When added to sensitized cells it elicited production of MIF. However, when cells sensitive to α-DNP-(lys)$_{8.4}$ were challenged in vitro with a different antigen, in this case ϵ-DNP-(lys)$_{14}$, no inhibitory supernatants resulted. When the reciprocal experiment was performed, with ϵ-DNP-(lys)$_{14}$ being the immunogen, migration inhibitory supernatants were obtained only when the cells were challenged in vitro with ϵ-DNP-(lys)$_{14}$, and not with α-DNA-(lys)$_{8.4}$. The strain 13 animals, referred to as non-responders were incapable of responding to either of these immunogens as test antigens.

Instead of looking for the production of MIF, the experiment can be performed using the incorporation of tritiated thymidine into DNA as the indicator of lymphocyte activation. The results of such an experiment are given in Table 28.

TABLE 28

Indirect Assay for Migration Inhibition. Capillary Tube Migration Indexes Using Lymph Node Cell Suspensions* from Sensitive Strain 2 or Non-Responder Strain 13 Guinea Pigs

Strain of Guinea Pigs	Immunogen	Test Antigen	Migration Indexes					Mean M.I.
2	α-DNP (lys)$_{8.4}$	α-DNP ϵ-DNP	37 114	54 93	50 96	61 104	31 95	46.6 100.4
2	ϵ-DNP (lys)$_{14}$	ϵ-DNP α-DNP	38 107	42 102	49 105	36 98	30 97	39.0 101.8
13	α-DNP (lys)$_{8.4}$	α-DNP ϵ-DNP	102 110	95 104	99 90	92 96	109 98	99.4 99.6
13	ϵ-DNP (lys)$_{14}$	ϵ-DNP α-DNP	103 106	108 93	101 95	111 97	105 91	105.6 96.4

* Suspensions incubated in the presence of antigen represented the potential M.I.F. supernatant fluids to be added to the Sykes-Moore closed chambers containing the indicator cell population. Indicator cells were non-sensitive guinea pig peritoneal exudates from the same strain placed in capillary tubes.

Lymph node test suspensions were incubated with homologous and heterologous antigens. When the cells were cultured with the antigen used for sensitization there was a considerable increase in incorporation of thymidine relative to the non-stimulated controls. Again, the heterologous antigen, for example α-DNP-(lys)$_{8.4}$ tested on cells sensitive to ε-DNP-(lys)$_{14}$ was without effect and the results did not differ from non-stimulated controls. We have thus been able to stimulate lymphocytes of strain 2 guinea pigs sensitized to different DNP-oligolysines to make MIF or incorporate tritiated thymidine in response to homologous antigen. Strain 13 animals could not be sensitized by either of these immunogens and their cells were non-reactive *in vitro* to challenge with each immunogen.

Table 29 shows the results of further experiments in which RNA isolated from lymph node cells of responder strain 2 guinea pigs, immunized to either antigen, was transferred to normal lymph node cells of either strain. Non-sensitive lymph node cells were incubated for 30 minutes at 37°C with 200 µg RNA. When the RNA-treated normal cells were exposed to specific antigen they were found to elaborate into the medium a factor which inhibited migration of normal macrophages. This material was eluted from sephadex G-100 in the second peak and thus resembled MIF. In addition, normal lymphocytes treated with specific RNA, incorporated more tritiated thymidine after exposure to specific antigen than to the heterologous antigen. However, there may be some non-specific effects produced by the ε-DNP-(lys)$_{14}$ which we are now investigating.

Table 30 shows the effect of addition of RNA obtained from sensitized responder animals to non-responder normal lymphocytes. I have indicated that we were unable to find any effect in strain 13 guinea pig using these two antigens as immunogens. RNA extracts from sensitized strain 2 lymphocytes were fractionated into the 5s-20s species on sucrose or cesium sulfate gradients. When 20-100 µg of this RNA was incubated with normal non-responder strain 13 lymph node cells, these cells then produced a MIF-like substance upon exposure to the specific antigen; antigen alone and RNA alone were ineffective. Non-responder cells treated with RNA from strain 2 animals sensitized to α-DNP-(lys)$_{8.4}$, responded when challenged with the homologous antigen, but not to ε-DNP-(lys)$_{14}$.

IV. BIOLOGICAL ACTIVITIES OF LYMPHOCYTE PRODUCTS

TABLE 29

Migration Index Using the Indirect Assay for M.I.F. Production and Radioactive Incorporation* of Non-Sensitive Strain 2 Guinea Pig Lymph Node Cells** Following Incubation with RNA Extracts Obtained from Sensitive Strain 2 Lymph Nodes.

IMMUNOGEN	α-DNP (LYS) 8.4		ε-DNP (LYS) 14		CONTROL CPM
	Ave. CPM	M.I.	Ave. CPM	M.I.	
ε-DNP (LYS) 14	2,032	90	39,360	32	874
α-DNP (LYS) 8.4	31,778	42	1,070	104	1125

* Radio incorporation as a measure of blast transformation was studied using tridiated thymidine.

** Values shown in the table represent the averaged findings of 5 recipients and 5 donors.

TABLE 30

Migration Index Using the Indirect Assay for M.I.F. Production and Radioactive Incorporation of Non-Responder Strain 13 Guinea Pig Lymph Node Cells Following Incubation with RNA Extracts Obtained from Responder Strain 2 Lymph Nodes*

IMMUNOGEN	α-DNP (LYS) 8.4		ε-DNP (LYS) 14		CONTROL CPM
	Ave. CPM	M.I.	Ave. CPM	M.I.	
α-DNP (LYS) 8.4	19,010	54	752	105	691
ε-DNP (LYS) 14	2,371	97	54,223	41	719

* Values given in the table represent the averaged values of 3 strain 13 studies incubated with RNA from 3 strain 2 animals.

IV. BIOLOGICAL ACTIVITIES OF LYMPHOCYTE PRODUCTS

DR. TURK: Could you briefly tell us how you prepared your RNA.

DR. THOR: The RNA that I referred to is extracted by a modification of the Sherrer and Darnell procedure using phenol-saturated acetate buffer (0.01M), extracting the buffer phase with hot phenol, and precipitating the RNA from the acetate buffer by 95% ethanol. The RNA can be re-extracted until the 260/280 O.D. ratio is equal to or greater than 2. This method extracts essentially all cellular RNA. The various species can then be separated either on sucrose or cesium sulfate density gradients. We have found activity in those parts of the gradient containing RNA's ranging in size from 4 to 18S. The highest activity seems to be associated with the fraction containing 5-10S RNA's.

DR. UHR: The RNA-rich preparations used in Dr. Thor's studies are of higher molecular weight than transfer factor, so the question arises as to whether their effects can be explained by a messenger RNA transmitting immunologic information to nonsensitive cells. In that regard, I would like to make two points: one, lymph node extracts have very high levels of RNAase activity. Unless heroic measures are taken to inhibit RNAase activity, any messengers present would be expected to be partially degraded.

The second point is that if there are intact messengers present that can penetrate plasma membranes analogous to DNA transformation of bacteria, the problem of assembly and transport in a compartmentalized mammalian cell must still be considered. For example, one would have to postulate that both the light and heavy chain messengers penetrate, that these messengers bind ribosomes, and that the resultant polyribosomes then attach to the proper sites on endoplasmic reticulum, in contrast to taking up residence in the cell cytoplasm where polyribosomes that are making non-secretory proteins are usually found. In addition, there may be further regulations of the assembly process. For example, light and heavy chain polyribosomes may have to be juxtaposed for efficient assembly. In other words, if we understood the processes of assembly, transport and secretion, there might be even more restraints about the possibility of messenger RNA's penetrating from the outside being responsible for IG synthesis and transport. I think it is much more likely that these RNA-rich preparations represent a special type of immunogenic situation.

DR. COHN: Dr. Thor gave us the controls for the specificity as regards the immunogen, but what were his controls for the specificity regarding the RNA?

DR. THOR: The RNA derived from tuberculin-sensitive outbred guinea pig lymphocytes can induce MIF production by normal lymphocytes as we have reported (J. Immunol., 101, 828, 1968). We have also reported on a similar situation in the human system with RNA from sensitized donors conferring the capacity for MIF production on non-sensitive recipient lymphoid cells (J. Immunol., 101, 469, 1968). In the controls that were listed in Table 30 which concerns the nonresponder strain 13's, these cells were incubated with strain 2 RNA, but without the antigen. The controls were four: (1) RNA from strain 13 animals, immunized but not responding in the presence of antigen, (2) RNA from strain 2, not immunized and without antigen, (3) RNA from strain 2, not immunized but with antigen, and (4) RNA from non-immunized strain 13's with and without antigen. None of these controls initiated MIF production.

DR. COHN: Therefore, you conclude that this is an RNA, which results from the induction by immunogen during immunization.

DR. THOR: Induction of some process within the immune mechanism. I do not believe the test necessarily implies an informational "RNA".

DR. BRAUN: I want to concur in Dr. Uhr's statement. I am glad to know that Dr. Thor likewise does not consider this to be an informational RNA.

DR. BACH: In his compilation of effector molecules Dr. Bloom included a blastogenic or mitogenic factor. I think it would be useful to review this story as it appears in the literature relating primarily to the phenomenon observed in mixed leucocyte cultures (MLC) and to summarize for you our recent results in relation to this factor. This activity was first described by Gordon and McClain and by Kasakura and Lowenstein almost simultaneously, and the

IV. BIOLOGICAL ACTIVITIES OF LYMPHOCYTE PRODUCTS

latter group suggested that the factor might in fact be a histocompatibility antigen. The factor is prepared in the following way: one person's peripheral blood leukocytes cultured either alone or as an MLC between two individuals. After varying periods of time, usually four days in our experience, the cell-free supernatant is obtained from these stage I cultures and tested for its ability to stimulate fresh cells of one individual in a stage II culture. The original authors had found that if cells of one individual alone were cultured, blastogenic factor was produced. It was reported that this blastogenic factor stimulated only cells of other individuals and not the cells of the same individual. It was for this reason that the conclusion was reached that this activity might be due to transplantation antigens released into the medium. It was also suggested that MLC's produced more of this blastogenic factor than individual cultures.

Together with Dr. Martin Janis, we have repeated these experiments and while confirming some of the findings we differ on other points made in the original studies. The amount of blastogenic factor activity in MLC is indeed more than that found in the culture of the cells of one individual alone. When one individual's cells are cultured alone, though much less activity is found in the supernatant, it will on the average stimulate isogeneic and allogeneic cells to the same extent. That is, we find the same degree of stimulation of isogeneic cells (i.e. cells from the same donor used in the stage one culture), as with allogeneic cells. In this important respect we cannot find any evidence for specificity of the supernatant factor, a finding which also argues against the activity being due to histocompatibility antigen.

In the MLC the maximum blastogenic factor activity is found at about four days and is present in the 105,000 G supernatant. The factor is excluded on G-25 sephadex; is trypsin sensitive; but is unaffected by treatment with DNAase or RNAase. We have sought to determine the specificity of the factor in unidirectional MLC. In the experimental mixture, a supernatant of a culture in which one person's untreated cells which had responded to the mitomycin C treated cells of another individual, is tested for blastogenic activity. Such findings may be criticized on the grounds that the mitomycin C treated cells of both reactors do not constitute a valid control. We have thus tried to get at the issue of specificity in another way with the following results: Cells of one individual stimulated with PHA, and put in contact with PHA for 12 to 16 hours, washed five times and then reincubated with fresh PHA - free medium for three to four days, yields maximum amounts of blastogenic factor.

Finally, the kinetics of release of blastogenic factor by PHA are strikingly similar to the kinetics of release in the MLC reaction. These considerations suggest that blastogenic factor is not PHA, and is moreover non-specific since cells isogeneic to those producing the factor are stimulated by it. Accordingly, it seems unlikely that blastogenic factor is a transplantation antigen. We are inclined to view it as a non-specific recruiting agent. There are obvious contrasts between the physical characteristics of blastogenic factor and dialysable transfer factor, although I am not sure there are differences between this factor and the factor that Drs. Valentine and Lawrence described earlier which is produced by sensitive lymphocytes incubated with tuberculin.

DR. VALENTINE: My question to Dr. Bach is for a point of information. My memory of the Kasakura and Lowenstein experiments is that by centrifugation at 100,000 X G, they could, in fact, sediment a good bit, if not a majority of their activity, even though they then referred to some remaining in the supernatant. This is of importance in our own experiments because our material, cannot, in fact, be sedimented; full supernatant activity remains after 100,000 X G centrifugation.

DR. BACH: Your memory is quite correct. They did have some activity left. This is another of their observations we cannot confirm. In our experiments, which involve conditions different from yours, we have subjected blastogenic factor to centrifugation at 105,000 X G and find that most of the activity remains in the supernatant. Let me make one thing clear; it is other authors who have regarded blastogenic factor as stimulating only allogeneic cells and not isogeneic ones. Dr. Janis and I think we see blastogenic factor produced by the cells of one individual affecting equally isogeneic and allogeneic cells.

IV. BIOLOGICAL ACTIVITIES OF LYMPHOCYTE PRODUCTS

DR. OPPENHEIM: I would like to identify another role for some of these factors such as MIF. The observations are non-quantitative and evident in in vitro cultures. It has been observed that separated lymphocytes, in the absence of the macrophages, in response to antigen manifest considerably less blastogenesis than in the presence of the macrophages. I would therefore suggest that MIF or lymphotoxin production may also relate to this phenomenon. The pictures shown by Dr. Salvin are intriguing, in this regard, because it does look as though cells become rather sticky and the so-called rosette formation ensues with lymphocytes adhering to and concentrating at the surface of the macrophages.

We approached this matter in inbred guinea pigs by experiments using mixtures of peritoneal macrophages and purified lymph node lymphocytes from immune versus non-immune animals. Dr. Seeger in our laboratory is determining whether immune macrophages can stimulate non-immune lymphocytes or whether non-immune macrophages can stimulate immune lymphocytes, and has obtained the following results. Only the immune lymphocytes (i.e. lymphocytes of sensitized animals), can be stimulated. However, under optimal circumstances they are stimulated equally well by macrophages pre-exposed to antigen, whether or not these macrophages are derived from immune or non-immune animals.

This would argue that the role of the macrophage in this system, is a non-specific one, and that it has no informational or direct instructional role. This may in turn be promoted in lymphoid cells by the effects of lymphocyte products on the macrophage such as MIF immobilization, increased aggregation, stickiness and rosette formation. Such a mutual interaction of lymphocytes and macrophages would produce a rapid amplification of an immune response.

DR. MOLLER: I would like to report some findings made by Dr. Falk in our laboratory, who has been successful in releasing factors from mouse, human and rat lymphocytes by means of corpuscular antigens (sRBC) and histocompatibility antigens. He tests these supernatants for migration inhibition but using spleen cells and peripheral blood lymphocytes rather than macrophages. The cells release a factor that inhibits the migration of lymphocytes; it is noteworthy that the same supernatant will also stimulate the lymphocytes to divide. Obviously inhibition of lymphocyte migration is entirely compatible with stimulation of lymphocytes. Perhaps in this case inhibition is due to stimulation of the lymphocytes which we believe results in cell agglutination.

Since Dr. Falk works with particulate antigens, he is able to remove the antigen by centrifugation, and add the supernatant to syngeneic cells. Even in that situation the factors work equally well; consequently, it does not appear to be antigen dependent. I would point out that this factor, added to fibroblast cultures, causes no cytotoxic effect. However, if lymphocytes are present on the fibroblasts, and the factor is added, the lymphocytes transform, become cytotoxic and the fibroblasts are killed. The phenomenon is also operative in completely autologous situations, that is, the patient's lymphocytes can be caused to act on his own fibroblasts, i.e. if the lymphocytes are triggered they become cytotoxic. Moreover, antisera to these supernatants can be raised. Such antisera, injected into rats, will prolong skin graft survival from control values of ten days up to as long as 25 days.*

---

* EDITOR'S FOOTNOTE: A cautionary comment is in order. A consensus has already been reached that activated lymphocyte culture supernatants contain a multiplicity of factors capable of mediating a variety of different effects. Experiments based on the use of neat, unfractionated supernatant culture fluids are therefore difficult if not impossible to interpret with respect to any single biologic activity.

Lymphocyte culture supernatants surely contain a host of newly synthesized proteins among which are the effector molecules that concern us here. Moreover, it is also likely that membrane antigens are also present in such supernatants either in soluble form or as small fragments. Viewed in this context, antisera prepared by immunization with unfractionated lymphocyte culture supernatants could be, among other things, anti-lymphocyte sera. In that event the action of such antisera would be directed against the lymphocytes themselves as well as their effector molecules.

IV. BIOLOGICAL ACTIVITIES OF LYMPHOCYTE PRODUCTS

DR. LAWRENCE: I would like to organize a schema of the activities either liberated from or produced by sensitive lymphocytes incubated with specific antigen. This family of molecules appears in the culture supernatant after varying periods of incubation, particularly, when human blood lymphocytes are used; activity is found to vary depending on the experimental assay model. We are now faced with the decision of which molecule or molecules are identical and which are different. Since they all seem to appear in the same supernatant simultaneously I would suggest that their susceptibility to inactivation by exposure to $56°C$ for 30 minutes be applied as a crude initial step in the separation of these activities; this despite the probability that there occurs a varying concentration of each activity in the undiluted medium.

As we have discussed earlier, and is shown in Fig. 36, transfer factor is liberated from sensitive cells after as short as one hour incubation with antigen as shown by in vivo transfer of sensitivity with such supernatants.

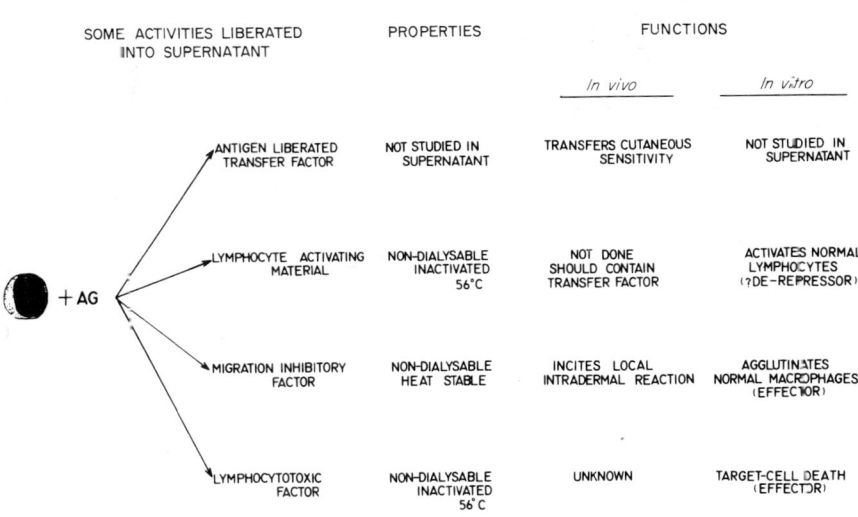

Fig. 36 Activities produced by or liberated from antigen-responsive human blood lymphocytes following interaction with specific antigen. Transfer Factor - liberated after 1 hr. incubation with antigen (Lawrence and Pappenheimer, 1956, 1957); Lymphocyte Activating Material - produced after 24 hrs. incubation with antigen (Valentine and Lawrence, 1968, 1969); Migration Inhibitory Factor - produced after 24 hrs. incubation with antigen - heat-stable MIF is produced by human lymphocytes, (Thor et al, 1968) some properties listed in this figure were obtained in the guinea pig (Bloom and Bennett, 1966; David, 1966); Lymphocytotoxic Factor - produced after 36 hrs. incubation with antigen (Kolb and Granger, 1968; Lebowitz and Lawrence, 1969).

(Reproduced with permission Advances in Immunology, 1969)

If this is the same molecule as that separated from leucocyte extracts by dialysis, the latter is inactivated by $56°$ for 30 minutes.

It must be stressed at this point that transfer factor differs markedly from the other materials present in the same supernatants (i.e. the effector molecules such as MIF and LT) in at least three distinctive properties: 1.) Transfer factor is not an effector molecule, but rather functions to convert non-sensitive lymphocytes to an antigen-responsive state. 2.) This conversion is immunologically specific and only very few cells are engaged. 3.) Lymphocytes converted to a sensitive state by transfer factor have been shown in the presence of specific antigen to produce an effector molecule (e.g. MIF produced in the presence of Candida antigen, see David's discussion, Session III this volume).

The next activity to consider is the material detectable after 36 hours incubation, that Valentine and I have studied, that causes non-sensitive lymphocytes to respond to antigen by transformation and clonal proliferation. This lymphocyte activating material is non-dialysable; not sedimented at 100,000 X G; and inactivated by $56°$ for 30 minutes. I would ask Dr. Bach is the blastogenic factor he is studying inactivated at $56°C$?

IV. BIOLOGICAL ACTIVITIES OF LYMPHOCYTE PRODUCTS

DR. BACH: We are not yet sure.

DR. LAWRENCE: The next activity to consider is the MIF of Dr. Bloom and Dr. David. This material of guinea pig origin is non-dialysable and unaffected by heat at $56^\circ C$ for 30 minutes. I would ask Dr. Thor whether the MIF produced by human lymphocytes is inactivated by heating at $56^\circ C$?

DR. THOR: The guinea-pig MIF is not inactivated, the human MIF is not inactivated and the rabbit MIF is not inactivated by heating at $56^\circ C$. Moreover, MIF activity produced by the lymphocytes of any of these three species can affect migration of macrophages from any of the others.

DR. LAWRENCE: Our next consideration is the cytotoxin produced by antigen-responsive human lymphocytes. Lebowitz and I have found this material is detectable after 36 hrs. incubation and it is non-dialysable and it is inactivated by heating at $56^\circ C$ for 30 minutes (Fed. Proc., 28, 630, 1969). I would ask Dr. Granger whether his lymphotoxin is inactivated by heating at $56^\circ C$ for 30 minutes?

DR. GRANGER: This depends on what species it is derived from.

DR. LAWRENCE: I agree, but is the material you have liberated from human cells incubated with tuberculin inactivated at $56^\circ C$ for 30 minutes?

DR. GRANGER: I can't answer that because we heat for 15 minutes.

DR. LAWRENCE: I would suggest heat lability as a relatively simple starting point to sort out the biological activities which appear in the same supernatants and are produced by the same responsive lymphocytes.

DR. LANDY: While appreciating the kind of organization of findings Dr. Lawrence is seeking, I want to re-emphasize a point raised by Dr. Granger. Heat lability need not be an absolute inasmuch as the lymphotoxin derived from various species differs markedly in this respect. This criterion would, therefore, be useful provided we restrict our comparisons to such data within a species.

DR. ROSENAU: I think that we should also be cautious in using differences in temperature sensitivity to conclude that various fractions are really different. Preparations of the same material but of different degrees of purity may show different temperature sensitivity.

DR. LANDY: Dr. Granger, do you have anything to add about the properties of lymphotoxin derived from murine cells?

DR. GRANGER: We have done extensive studies on the material released from PHA-stimulated normal mouse and human lymphocytes. Mouse lymphotoxin is stable up to $100^{\circ}C$ in MEM containing 10% serum. However, human lymphotoxin is inactivated by heating up to $85^{\circ}C$. Dr. Rosenau has raised a salient point; namely that heat sensitivity is influenced by the presence of other proteins in the medium. Before we can arrive at any firm conclusions regarding heat sensitivity, we will need some standard procedures of time, temperature and milieu.

DR. LAWRENCE: Of course, I agree with Dr. Granger's and Dr. Rosenau's cautionary note. However, until clean fractions of each lymphocyte activity are isolated, reasonably well purified and separable from the other activities, heat sensitivity of some but not other molecules present in the same supernatant can be applied as a crude measure of separating the various functions.

For example, the same supernatant prepared from antigen incubated human lymphocytes containing both MIF and lymphocyte activating material, when placed on non-sensitive lymphocytes causes their transformation, while supernatant heated at $56^{\circ}C$ for 30 minutes does not. This result at the very least affords suggestive evidence, even allowing for differences in concentration of each activity, that heat stable MIF is not the moiety causing non-sensitive lymphocytes to undergo transformation.

EDITOR'S FOOTNOTE: The kind of comparisons being made are clearly influenced to a major extent by the number or proportion of lymphocytes in the total population responding to antigen *in vitro*. This in turn is a consequence of the

IV. BIOLOGICAL ACTIVITIES OF LYMPHOCYTE PRODUCTS

DR. CHESSIN: I think another issue that can be brought up at this time is whether cells involved in immune reactions can be engaged in more than one function simultaneously. We have reported (Chessin et al., Ann. Int. Med., 69, 333, 1968) that continuous lymphoid cell lines derived from human blood are composed of a heterogeneous population of lymphoblastic cells capable of synthesizing, among other things, immunoglobulins, interferon and C'3. In addition, these cell lines contain cells capable of phagocytosis. In view of the growing list of the activities associated with cell mediated immunity (i.e. transfer factor, migration inhibitory factor (MIF), lymphotoxic factor, skin-reactive factor, chemotactic factor, mitogenic factor and interferon) it will be important to determine whether cells synthesizing immunoglobulins also make any or all of these effector molecules.

DR. TURK: I would like to comment on the skin reactive aspects of these mediators. The point at issue is, are the reactions produced in the skin by these mediators analogous to delayed type hypersensitivity as a large number of us

---

degree of sensitivity of the donor of sensitive cells. As previous discussions have already brought out the maximum figure for specific immune responses would not exceed two percent of antigen-responsive cells. Donors possessed of this degree of exquisite sensitivity are infrequently encountered and it is more likely that much of the results discussed have been obtained using cell populations in which the percentage of specifically reactive cells is actually far less than this figure.

At the other extreme we have discussed results obtained using mitogen-activated normal lymphocytes where it is now well-established that the overwhelming preponderance of cells from normal donors are in fact responding. This figure may range from as little as 60% to virtually all cells present.

Perhaps the point to be made is that under these contrasting conditions, culture supernatants vary so greatly in potency that marked quantitative differences could understandably be misconstrued for qualitative distinctions.

have been studying it in actively sensitized animals and in animals after passive transfer. The first type of reaction of this type was produced by Metaxas, many years ago by mixing peritoneal exudate cells with antigen and injecting them intradermally or by injecting the peritoneal exudate cells intradermally followed by antigen intravenously. Following this, we and others found that if we took purified lymphocytes from inbred animals, administered them with antigen, we could still produce this type of reaction. However these reactions develop between three and six hours after the intradermal injection -- thus differing markedly in their time course from the reactions produced in animals following systemic passive transfer or the reaction in the actively sensitized animal.

I think it might be profitable to illustrate some of these reactions that have been produced in my laboratory by Drs. Pick and Krejci by the intradermal injection of supernatants prepared from cultures of sensitized lymphocytes incubated with antigen (Fig. 37). These reactions at three to six hours are strikingly raised above the skin surface, and the induration and erythema is most marked (Fig. 37a).

In histologic sections of these lesions we have paid particular attention to the infiltrate around blood vessels. The appearance of the skin following the injection of the supernatant from a culture without antigen, is the same as that following injection of saline intradermally; just a few polymorphonuclears infiltrate the blood vessels (Fig. 37b). Six hours after the intradermal injection of the purified culture supernatant from the incubation of sensitized lymphocytes with antigen, the markedly indurated lesions contain a large number of polymorphonuclear cells and these persist for 24 hours. Mononuclear cells are noted to be in a minority. The presence of polymorphonuclear cells is not of particular concern as they are always present in the test sites of actively sensitized guinea pigs until about 48 hours (Fig. 37c,d).

IV. BIOLOGICAL ACTIVITIES OF LYMPHOCYTE PRODUCTS

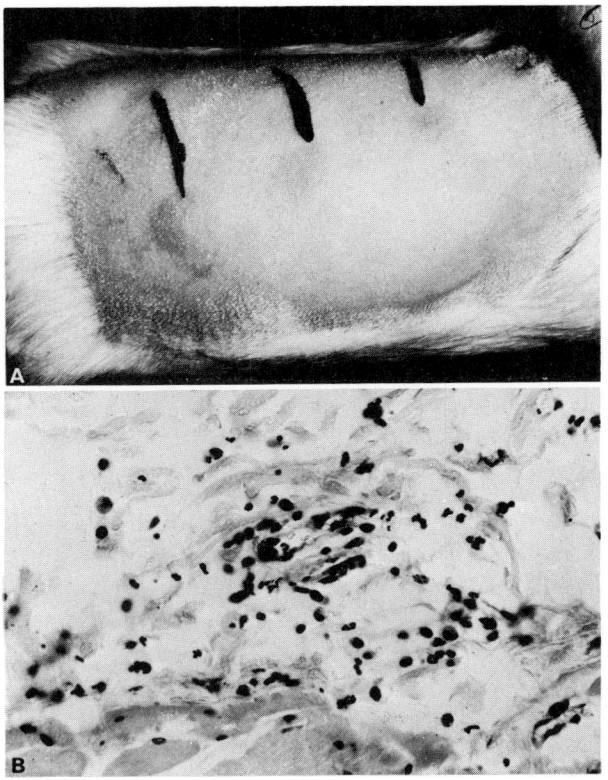

Fig. 37 Macroscopic aspect and histology of skin reactions induced by the intradermal injection of cell-free supernatants of sensitized peritoneal exudate lymphocytes cultured in the presence of specific antigen or PHA.

a) 6 hours skin reactions induced by (from left to right): supernatant of a culture containing 10 µg PPD/10^7 lymphocytes, containing 0.2 µg PPD/10^7 lymphocytes and supernatant of lymphocytes cultured without PPD.

b) Skin of a normal guinea pig 6 hours after the injection of 0.1 ml of supernatant of sensitized lymphocytes cultured without PPD (Haematoxylin eosin, X 250).

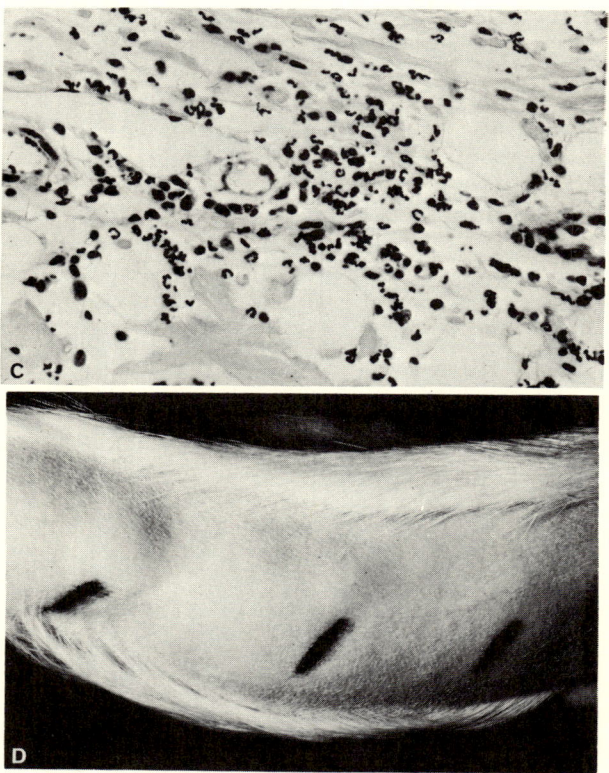

c) Skin of a normal guinea pig 6 hours after the injection of 0.1 ml of supernatant of sensitized lymphocytes cultured in the presence of PPD, 10 µg/10^7 cells (Haematoxylin eosin, X 250).

d) 6 hours skin reactions induced by (from left to right): supernatant of a culture of lymphocytes incubated with PHA, PHA alone and supernatant of lymphocytes cultured without PHA.

Fig. 38a depicts the sephadex G-200 fractionation of the supernatants and shows that our material is localized in a very concentrated peak corresponding to Dr. Bloom's peak for MIF. On DEAE cellulose, the material purified on

IV. BIOLOGICAL ACTIVITIES OF LYMPHOCYTE PRODUCTS

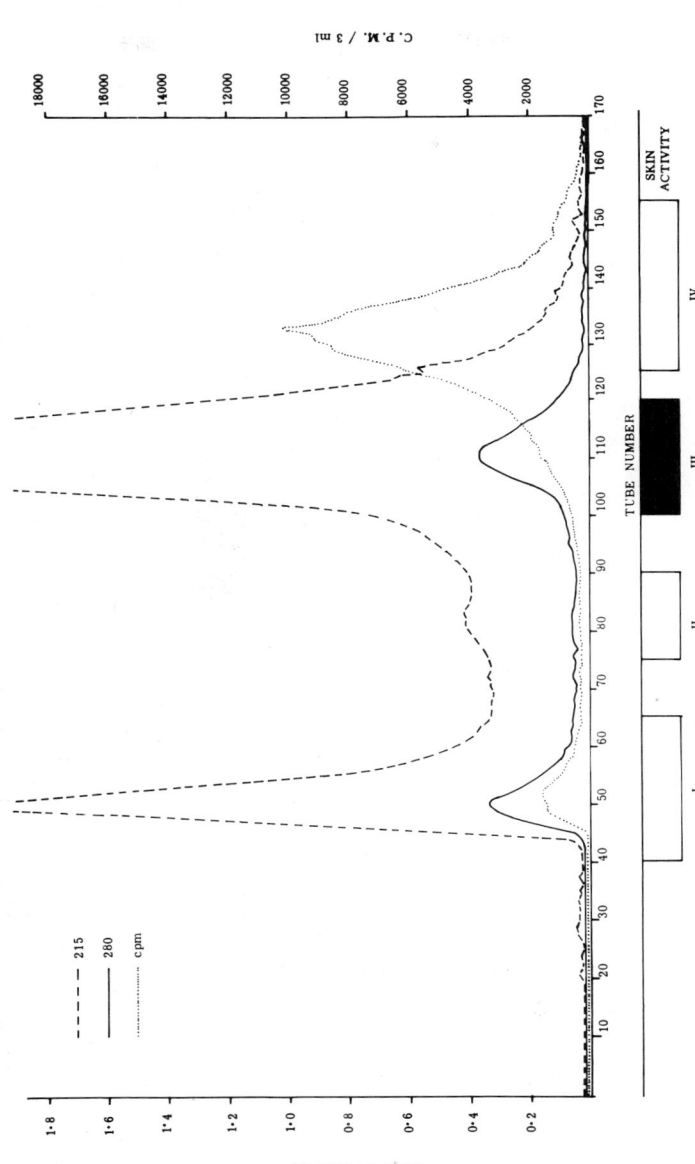

Fig. 38a Sephadex G-200 fractionation of supernatant from a culture of peritoneal lymphocytes incubated with ^{125}I-PPD, 10 μg/10^7 cells. Elution patterns show O.D. at 215 mμ, O.D. at 280 mμ and amount of ^{125}I-PPD as counts per minute. Skin activity, indicated by the shaded rectangle, was limited to peak III.

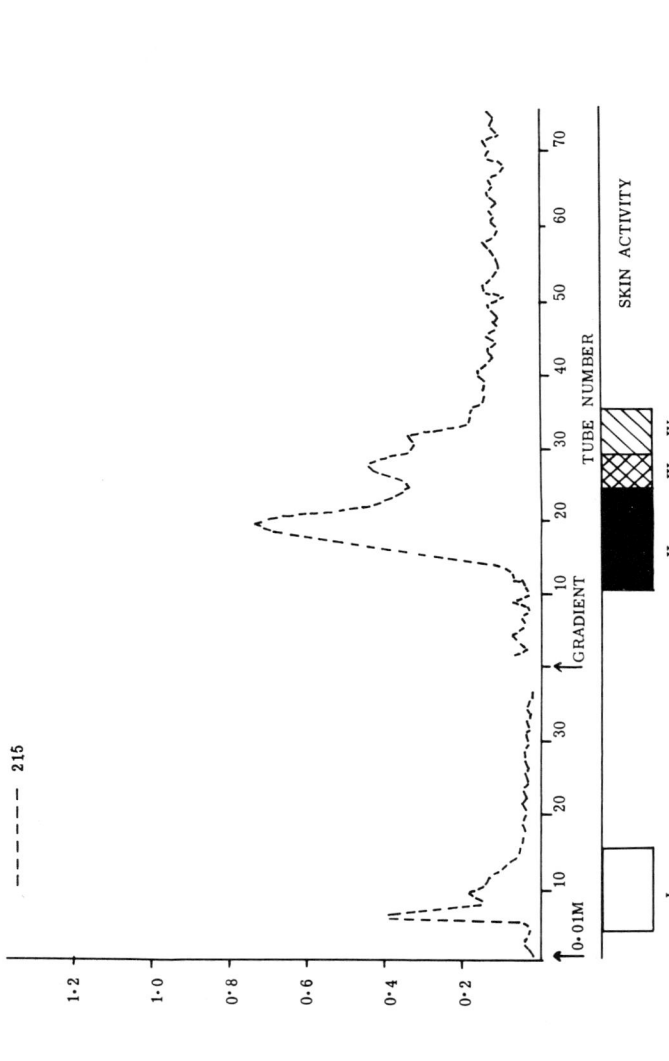

Fig. 38b DEAE-cellulose chromatography of peak III obtained by gel filtration on Sephadex G-200 of PPD incubated peritoneal lymphocytes culture supernatant. Eluants were 0.01 M potassium phosphate buffer pH 8.0 which was followed by a linear gradient (0.01 M – 0.3 M) of the same buffer. Elution pattern shows O.D. at 215 mμ. Skin activity, as indicated by the shading of rectangles representing the peaks, was maximal in peak II, moderate in peak II and slight in peak IV.

IV. BIOLOGICAL ACTIVITIES OF LYMPHOCYTE PRODUCTS

sephadex G-200 runs in a position with the more highly charged molecules (Fig. 38b)

"Table 31 shows the influence of inhibitory drugs on the formation of skin active culture supernatants. The formation of skin active culture supernatants. The inhibitors were present during the 24 hours incubation of sensitized lymphocytes with specific antigen. This table summarizes evidence that the production of this agent in culture being depressed by actinomycin, and ingibited by puromycin, whereas neither chloraphenicol nor EACA, nor soybean trypsin inhibitor have any significant effect."

TABLE 31

Influence of Inhibitory Drugs on the Formation of Skin Active Culture Supernatants. The Inhibitors Were Present During the 24 Hours Incubation of Sensitized Lymphocytes with Specific Antigen. SRF = Skin Reactive Factor, EACA = $\mathcal{E}$-Aminocaproic Acid, SBTI = Soya Bean Trypsin Inhibitor.

Drug Added to Culture	Concentration	Effect on Formation of SRF
Actinomycin D	2 μg/ml	Depression
Puromycin	50 μg/ml	Total inhibition
Chloramphenicol	50 μg/ml	No effect (Potentiation?)
EACA	10 mg/ml	No effect
SBTI	5 μg/ml	No effect
SBTI	50 μg/ml	No effect

It has not been possible completely to exclude the presence of antigen in our active supernatant. If we use radioactive tuberculin, we always find a trace of radioactive tuberculin in our active peak from the sephadex. However, the majority of the antigen is localized in other peaks. As is shown in Fig. 39, whole culture supernatants, or the material from active peak itself, developed in immunoelectrophoresis with an anti-immunoglobulin serum, and followed by autoradiography, discloses the radioactive antigen bound to a material which cross-reacts with immunoglobulin migrating in the beta region. We are not certain precisely what this material is; it could be an immune complex. If it were a globular protein based on its behavior on sephadex G-200 the material would have a molecular weight of about 68,000. This might, in fact, be a peptide chain, a heavy chain linked to antigen.

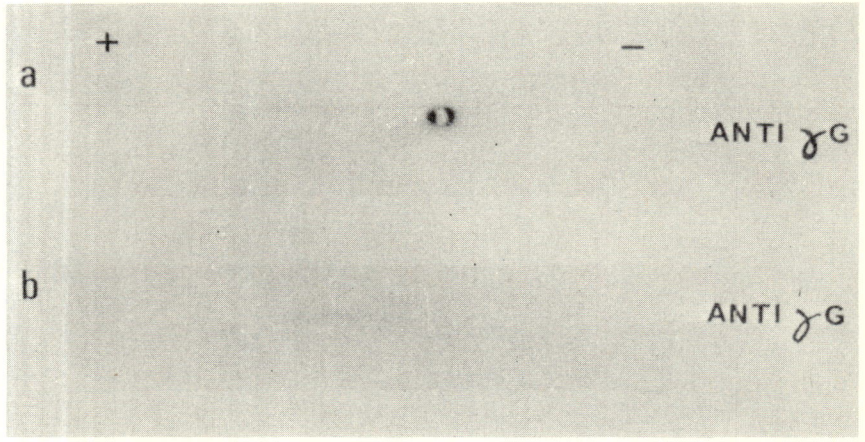

Fig. 39 Radioimmunoelectrophoretic pattern of the supernatant of sensitized lymph node cells cultured in the presence of ^{125}I-PPD (10 µg/10^7 cells).

a. Whole supernatant in the well, anti-slow and fast γG in the trough.

b. Peak III of Sephadex G-200 fractionated supernatant in the well, anti-slow and fast γ-G in the trough.

IV. BIOLOGICAL ACTIVITIES OF LYMPHOCYTE PRODUCTS

The other rather remarkable finding is that we have released a similar skin reactive factor from normal lymphocytes cultured with PHA. This cell product results in an indurated lesion in the skin, maximal three to six hours after injection. The latter is far greater in size than that produced by the trace of PHA present in the culture fluid alone. The latter is capable of producing only a minute amount of erythema without induration. This material has yet to be characterized.

Finally, when we take our active sephadex peak from the culture of sensitized lymphocytes incubated with antigen and we put it on preparative polyacrylamide gel electrophoresis, we get an active peak which contains hemoglobin, and two other bands. Thus, our active material runs electrophoretically with hemoglobin, but we can also see two other bands in the fraction in addition. We have not fully excluded the possibility that this material is an immune complex. However, if this were one it would not be a typical complex. These are, I believe matters that require consideration as fundamental questions, because when we talk about *in vitro* correlates, we are all too frequently not really sure whether we have *in vivo* correlation.

DR. CHASE: I think this is most important and interesting work. The threads may still be somewhat tangled at present, but they certainly are going to be straightened out in the near future. While I am not inclined to think these reactions are clearly delayed hypersensitivity, it is not surprising that materials produced *in vitro* and injected "preformed" would lead to far more prompt reactions than in the situation of the actively sensitized animal in which antigen must first mobilize the right cells, and then activate them to elaborate and release the mediators.

There has been a recent report from Dr. Mackaness' laboratory relative to this particular issue, that he should be able to discuss in more informative detail. In effect, it was found that if cells have been pre-accumulated in a site before the test antigen was applied, a rather prompt response occurred.

DR. MACKANESS: In common with the work of Lubaroff and Waksman, Dr. Volkman, in our laboratory, has found that

the great majority of cells that migrate into the site of
delayed hypersensitivity reaction are bone-marrow derived
cells belonging to the monocyte-macrophage series. Inasmuch
as Volkman has previously shown that bone marrow contains
a radiosensitive precursor of the circulating blood monocyte, he asked what would be the effect of X-irradiation
upon the expression of delayed hypersensitivity. Here we
are addressing ourselves to a different question from the
one which was raised in an earlier session concerning the
radio-sensitivity of the induction of delayed sensitivity.
We learned then that perhaps the induction of delayed
type hypersensitivity is perhaps more resistant to X-
irradiation than is the induction of antibody formation.
On the other hand, Volkman and Collins found that the
expression of pre-existing delayed sensitivity is radio-
sensitive in both the mouse and the guinea pig. Exposure
to approximately one LD_{50} of whole body irradiation
abolished sensitivity to antigen given within 24 hours of
irradiation. They also showed that coincident with the loss
of sensitivity there was a disappearance of monocytes from
the blood. They found, moreover, that reactivity to
tuberculin reappeared at a time when monocytes began once
again to emerge again from the bone-marrow. Although they
are not found in the blood at this time, cells with the
appropriate labelling characteristics turn up in the
reaction site in the animals recovering from irradiation.
These findings suggest that the circulating monocyte may be
necessary for the expression of a delayed hypersensitivity
reaction, just as the polymorphonuclear is for the expression of Arthus reactivity. The findings of Coe,
Feldman and Lee also support this view. They showed that
X-irradiated recipients that are given thoracic duct lymphocytes from a tuberculin sensitive donor, do not display
delayed hypersensitivity to tuberculin. By all accounts
the recipient animal should have been sensitive, unless a
radio-sensitive component in the recipient is necessary for
the expression of delayed sensitivity.

Accordingly, Dr. Hill suggested that if circulating monocytes are necessary for the expression of delayed sensitivity, it would be of interest to study the effect of
inducing a cellular exudate in the skin at the site of a
prospective skin test with specific antigen. Therefore,
Hill performed the experiments which were reported recently

IV. BIOLOGICAL ACTIVITIES OF LYMPHOCYTE PRODUCTS

(J. Exp. Med., 129, 363, 1969). He found that prior injection of a very mild irritant such as saline, followed twenty-four hours later by injection of antigen into the same site gave an accelerated delayed hypersensitivity reaction; it was often quite explosive. If we compare what happens at a prepared site with the progression of events at a normal reaction site elsewhere on the same animal, one finds an immediate reaction which reaches 50 percent of its maximum within one and a half hours, attaining its peak in eight to ten hours and persisting much longer than it does at an unprepared site.

Thus, having prepared a skin site by an inductive process which involves the accumulation of cells at random from the circulation, all of the ingredients necessary to set a delayed reaction in motion have been assembled and are ready to react promptly just as soon as antigen is introduced. This implies that the reaction is normally delayed because it takes a certain length of time for an effective concentration of cells to accumulate at random in the reaction site.

DR. UHR: Have you tried doing this special type of skin testing on animals that have been sensitized but have not yet reached the point in time when they show conventional delayed skin reactivity, for example, a day or two after sensitization?

DR. MACKANESS: No. I think the earliest time at which Hill has tested for sensitivity was one week after immunization. Tests for accelerated delayed reactions have included contact sensitizing chemicals, infectious agents and protein antigens in complete Freund's adjuvant.

DR. UHR: The point is this technique might be a tremendous magnifier of the delayed hypersensitivity state. This observation might have implications for the problem of transfer factor.

DR. MACKANESS: I agree that it is a tremendous amplifier of the phenomenon. The mouse is not an ideal animal in which to study delayed sensitivity; but it can be done nonetheless in the footpad, as first described by Fenner. In Hill's experiments the foot of the animal swells up to several times its normal size within an hour and a half; it is an impressive phenomenon which has all the correlatives of delayed-type hypersensitivity; it can be transferred with cells, is specific for the antigen, and resembles conventional delayed reactions histologically.

DR. LAWRENCE: Consonant with Dr. Mackaness' comments we have observed a similar phenomenon when we employ the local technique of transfer in humans, as originally described by Metaxas for guinea pigs. When a local skin site is prepared with sensitive viable cells, leucocyte extracts, or dialysable transfer factor and the specific antigen injected atop the prepared site 24 hours later, an intense local delayed-type reaction results as well as a marked degree of cutaneous reactivity occurs in remote sites of antigen injected simultaneously in unprepared skin sites. The local site begins to react in a matter of hours (Proc. Soc. Exp. Biol. Med., 71, 516, 1949; also in: Cellular and Humoral Aspects of Hypersensitive States, ed. Lawrence, Hoeber, p. 279, 1959). Moreover, if sensitive leucocyte extracts are pre-incubated with specific antigen and this mixture injected intradermally, there also results an accelerated appearance of the delayed cutaneous reaction to coccidioidin at that site (Rapaport et al., J. Immunol., 84, 358, 1960).

DR. CHASE: Two comments may be in order about the Metaxas experiment: two types of operations were performed. In one, the cells were injected intradermally with the usual result; namely, production of an area of moderate inflammation and then on the next day, if my memory serves, tuberculin was injected intradermally. This reaction is indeed feeble, with a small center of injury but without other evident earmarks as to the type of reaction.

The other Metaxas experiment was to inject the cells intradermally but on the following day to inject a large amount of old tuberculin intraperitoneally. I carred out such tests. A reaction wholly typical of the Shwartzman reaction developed in the local dermal site, as described for the guinea pig by the late Jules Freund. Consequently, we are perhaps overstressing the Metaxas experiment and its meaning, even though the procedure deserves study on its own.

IV. BIOLOGICAL ACTIVITIES OF LYMPHOCYTE PRODUCTS

DR. LAWRENCE: I neglected to add one additional bit of evidence in concurrence with Dr. Mackaness' statement. If the local technique of transfer is used, the dose of cells required can be decreased tenfold (i.e. from 85 to 8.5 x 10^8) and still effect the transfer of an equivalent degree of systemic sensitivity. The local reaction is always most intense. Thus the juxtaposition of soluble antigen or a skin homograft and transfer factor, increases the intensity of the transfer both locally and systemically.

DR. TURK: There is always one problem that worries me with the Metaxas type transfers, and that is, as Dr. Chase indicated, one never gets as large a reaction as one can in the truly passively sensitized animal or in the actively sensitized animal. One rarely gets a reaction greater than 12 millimeters diameter even when the lymphocytes are actually mixed with antigen and given directly in inbred animals. This is getting both reactants together, and even under these ideal conditions one does not see a reaction larger than 12 millimeters in diameter. We actually have observed more intense reactions with the culture supernatants containing MIF, than we do with the mixture of the cells with antigen.

DR. WAKSMAN: A number of findings in the literature suggest that vascular injury of <u>any kind</u> leads to intensification and acceleration of a delayed reaction elicited at the same site. I would therefore ask Dr. Mackaness what type of controls were done to establish that the role of the macrophages that were put in was not simply to produce vascular damage. He concluded from the experiment, that since delayed reactions have an accumulation of mononuclear phagocytic cells, that putting these in early intensified the lesion because they were already there, instead of having to be accumulated. My point is that any vascular injury in a sensitized animal enhances elicitation of the specific delayed reaction, and for this reason I am interested in what your controls were.

DR. MACKANESS: I don't think there can be a control to cover such a possibility. I suppose one could cause vascular injury and then inject antigen before cells have had time to accumulate. However, I would warrant that an accelerated reaction would not occur in such circumstances.

It seems to me that the answer to your question rests with the observations of Coe, Feldman and Lee, as well as those of Volkman and Collins, whose evidence suggests that the state of reactivity to antigen is lost when levels of circulating monocytes are depressed.

I think there is another situation in the literature which is essentially analogous to this. It is impossible to elicit a delayed reaction in the footpads of cortisone-treated mice, yet you can passively transfer sensitivity to a normal recipient with spleen cells from cortisone-treated donors. Conversely, you cannot transfer delayed sensitivity to recipients that have been treated with cortisone. A likely explanation for this is the well known fact that cortisone prevents the emigration of blood leucocytes. I suspect, therefore, that the reason one cannot elicit a delayed reaction in cortisone-treated mice is that cells fail to accumulate in the site of antigen deposition, again emphasizing the ancillary role of monocytic cells in delayed hypersensitivity.

DR. SILVERSTEIN: Insofar as MIF and other effector molecules have been described as models of a system, I would like to describe a model of a model, which I think has some interest and perhaps only a few of you have heard about. We have been discussing the stimulation by specific triggers leading to release of essentially non-specific mediators of inflammatory reaction. These are, in the main, the same types of inflammatory reactions that one sees in invertebrates that have not got the advantage of these specific and efficient signals.

I would like to describe to you some work by Drs. Prendergast and Suzuki at Johns Hopkins, using the marine starfish, whose coelomic fluid contains a mononuclear cell with some very interesting properties. One can extract from this mononuclear cell, fully formed, a variety of protein substances, some eight or ten of which can be well separated and well defined. One of these, at least, is an agglutinating factor for the macrophages of the sea star, but has no effect on mammalian cells. Another, different factor, acts even in the mammals, with the attribute of inhibiting migration. It is a protein of molecular weight about 32,000, can be purified and apparently mono-specifically by a simple three-step procedure. It is

IV. BIOLOGICAL ACTIVITIES OF LYMPHOCYTE PRODUCTS

highly immunogenic in the rabbit. It has the additional advantage that it can be obtained in milligram amounts. This protein will inhibit guinea pig macrophage migration *in vitro*, with or without lymphocytes, just as does the mammalian factor we have been referring to as MIF. Interestingly enough, this protein injected intradermally in microgram amounts into mammals (and some half dozen mammalian species have been tried) gives rise to an inflammatory reaction indistinguishable, by both temporal and cytologic criteria, from the delayed hypersensitivity reaction.

This is intriguing from several points of view. First, because I think it indicates that some of the non-specific factors that we have heard described are likely to have persisted in evolution, having been necessary quite early. Secondly, it is the only substance I am aware of that will give rise in the mammal to this type of cellular infiltrate on a non-immunologic basis.

CHAIRMAN BILLINGHAM: There is a recent report by Dr. Good and his associates we should have a chance to discuss. As I recall the work, guinea pigs that had been rendered delayed hypersensitive to a specific antigen and then heavily irradiated, have some kind of specific effector agent liberated into their plasma.

DR. GOOD: The observations Dr. Billingham refers to stem from an experiment that arose from our concern with whether or not kidney homograft rejection in the dog was mediated by antibody or by some cellular mechanism.

Dr. Scott Clark designed an ingenious model to separate the effector processes from the sensitizing processes. What he did was to take three dogs: A, B, and C; take one kidney from A, put it into B, and leave it there for three to four days, then removed and discarded the kidney, following which the animal was given lethal irradiation. After the circulating lymphocytes had disappeared completely from this irradiated animal, Clark took the second kidney from A, put it into the circulation of B, and left it there for just two to four hours.

He studied the kidney at that juncture and found it to be functioning normally at this time; he also examined it histologically and found it normal. There was no detectable abnormality. He then put this same kidney back into A and found it was rejected within 12 hours, almost like some heterografts are rejected. The rejection process he found to be rather complex and with Drs. Foker and Varco, he dissected this complex phenomenon. They treated dog A with large enough doses of cobra venom inhibitor, to reduce drastically the complement system and found that they could delay rejection and eliminate polymorphonuclear infiltration and platelet vascular occlusion. In this way they revealed an underlying mononuclear rejection process that appeared to be relatively independent of complement.

This rapid rejection was due to a highly specific phenomenon which had occurred in B, because C's kidney was put into B at the same time when the animal was sensitized to A and after two to four hours that kidney was retransplanted back into C, it survived without evidence of rejection in 70% of the instances. The 30 percent incidence of rejection reactions we believe can be attributed to cross-reacting antigens shared by dogs A and C in this outbred population.

Dr. Perey, Dupuy and I thought it might be informative to use this approach in other systems. We immunized guinea pigs with BCG until they developed strongly positive tuberculin reactions. Then we administered a dose of lethal irradiation to the guinea pigs, took their serum four days later at a time when their lymphocytes had completely disappeared from their lymphoid tissue and circulation. We injected this plasma into non-sensitized guinea pigs and found that by giving a big enough dose we could specifically sensitize these guinea pigs to tuberculin.

This was not an immediate sensitization and it required essentially the plasma volume of one fatally irradiated guinea pig to successfully transfer tuberculin sensitivity. The earliest we have been able to demonstrate what we considered significant delayed-allergy after such a transfer, was about four days. The best results were achieved seven to nine days after transfer. We interpreted this transfer with plasma to be due to transfer of an antibody or "IgX"

IV. BIOLOGICAL ACTIVITIES OF LYMPHOCYTE PRODUCTS

from the sensitized donor to the non-sensitized recipient. The best evidence for this interpretation is that the transferring material is a protein; it is non-dialysable and transferable to normal lymphocytes converting them to cells capable of transferring the same hypersensitivity. These observations have been described in detail recently (Dupuy et al., Lancet, 1, 551, 1969).

We have also applied these findings to the homograft system in the mouse and have been able to passively transfer specific immunity both of the white graft rejection type as well as the accelerated rejection type by means of plasma from mice previously sensitized to reject a skin homograft. In both the guinea pig system and in the mouse system, something appears in the plasma that will transfer this sensitivity reaction.

Here again, if we take normal lymphocytes from either the guinea pig in the tuberculin system or the mouse in the homograft system, put these cells into the plasma bearing this transfer factor, they become sensitized and capable of transferring tuberculin sensitivity or the homograft rejection reaction respectively and the plasma then loses at least some of this capacity. We have not yet made exhaustive absorption experiments but I believe that there is no question but that the lymphocytes have a receptor which allows them to deplete this material from plasma.

With this same model, we have also been able to completely immunize mice to one form of leukemia. We worked first with the C57BL Friend virus system. These animals are very resistant to the Friend virus and do not develop leukemia following infection with this virus. If we take these animals and inject Friend virus into them and wait three weeks or so, and then take their plasma at this time, we are unable to transfer resistance to DBA_2 animals. However, if we give similarly treated animals fatal irradiation, their plasma now protects completely against the development of leukemia in this system.

We have begun to do fractionation experiments. Whatever is active in that plasma is not a gamma globulin, neither Ig G. nor Ig M. Our activity is present in that difficult area for definition, among the proteins that migrate more rapidly on starch gel. It does not migrate with IgG, but rather closely to albumin.

To me the real question about this system is whether we are transferring antigen or immunogen. There is no question that the reaction we transfer is specific and we feel strongly it is cellular immunity. The lesions in neither our sensitized animals nor our recipients are as large as those lesions that Dr. Chase showed us. Maximal lesions are about 12 to 15 millimeters across, they contain a predominance of mononuclear cells at 48 hours.

It is now essential to identify this material. We don't want to claim that we have any of the transfer factors, that have been discussed at this meeting until we have precisely identified the compound effecting the transfer. But, at least we have got something in the plasma that will be possible to identify precisely. We have also begun to work with DNP protein system, but it is too early to determine whether we transfer carrier specificity. Dr. Perey has, however, transferred homograft immunity from agammaglobulinemic to normal chickens.

CHAIRMAN BILLINGHAM: Have you tried to abolish tolerance in homografts in mice?

DR. GOOD: No, we have not done that yet. I think this certainly should be done and it will be.

DR. CHASE: Does your transfer of sensitivity to DNP similarly require days to become apparent after the transfer?

DR. GOOD: All of the transfers have been similarly delayed. I think the earliest we have been able to get the degree of sensitivity we have described, has been about four days following transfer so it could surely reflect active sensitization.

DR. CHASE: Do you tend to identify the factor now described with the one Cole and Favour reported some years ago?

DR. GOOD: It could be the same thing only released by irradiation. I know we are working in a difficult area where people have foundered in the past. Perhaps, we will

IV. BIOLOGICAL ACTIVITIES OF LYMPHOCYTE PRODUCTS

too, but I think that the model is basically a good one and we should soon be able to tell if we have an antigen, superantigen, IgX, or a transfer factor for animals. The fact that this material goes on board the lymphocytes and renders them sensitive makes me think we may be dealing with the "antibody" of the thymus dependent system.

DR. LAWRENCE: Once you get your activity bound to the lymphocyte, can you liberate it in turn by irradiation of those "passively" sensitized cells?

DR. GOOD: We have not done that particular experiment. We have tried earlier to release something of this sort from lymphocytes of sensitive animals by irradiating the lymphocytes and we couldn't demonstrate anything in this system. However, we haven't done the experiment Lawrence suggests. It might be a good one.

V

VARIED EFFECTS OF LYMPHOCYTE PRODUCTS RANGING FROM DESTRUCTION OF TARGET CELLS TO ACTIVATION OF LYMPHOCYTES AND MACROPHAGES

Agents, specific and non-specific, that activate lymphocytes result in release of LT — LT cytotoxicity for target cells is independent of cell type or species of origin — LT production blocked by inhibitors of protein synthesis; unaffected by inhibitors of cell-division — Physicochemical properties of human versus murine LT — Characteristics of target cell destruction by LT — Membrane destructive effects of LT — Relative insensitivity of lymphocytes to LT — Evidence for identity of LT and MIF; dose-dependent effects — Lymphocyte target cell contact; is it obligatory for cytotoxicity — Concentration gradients and the microenvironment limit cytotoxicity of LT — Role of macrophages in recovery from infections caused by intracellular microbes — Specific and non-specific events in allograft rejection — Immunologically induced cytotoxicity versus allogeneic inhibition — Secondary tissue damage in the vicinity of delayed reactions — Cellular immunity and recovery from intracellular microbial and viral infections.

V. CYTOTOXICITY OR STIMULATION BY EFFECTOR MOLECULES

CHAIRMAN SILVERSTEIN: It has always seemed to me that the principal biological significance of immunologic mechanisms lay in their contribution to the defense of the host against pathogenic infections. I personally would think that this is by far the more important mechanism, rather than the surveillance function against somatic mutation which has been suggested elsewhere. The most effective and efficient mechanism for this defense system is, I think, accepted to be the inflammatory reaction in its most general manifestations as defined by Cohnheim, Metchnikoff and many others. I would think that the main thrust of immunologic evolution has probably been to contribute, in the vertebrate species, the specific trigger mechanisms and signals that have been the subject of our discussions, to attain more rapid and efficient mobilization of the non-specific factors that are involved in the inflammatory reaction. During the past ten years or so, we have learned how antibodies are involved not only in opsonization but also, where they meet antigen and complement, in the mediation of the factors involved in the acute inflammatory reaction. We have learned how the Arthus and anaphylactic reactions serve to mobilize an array of essentially non-specific pharmacologically active materials.

It is becoming more apparent from our discussions here that the mechanism that we designate delayed hypersensitivity may well serve the role for chronic inflammatory reactions involving mononuclear cells that antibodies are known to serve for acute inflammatory reactions involving PMN leucocytes. We heard at preceding sessions that delayed hypersensitivity is at last developing a real measure of respectability, in that some of those factors involved in the effector limb are now being isolated and characterized, and the way they are involved in the mobilization by the host of defense mechanisms are being defined. But just as antigen-antibody interactions involve not only the destruction of pathogens but also a certain damage to host tissues, so we must suspect that delayed hypersensitivity may involve the destruction of microbial pathogens as well as its more notorious involvement in the embarrassment of the host.

CELLULAR IMMUNITY

Accordingly, the issues that we will want to explore at this session are the following: First, what are the non-specific mediators of damage to pathogen and host that are released by the interaction of sensitized lymphocyte with antigen, and how these factors operate? Secondly, are there any *specific* mechanisms of damage to either microbe or host other than the simple trigger event itself? Finally, what are the biological implications or consequences of the cell-mediated mechanism, whether beneficial or deleterious?

DR. GRANGER: The demonstration *in vitro* of cell-mediated immune reactions had its origin in the development and refinement of tissue culture techniques by Govaerts (J. Immun., 85, 516, 1960) and by Rosenau and Moon (J. Nat. Canc. Inst., 27, 471, 1961). Their work marked the beginning of a shift from the extreme complexity of animal studies to the more manipulatable *in vitro* models. I have sought, in Table 32, to summarize and relate the results of some of the important studies that emerged from their pioneering efforts, considering these data in three categories, based on the status of the aggressor lymphocytes and the character of the antigens employed.

TABLE 32

In Vitro Systems in which Aggressor Lymphocytes Induce Target Cell Destruction

Status of Aggressor Lymphocytes	Induction	Aggressor Cell Response	Cell Destruction
Immune to cellular antigens	Specific cell contact & membrane interaction	Protein biosynthesis Transformation	Specific & Nonspecific
Immune to soluble antigens	Specific interaction with antigen	Protein biosynthesis	Nonspecific
Normal	Nonspecific interaction with mitogens	Energy metabolism Transformation	Nonspecific

V. CYTOTOXICITY OR STIMULATION BY EFFECTOR MOLECULES

It is well documented that the first category shown in Table 32, i.e., lymphoid cells from presensitized animals and man, is capable of initiating in vitro cytolysis of either normal or neoplastic donor target cell monolayers. Moreover, depending on the systems studied, either target and aggressor cells or target cells alone are destroyed during the course of the interaction. Neither antibody nor complement are involved in these situations, but close physical contact between the target and aggressor cells is an essential first step. This aggregation is considered to be immunologically specific and is probably promoted by an immunoglobulin receptor present on the surface of immune lymphocytes. It is now apparent that steps subsequent to cell contact, probably an interaction of target and aggressor-cell membranes are also necessary. It was proposed more or less simultaneously by two separate groups that membrane interaction between the aggressor and target cell directly causes cell destruction (Möller, Science, 147, 873, 1965 and Hellstrom et al., Nature, 208, 458, 1965). However, recent reports from a number of laboratories, including our own, do not support this concept but suggest instead that membrane interaction, subsequent to contact, serves primarily to trigger additional essential steps that involve aggressor lymphoid cell biosynthesis and perhaps morphologic transformation. Once initiated, the destructive reaction requires active aggressor cell metabolism and protein biosynthesis. However, the exact mechanism by which cell destruction occurs is still uncertain. Our studies have led us to the conclusion that the principal means by which this can be effected is by contact - "activated" immune lymphocytes secreting a nonspecific cell-toxin.

In the second category are lymphoid cells from experimental animals and man, hypersensitive to various soluble antigens such as BSA, ovalbumin, and PPD, that can cause in vitro destruction of neighboring cells when cultured together in the presence of antigen. The initial steps which trigger cytolysis are specific for the sensitizing antigen and set in motion by the interaction of immune cells with antigen. However, cell destruction occurs via a nonspecific mechanism not dependent on cell contact. It has been reported first by Ruddle and Waksman (Science, 157, 1060, 1967) and subsequently by our group (Granger et al., Nature, 221, 1155, 1969) that this destruction is mediated by a soluble cell-free toxin released by antigen-activated immune lymphoid cells. Information is incomplete on the formation of the cell toxin in these systems, but our initial studies indicate that lymphocyte protein biosynthesis is required.

The last of the three categories is that of lymphoid cells from normal animals that in the presence of PHA, as first shown by Holm and co-workers (Nature, 203, 841, 1964), cause destruction of allogeneic target cells in vitro. Subsequently these findings have been extended by numerous investigators to include lymphocytes from various animal species and other inducing agents, i.e., streptolysin O, staphylococcal filtrate, xenogeneic antibody. The cytolytic reactions typical of these systems display certain features that parallel immune target-cell in vitro systems. Initially, it was assumed that the mechanism by which these various agents induce cell destruction was by promoting aggressor-target cell membrane contact. Instead it now appears that these agents may act by interaction with natural lymphoid cell membrane triggers to cause direct activation and thus completely bypass the initial contact step which normally activates immune lymphocyte-target cell interactions. The correlation of lymphocyte transformation with the subsequent effects on target cells has been brought out by the in vitro studies of Ginsberg and Sacks (J. Cell and Comp. Physiol., 66, 199, 1965), of Holm and Perlmann (J. Exp. Med., 125, 721, 1967) and ourselves. It is apparent that once activated in vitro by mitogen, aggressor lymphocytes can induce a rapid destruction of target cells, irrespective of genotype, which may or may not require cell contact. For target cell cytolysis mediated by PHA stimulated murine or human lymphocytes, aggressor cell DNA synthesis is not required, but active cellular metabolism is essential. A recent study by Holm (Exp. Cell Res., 48, 334, 1967) suggests that nucleic acid and protein biosynthesis are not required for some degree of early cell destruction; however, this remains to be confirmed.

Our own earliest in vitro studies (J. Immunol., 101, 111, 1968) provided strong indications that destruction of target L cells by either immune or PHA-stimulated normal mouse lymphocytes was not the direct result of aggressor-target cell contact, but was instead associated with contact-induced lymphocyte activation and consequent secretion by

V. CYTOTOXICITY OR STIMULATION BY EFFECTOR MOLECULES

lymphocytes of a soluble nonspecific cell-toxin that we have designated Lymphotoxin (LT). Accordingly studies were initiated on a broad scale to examine the following questions: (a) What cells release LT?; (b) What treatments or agents will trigger its release?; and (c) Is the release of LT by activated mouse lymphocytes a restricted biological event or is it an example of a general biologic phenomenon shared by the lymphoid cells of many animal species? Numerous experiments in a continuing series of studies revealed that lymphoid cells from a variety of animal species i.e., mouse, rat, cat, rabbit, human, could be induced with PHA to release LT in vitro, in the absence of target cells (Williams and Granger, Nature, 219, 1076, 1968). Furthermore, it became apparent that only viable, metabolically active cells, and only those of lymphoid origin could be stimulated in vitro to release LT (Granger and Williams, Nature, 218, 1953, 1968). Thus far we have been able to initiate via PHA the release of LT from lymphocytes obtained from a variety of tissue sources; however exceptions to this are neonatal or adult murine thymic lymphocytes or the small lymphocytes obtained from human patients with chronic lymphocytic leukemia or Hodgkins disease (Granger and Kolb, in preparation). Whether this lack of response is due to absence of appropriate membrane receptors, a deficit of the cellular components to respond, or suboptimal conditions of cell culture remains to be determined. In any event, it is noteworthy that these cells are also incapable of inducing in vitro target cell destruction.

Additional studies revealed lymphocytes can release LT when cultured in vitro with any of an extensive and varied array of agents that induce transformation (Williams and Granger, J. Imm., in press, 1969). A summary of the results of these studies is given in Table 33 and shows that there are indeed many situations, both specific and nonspecific, that trigger the induction of LT release. Specific initiation and lymphotoxin release occur when immune cells contact soluble or cellular antigens. In contrast, the situations that lead normal lymphocytes to release LT are nonspecific in the sense that no prior immunologic sensitization of the lymphocyte donor is required. The amount of LT released in these situations appears directly related to the magnitude of the activation induced by the stimulant in the test lymphocyte population.

TABLE 33

Agents and Situations that Induce <u>In Vitro</u> Release of LT from Lymphocytes

Species Lymphocytes	Nonspecific					Specific	
	Normal Lymphocytes					Immune Lymphocytes	
	A L S (1)	X A B (2)	P H A	P W M (3)	S L O (4)	M L C (5)	P P D	Histo-Plasmin	Cellular Antigens
Mouse	+	+	++	++		++	+		++
Human			++++	++++	++	+++	++	++	
Guinea Pig			++				+		

Scoring

+	⁕	Toxic at 1:1 dilution
++	"	1:1 to 1:4
+++	"	1:5 to 1:10
++++	"	1:10 to 1:50

Key

(1) anti-lymphocyte serum
(2) xenogeneic antibody
(3) Pokeweed mitogen
(4) streptolysin O
(5) mixed lymphocyte culture

(Data reproduced with permission of Journal of Immunology)

V. CYTOTOXICITY OR STIMULATION BY EFFECTOR MOLECULES

Although the agents or situations which induce LT release in vitro are known to cause lymphocyte transformation, and an overall relationship was thus indicated, it was sought to determine whether an active cellular process was responsible for the appearance of LT in the culture medium. To this end we examined the kinetics of release of LT in vitro by PHA-activated normal human lymphocytes with the results shown in Fig. 40. It is apparent that upon activation, release begins quickly and seems to plateau after 24 hrs. However, this plateau really reflects limiting numbers of target cells in the assay cultures since levels of toxicity, as determined by end point dilution of the toxic medium obtained after 24 hrs., continues to increase for many days in culture. Moreover, these cells continue to release LT as evidenced by the continued reappearance of LT when lymphocytes are washed and resuspended in serum-free medium; this procedure can be repeated sequentially.

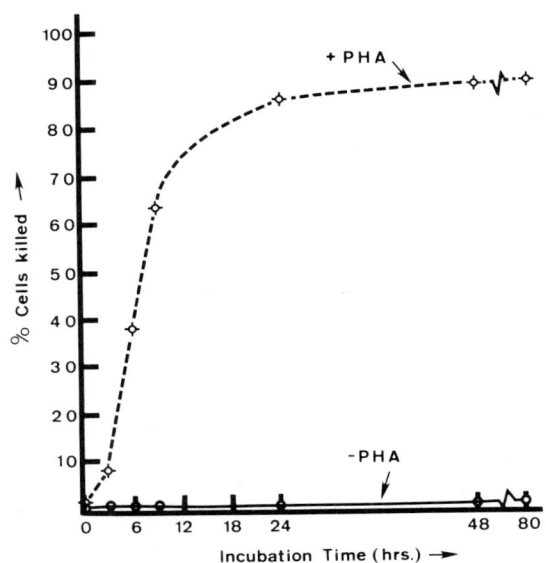

Fig. 40 The kinetics of in vitro human LT release by PHA-activated normal human lymphocytes.

Studies of this same in vitro system employing metabolic inhibitors, revealed that the elaboration of LT involves a triggering or initiating step, then active lymphocyte metabolism and protein biosynthesis. The effect of various inhibitors was tested at these separate phases, i.e., during the initiation phase and at 24 hrs. post activation, when the cells were actively engaged in biosynthesis. Except for actinomycin D, exposure to the various inhibitors was not toxic to the cells. The results presented in Table 34

TABLE 34

The effect of metabolic inhibitors on in vitro release of LT from PHA-activated human lymphocytes

Agents that inhibit release	Effective concentration
2,4-Dinitrophenol	5×10^{-3} M
Puromycin	50 µg/ml
Cyclohexamide	50 µg/ml
Low Temperature	4°C
Hydrocortisone acetate	10-25 µg/ml
Agents that do not block release	Concentration tested
X-irradiation	300-2,000 rads
Actinomycin D	1-50 µg/ml*

*Slowed but did not stop release

(Data reproduced with permission of Journal of Immunology)

show that interference with protein synthesis or general cellular metabolism blocked LT release; additionally the immunosuppressant cortisone also inhibited. In contrast, blocking RNA and DNA biosynthesis reduced but did not stop release. This is of particular interest as LT mRNA must either be stable or continuously turning over to be

V. CYTOTOXICITY OR STIMULATION BY EFFECTOR MOLECULES

available to ribosomes for transcription upon cellular activation. These data, taken together with the findings that release continues upon transfer of activated cells to fresh medium, are strongly indicative of de novo synthesis. Since LT release begins rapidly upon initiation, long before evidence of cell division, it will also be of some importance to determine the relationship of LT-secreting cells to the cells that go on to DNA synthesis and cell division.

We have been progressively delineating the physical properties of LT released in vitro by PHA-stimulated normal murine and human lymphocytes (Kolb and Granger, PNAS, 61, 1250, 1968; Fed. Proc., 27, 2653, 1968). These systems were utilized because they permit a comparison of the toxin from different animal species and because PHA induces LT in amounts which facilitate biochemical study. The findings, summarized in Table 35, show that there are both

TABLE 35

Physical Characteristics of Lymphotoxin

Treatment	Murine LT	Human LT
Heat sensitivity	$100°C$	$85°C$
pH	Stable over range of 2-12	Stable over range of 5-8
Phenol extraction	Sensitive	Sensitive
Ether extraction	Resistant	-
DNAse RNAse Trypsin	Resistant " "	Resistant " "
Molecular weight	85-95,000	80-85,000
Buoyant density in CsCl equilibrium density gradient centrifugation	1.33(protein)	1.33(protein)

(Data reproduced with permission of Proceedings of National Academy of Sciences)

similarities and differences between the toxins released by lymphocytes of these two animal species. While differing with respect to their sensitivity to heat and pH, both are inactivated by phenol and, as determined by CsCl buoyant density gradient centrifugation, display a density characteristic for protein uncomplexed to other moieties. In addition both toxins pass through sephadex G-25, 50 and 75 but are retained by G-100. They elute from sephadex, albeit with slight differences in position, as single symetrical peaks closely associated with an alkaline phosphatase enzyme marker of 80,000 MW. Various measurements reveal that mouse LT possesses a high negative charge at pH 8.6 and migrates in association with serum albumin; in contrast human LT is weakly charged and behaves as a slow moving beta or fast gamma globulin. In addition, they appear to be antigenically distinct since rabbit antiserum made against mouse LT does not neutralize human LT and vice versa (Granger et al., Fed. Proc. 28, 2071, 1969).

Our studies to date suggest that although induced by the same agent the toxins from murine and human cells differ in physical properties. On the other hand, LT appears similar or very closely related within the same animal species as judged by physical and immunologic criteria, even though it has been induced by various and quite different means. The size, specificity and physical properties of these toxins suggest they are quite unrelated either to antibody or to complement.

We have been particularly concerned with elucidating the mechanism by which these toxins effect cell destruction. I would emphasize that the kinetics and extent of cell destruction are markedly dependent upon the concentration of LT in the culture medium. The higher the concentration the more rapid, dramatic, and complete are the cytolytic effects. In contrast, at lower dilutions the cells are visibly affected for an interval of time, but they can and do recover. The destructive events are not immediate but occur over a finite time span and involve a dynamic interaction between the toxin molecule and the target cell. When LT from activated lymphocytes is placed on fresh target monolayers cytolysis occurs irrespective of cell genotype. The spectrum of species and cell types affected by PHA induced murine LT is shown in Table 36. It is lytic for both normal cells,

V. CYTOTOXICITY OR STIMULATION BY EFFECTOR MOLECULES

TABLE 36

Cytolysis Induced by Murine Lymphotoxin

In Vitro Sensitivity of Various Continuous and Primary Cell Lines

Human - Hela, Hep-2, erythrocytes
Monkey - Cv-1.
Cow - MBK.
Rabbit - MA-111, erythrocytes
Goat - erythrocytes
Hamster - Ad-7, BHK
Mouse - L cells, Fetal Fibroblasts, Peritoneal Macrophages.

Chicken - Embryonic Fibroblasts.
Fish   - Fat head minnow

(Data reproduced with permission of Journal of Immunology)

including erythrocytes, and neoplastic cells as well; affected more or less equally are cells from a variety of different tissues and animal species. In general, the array of susceptible cells is similar for human LT, however, the sensitivity of erythrocytes from various species to mouse LT differs appreciably from that of human LT. Lymphocytes themselves are also susceptible to the toxin; however, the human lymphocyte appears more refractory than murine. This susceptibility is however of a different order of magnitude from that of non-lymphoid cells.

The first visible morphologic indication of cellular destruction in toxin-treated cells is cytoplasmic vacuolation; the plasma membrane then begins to bleb and actual shedding of cell processes into the medium occurs. The cell then rounds up, cytoplasmic vacuoles increase in size and rupture leaving, attached to the glass, a bare intact nucleus which then may burst. It is noteworthy that in these cultures destruction is not entirely synchronized, but is instead a series of random events destroying individual cells until the entire culture is eliminated. Our colleague, Mr. Sundesmo has been examining by electron microscopy mouse L cells and HeLa cells exposed to human LT; these cells undergo a period of intense membrane activity apparent as plasma membrane blebbing and extension of many cytoplasmic processes. Painstaking examination has revealed what appear to be small partial discontinuities in the cytoplasmic membrane around the membrane blebs which seem to leak cellular contents into the medium. The morphologic changes seen are generally similar for the many different types of target cells examined and for LT from lymphocytes of different species, supporting the concept that all may act on the cell in a similar manner.

On the basis of biochemical studies on LT-target cell interaction (Williams and Granger, J. Imm., 102, 911, 1969) the distinguishing characteristics of LT are listed in Table 37. The findings are consistent with the aforementioned direct electron microscope visualization, that LT derived from murine and from human lymphocytes induces target cell destruction by action on the plasma membrane. Moreover, LT-target cell interaction is a dynamic process in which the affected cell seems actively to resist degradation. This becomes apparent from studies in which Mr. Williams found that the inhibition of macromolecular biosynthesis and energy metabolism caused target cells to be destroyed 8-10 times more rapidly. We believe that cellular synthesis represents an attempt on the part of the target cell to repair and replace degraded membrane components. It has also become evident that unpurified toxin in subtoxic dilutions stimulates and increases protein synthesis of many cell types *in vitro*. Studies are currently underway with purified fractions seeking to verify that this stimulation is in fact due to LT rather than to different lymphocyte products.

It is thus evident that once activated, lymphocytes can release products which participate in and probably mediate a variety of important immunologic responses. In order to distinguish whether these various responses are the result of one, a few, or of many separate factors,

V. CYTOTOXICITY OR STIMULATION BY EFFECTOR MOLECULES

TABLE 37

Characteristics of In Vitro Target Cell Destruction Induced by Lymphotoxin

---

Cells exposed to either human or murine LT undergo cytolysis

Destruction is nonspecific; sensitivity of the target cell and rate of damage is concentration-dependent

LT does not seem to bind or enter the target cell

Various polyanions can compete with LT for membrane sites

Cells exposed to sublethal concentrations of LT actively resist cytolysis

---

we are utilizing refined preparations of human LT in various in vivo and in vitro experimental situations. Preparations of human LT have been preferentially precipitated with ammonium sulfate and then further refined by DEAE-cellulose column chromatography. Various fractions are being tested for their capacity to block migration of normal guinea pig peritoneal macrophages from capillary tubes. The results of one such experiment, shown in Fig. 41 attest to such inhibition by an LT fraction whereas control fractions representing medium from nonactivated lymphocyte cultures of medium alone were without effect. Thus far MIF activity has not been detected in any other fraction from such columns. This kind of evidence strongly suggests that purified human LT has MIF activity and that these are either the same or very closely related substances.

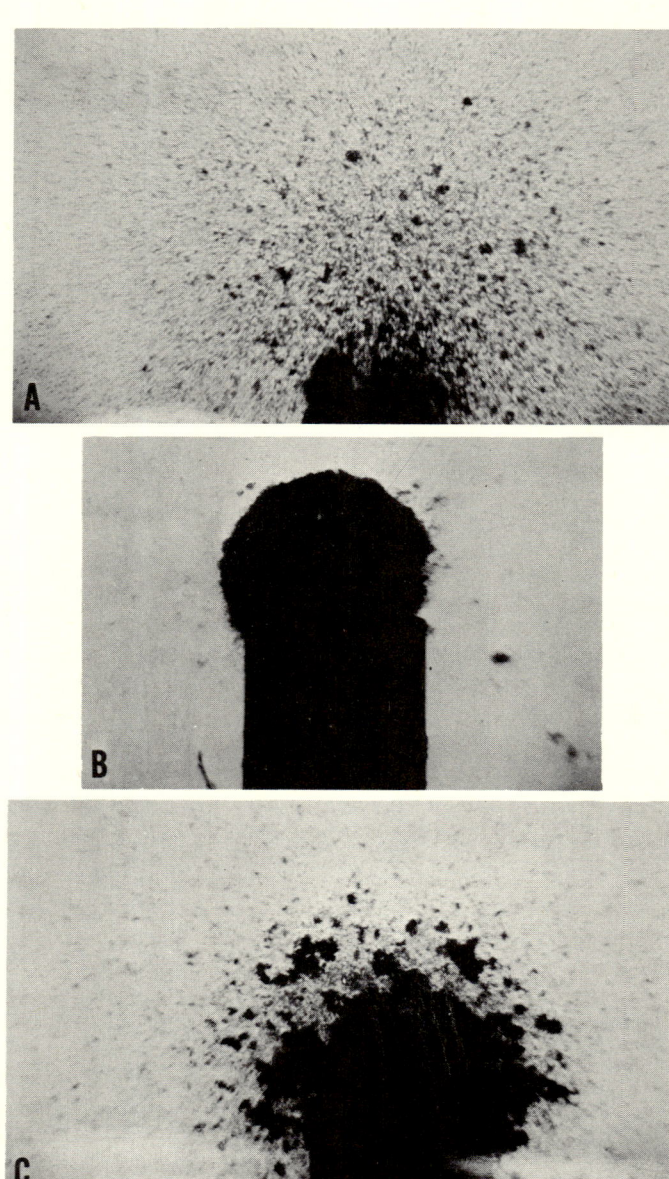

Fig. 41 The effect of DEAE-cellulose column purified human LT and control fractions on in vitro migration of normal guinea pig macrophages.

V. CYTOTOXICITY OR STIMULATION BY EFFECTOR MOLECULES

In retrospect it is not entirely surprising that the kind of cytotoxic effects evoked by LT were not reported heretofor by other investigators, although there have been no lack of attempts to detect culture medium cytotoxicity. Numerous experiments have finally made it clear to us that while a small number of activated immune cells (the experimental model most widely utilized by other workers) can release enough LT <u>locally</u> to dispatch target cells in their immediate vicinity, it is only when the maximum degree of initiation is attained that meaningful and readily detectible levels of LT appear in the cell culture medium. To this end many requirements have to be met, such as for example optimal levels of the appropriate lymphocyte stimulant, as in the case of the mitogens, adequate numbers of lymphocytes, appropriate culture techniques, etc. and finally, but most importantly, assay procedures that favor the detection and measurement of LT.

It is apparent that the array of distinctive attributes displayed <u>in vitro</u> by LT are entirely consistent with its being an important effector molecule of cellular immunity. Moreover, the secretion by derepressed lymphocytes of an agent like LT with nonspecific attributes represents a common response of lymphocytes to many and diverse stimuli, quite unrelated except that they are each capable of interacting with cell membrane. Clearly, lymphocyte membrane receptor sites are of central importance in these reactions. Our knowledge of the receptors is still very limited; suffice it to say that they must differ for most, if not all, of the stimulants used. Upon interaction of the stimulant with its distinctive membrane site or counterpart, a series of events, undoubtedly very complex, is set in motion resulting in release of LT. The magnitude of the response elicited must surely be related to the number, the orientation, and the spatial relationships of the membrane receptors for any given activating agent. In the very special situation represented by specifically immune cells these reactions are believed to be facilitated by IgX, that is presumed to make for specific aggregation and thus facilitate interaction with membrane sites. However, there are situations in which nonsensitized lymphocytes also react; cells from normal individuals are capable of recognizing and interacting with antigenically disparate lymphocytes as in the mixed lymphocyte reaction. Then, too, there is evident a degree of killing in nonimmune aggressor-target cell combinations. The latter phenomenon should be of considerable biological significance for it could act as a screening mechanism for destroying constantly emerging mutant cells by virtue of their acquisition of new, tumor-specific, antigens. The magnitude and effectiveness of cellular destruction would presumably be related to the number of cells activated to release toxin and especially to their proximity to the stimulating and sensitive cells. It is envisioned that around each activated lymphocyte, LT levels would be rather high, creating a toxic micro-environment capable of nonspecific destruction of adjacent cells. It is expected that as it diffuses out and becomes diluted, its effectiveness would be diminished. Moreover, it is conceivable that there exist host mechanisms exercising some form of control over the lethal cell-toxin once released.

Although the various kinds of membrane receptors I have alluded to remain to be characterized, it is already clear that in reactions involving them there is a basic overall similarity in situations where lymphocytes are the main effectors of tissue destruction. The difference between these grossly different phenomena such as delayed-type hypersensitivity, allotransplantation, tumor immunity, and autoimmune disease states, would seem most logically to relate primarily to the particular receptors on lymphocytes in each of these situations. Once triggered the mechanism for activation of these cells with consequent release of nonspecific effector molecules such as LT is similar and perhaps even the same.

DR. BLOOM: Can LT be made in culture medium that is serum-free?

DR. GRANGER: Yes it can.

DR. BLOOM: In that case could you tell me how much sephadex-refined LT, in terms of protein, would be required to wipe out an entire tissue culture? I ask this question solely since we get such a tiny amount of protein in MIF preparations. It would be interesting to know how much LT is required for cell death.

DR. GRANGER: As we prepare it, LT is extremely effective in very small amounts. Concentration of the order of less than

V. CYTOTOXICITY OR STIMULATION BY EFFECTOR MOLECULES

a microgram of protein/ml suffice to induce cell destruction. Even so our best preparations are still so dilute that we can't locate LT by optical methods as a discrete visible band on acrylamide gels. Moreover, studies of LT-target cell interactions suggest that very few, perhaps even a single molecule per cell, may suffice for damage or destruction. Dr. Kolb, in our laboratory, now has a C_{14} amino acid labeled DEAE column purified human LT fraction, which should greatly facilitate analysis of purity on acrylamide gels.

DR. OPPENHEIM: It has been noted for a number of years that in PHA-leucocyte cultures, the better the culture responds the more rapidly the monocytes and PMN present in such leucocyte cultures are apparently lysed and disappear. Dr. Granger's LT probably provides an explanation for this increased and more rapid cell death and destruction on non-lymphoid cells in that situation. I wonder, however, whether you actually have seen any evidence of destruction of the lymphoid cells in your assay system? Since this is not apparent in a PHA-stimulated culture, would you speculate about possible membrane differences between the lymphoid cells as opposed to the array of non-lymphoid target cells you have listed?

DR. GRANGER: Actually, the human lymphocyte appears to be relatively resistant to LT action. I would stress the adverb "relatively," as it is by no means excluded that higher concentrations of LT would not kill lymphocytes as well. Studies are currently under way to determine just what effects LT has on lymphocyte biosynthesis and the degree of transformation. However, the producing cell does seem to be resistant to LT action; whether this is due to resistance at the membrane level or local neutralization we do not know at this time. It is very interesting that in contrast to human lymphocytes, mouse lymphocytes are readily destroyed by LT. I report this observation with some reservations as mouse lymphocytes generally do not seem to grow well in culture. However, improved culture techniques such as the one reported here by Dr. Smith will give us an opportunity to see whether mouse lymphocytes are really more sensitive to destruction by LT.

As regards control, we must consider it at two levels: in terms of what turns off LT - the producing lymphocyte and, what inhibits the LT molecule itself. It is for me inconceivable that such systems would not exist in vivo. In view of its remarkable properties LT would be a dangerous material to have loose in the tissues and could cause extensive destruction if there were no means of checking either its production or its action.

DR. BACH: Was the material which you found stimulatory to protein and RNA synthesis in very high dilution (i.e. in low concentrations), one of your highly purified preparations or was this relatively crude? This becomes very important in trying to determine whether some of the effector products are really the same.

DR. GRANGER: This was a crude ammonium sulfate fraction and represents relatively dilute LT. But more highly purified material is now being subjected to similar tests.

DR. COHN: Have you been able to isolate any LT-resistant cell lines?

DR. GRANGER: We believe we may have isolated a resistant mutant, but at this point the results are preliminary and do not warrant more than a statement that this work is in progress. We have cultures of a few cells that manage to survive exposure to LT and they are being cloned. However, they must be tested in various situations and with different LT concentrations if we are to determine whether they are truly resistant.

DR. COHN: Why do you not assay LT by establishing the kinetics of the killing of target cells?

DR. GRANGER: We have in fact examined a number of different experimental situations. I won't enumerate them all, but dilutions do serve to equate different lots of LT medium. The standard assay is to incubate 200,000 cells in two ml of test or control medium for 48 hours. Cell viability is assayed both visually and more objectively by loss of the capacity of the cells to incorporate C_{14} amino acids into cell protein. The standard assay system is not done on a dilution basis, but with straight undiluted LT medium.

V. CYTOTOXICITY OR STIMULATION BY EFFECTOR MOLECULES

Purified fractions are tested directly off the columns at approximately two-fold concentration.

DR. LANDY: Dr. Granger, you have clearly established that the LT from lymphocytes of various animal species differs in performance and properties. My question is whether you have comparative data on LT production by peripheral vs. central lymphoid tissue, i.e., cells from peripheral blood, spleen, regional nodes, thoracic duct, etc. I would particularly want to know whether thymic cells perform in this regard, especially as thymocytes don't seem to transform in response to the plant mitogens.

Since you mentioned that some of the LT-induced profound changes in cell membrane have been followed by electron microscopy, would it be possible actually to see the distribution and character of these lesions?

DR. GRANGER: In answer to your first question. The immune cells that have been initiated specifically with antigens such as PPD and histoplasmin were from human peripheral blood. In the work with cells of guinea pigs and mice, lymphocytes were from spleen and lymph nodes. As regards immune mouse lymphocytes responding to target cell antigens, we used cells derived from spleen and lymph nodes. In the nonspecific tests with mitogens, which were the easiest to do, we examined mouse lymphocytes from thymus, bone-marrow, lymph nodes and spleen obtained from very young (three hours) to old (16 months) animals. Of all these varied lymphoid cells, only the thymocytes could not be initiated to release LT under our culture conditions. This could of course be due either to a lack of membrane trigger or may represent a basic lack of cellular capability to respond. I think that most of us would be inclined to favor the first of these two possibilities.

In response to your query regarding LT-induced cell membrane lesions, Fig. 42 illustrates the membrane ruptures seen by Mr. Sundesmo of our group, who has been following the ultrastructural changes in mouse L cells exposed to human LT *in vitro*. This electron micrograph was taken of L cells at various intervals following exposure to human LT. This particular cell shows multiple vents in the plasma membrane, presumably the result of LT action. Similar changes are observed in HeLa cells subjected to human LT.

CELLULAR IMMUNITY

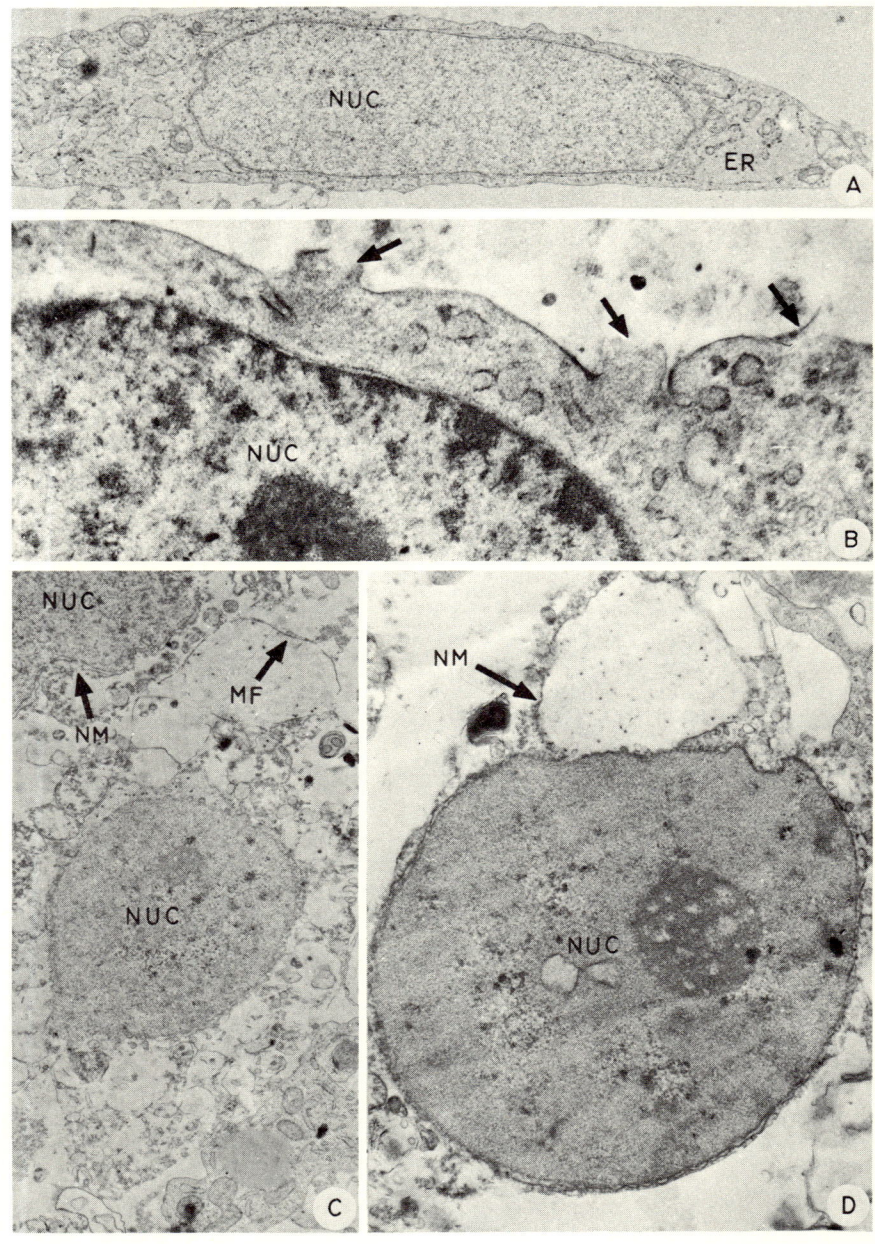

V. CYTOTOXICITY OR STIMULATION BY EFFECTOR MOLECULES

Fig. 42   Ultrastructural alterations in mouse L cells produced by human LT.

A.   Control L-cell, 67 hours after treatment with medium from non-stimulated lymphocytes supplemented with PHA. A prominent nucleus is visible and some swelling of endoplasmic reticulum is noted (ER). Fixation glutaraldehyde-osmium. Uranyl acetate and lead citrate stains. 8,550X.

B.   Twenty-four hours after treatment with cell-free medium from PHA-stimulated human lymphocytes (LT). Plasma membrane discontinuities are evident (arrows). Lead citrate stain. 18,000X.

C.   Sixty-seven hours after treatment with LT. Extensive depletion of cytoplasm has occurred, resulting in numerous isolated nuclei (NUC) delimited by intact or fragmented (arrow) nuclear membrane (NM), and surrounded by cell membrane fragments (MF). Uranyl acetate and lead citrate stains. 11,400X.

D.   Sixty-seven hours after treatment with LT. An intact nucleus with greatly distended nuclear membrane (NM) is evident. Remnants of cell membrane are still present closely apposed to some regions of the nucleus. Uranyl acetate and lead citrate stains. 15,000X.

DR. WILSON: We had better be clear about the finding of lack of LT production by thymus cells. Are you or are you not finding the production of LT under conditions where the thymus cells *are* responding to PHA?

DR. GRANGER: Under our conditions of cell culture we have not been able to activate thymocytes via PHA to release LT, nor have we been able with thymus cells to cause target cell destruction in the presence of PHA. Transformation of thymus cells by PHA has been reported. Consequently it is now essential that we repeat our work under such conditions; if we can activate thymus cells by PHA, the matter of LT release and target cell destruction by these cells would then be resolved unequivocally.

DR. THOMAS: How pronounced is the hemolytic property of your material? Why can't you simplify matters greatly by using hemolysis as a measure of activity?

DR. GRANGER: Dr. Thomas has identified an extremely interesting possibility. We are already utilizing a combination of techniques that include both cytotoxicity for nucleated cells and lysis of erythrocytes.

DR. THOMAS: Are you sure that LT is not a lysolecithinase?

DR. GRANGER: This possibility occurred to us and we are in fact looking by thin layer chromatography to see if it is indeed a lysolecithinase. In other words, LT could cleave the membrane liberating lysolecithin, which would then act on neighboring cells. However, present evidence does not support the role of lysolecithin in this process, for column chromatography and CsCl gradients demonstrate toxicity in one band or fraction. If lysolecithin were in the preparation, it should be resolvable from LT by these techniques since they separate by density and charge; moreover, toxicity is resolvable into single bands by sephadex molecular sieving techniques.

DR. EISEN: Is lymphotoxin bactericidal or bacteristatic?

DR. GRANGER: Thus far we have only studied effects on animal cells. It would be interesting and indeed important to determine whether microbial cell walls are likewise affected.

DR. VALENTINE: Dr. Granger, the sharpness of the fronts of the DEAE elution pattern which you showed us might suggest that this was a step-wise rather than a continuous gradient elution. If this were so it may prove a little less surprising if multiple activities appeared in the same tube, even if they were separate molecules.

DR. GRANGER: The DEAE separations were performed by continuous salt-gradient elution. A small degree of LT activity was noted on each side of the main fraction, but the great bulk of activity was restricted to the single fraction. As Dr. Valentine knows, the degree of separation achieved can be made maximal by adjusting the many parameters operative in this technique.

V. CYTOTOXICITY OR STIMULATION BY EFFECTOR MOLECULES

DR. UHR: Could you summarize the evidence bearing on the question whether LT and MIF are the same or dissimilar. I also am not clear about the status of your LT-antibody studies as preliminarily reported (Fed. Proc. $\underline{28}$, 630, 1969).

DR. GRANGER: In answer to your first question, we are not yet sure that MIF and LT are one and the same. What I am saying is that the single purified human LT fraction we elute from DEAE cellulose is toxic for target cells and is also able to inhibit macrophage migration. Thus, highly refined LT <u>can act</u> in biologic tests used to work with MIF. That does not necessarily mean they are the same. However, both activities do elute in the same single fraction of a total of 50 collected, which shows that whether they are identical or not they do possess very similar properties. Furthermore, it is clear that mouse LT migrates as a highly negatively charged molecule, closely associated with albumin, the very same area in which MIF activity is found in the guinea pig studies. These molecules thus show striking similarities in their physical properties.

In reply to Dr. Uhr's query on antiserum, we have prepared anti-LT by immunizing rabbits and goats with fractionated, concentrated LT derived from PHA-activated mouse lymphocytes. Rabbit anti-LT blocks mouse LT-induced target L cell cytolysis. Repeated absorption of antiserum with target cells or with murine lymphocytes does not diminish its effect against LT. Nor does prior incubation of lymphocytes with anti-LT reduce their capacity subsequently to cause target cell cytolysis. Parallel experiments with rabbit antiserum to mouse LT and to human LT indicated that the cytolysis blocking action of those reagents was species specific, i.e. anti-human LT did not block mouse LT.

CHAIRMAN SILVERSTEIN: You have indicated, as I understand it, that in lower doses, LT activates and in higher doses it is toxic - a not unusual biological situation. However, I would like to know the basis for your suggestion that the higher toxic dose represents a physiologic concentration.

DR. GRANGER: As shown in Table 33, the amount of LT present in the medium varies with the degree of activation achieved by the initiating agent. It therefore appears logical that the highest concentrations would be immediately adjacent to the cell releasing LT. The local concentrations attained in a micro-environment are likely to be far greater than those we achieve presently by biochemical methods. Thus, one could envision a gradient effect with highest concentration adjacent to the producing cell and decreasing proportionately with increasing distance from the cell. However, by high concentrations, I mean that amount released under optimal in vitro conditions, not as separated and concentrated by biochemical means.

We find that during the interaction of LT with the cell, the cell appears actively to resist or counteract its effect. This can be measured by increased protein biosynthesis which may result in membrane repair. Cells exposed to low levels of LT are stimulated to active protein biosynthesis, resist LT action and survive whereas at higher levels they are destroyed. It is conceivable that low levels of LT could stimulate lymphocytes by interaction with membrane triggers; this is in process of verification by studies with purified material.

DR. DAVID: The one thing I would like to emphasize is that with a cytotoxic factor such as described by Dr. Granger it would be not at all surprising that in killing cells they would lose the capacity to migrate. So if MIF were simply cytotoxic, capillary migration would be a poor way of measuring it. If MIF is doing something other than killing cells, that would be another matter. However I wouldn't be at all surprised that any time one is working with a factor cytotoxic for macrophages, their migration would be inhibited.

DR. GRANGER: I agree. The point is that if you have LT in your activated lymphocytes, as I believe you do, it would be capable of stopping macrophage migration. So unless you work with fractionated or refined MIF preparations it becomes difficult to know whether you are measuring the effects of MIF or of LT.

DR. MÖLLER: I think there is another very important issue involved here, and that is contact as opposed to absence of contact in effecting cytotoxicity. In this regard I would cite some of our previous data, obtained mainly by Dr. Lundgren. If you stimulate cells either nonspecifically

V. CYTOTOXICITY OR STIMULATION BY EFFECTOR MOLECULES

or specifically, they become cytotoxic. If it is non-specific stimulation with PHA, for instance, as illustrated in Fig. 43, cytotoxicity is very rapid; it does not require

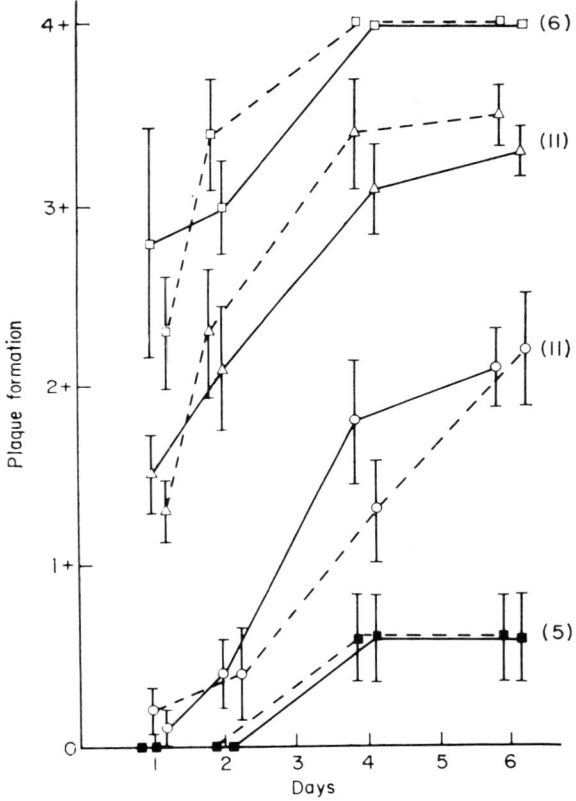

Fig. 43 Cytotoxicity of human lymphocytes on human fibroblasts in the presence of PHA. Destruction of the target monolayer at the site of addition of lymphocytes was graded from 0 to 4+. Solid lines indicate lymphocytes and target cells from the same individual and the broken lines allogeneic combinations. The number of experiments are given in parentheses. Symbols connecting lines indicate 10^5, 5×10^5, 10^6, and 5×10^6 lymphocytes per site of addition.

(Reproduced with permission of Clin. Exp. Immunology)

synthesis of DNA, RNA or protein, and it does not involve morphologic transformation. However, some kind of transformation obviously occurs since living and metabolically active cells are required. If cells are stimulated specifically, either by adding them to target cells having the antigen against which the lymphocytes are immunized, or by mixing lymphocytes from donors immunized to PPD or Salmonella and the corresponding antigen, both RNA and DNA synthesis is needed for cytotoxicity.

In the later case (Fig. 44) a magnification mechanism is

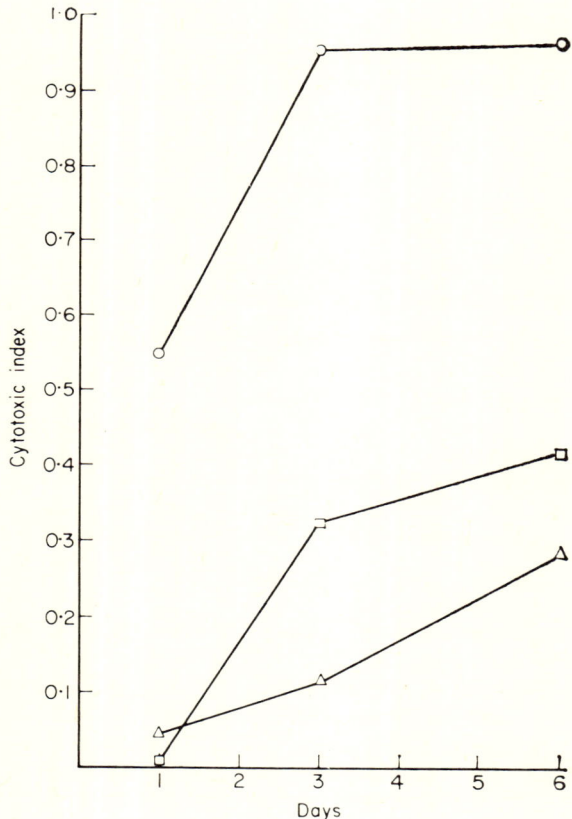

Fig. 44 Cytoxicity cf human lymphocytes for allogeneic Cr_{51} labelled fibroblasts in the presence of PHA. Fibroblasts

V. CYTOTOXICITY OR STIMULATION BY EFFECTOR MOLECULES

were labelled with Cr_{51} 48 hours prior to addition of lymphocytes. Supernatants were collected at various time intervals, the target cells washed and trypsinized. Supernatants and trypsinized fibroblast radioactivity was measured and the % of cytotoxicity determined as cpm in supernatant plus target fibroblasts. A cytotoxic index was calculated as % cytotoxicity in cultures exposed to lymphocytes plus PHA minus cpm in controls exposed to PHA alone divided by cpm in controls. Symbols indicate addition of 10^5, 5×10^5, 10^6 lymphocytes.

(Reproduced with permission of Clin. Exp. Immunology)

---

probably involved, only few cells initially reacting, which have to be increased in number for cytotoxicity to be expressed. As illustrated in Table 38, once lymphocytes

TABLE 38

Relation between HL-A antigens and cytotoxicity on various fibroblasts caused by human lymphocytes from skin grafted patients.

Donor of lymphocytes	Target cells	Reactive HL-A antigens	Cytotoxicity at day 1	4	6
ML	ML	-	0	0	0
	RF	HL-A1, HL-A7, 4C	0.5	1.4	3.2
	KL	HL-A7, 4C	0	1.0	1.5
	IA	HL-A1, HL-A7	0	1.5	1.3
	LL	HL-A1	0	1.0	2.3
	LA	HL-A7	0	1.0	1.0
	JF	-	0	0	0

acquire cytotoxicity it is expressed nonspecifically. However, there is very strong evidence that cell contact between the lymphocytes and the target cells is necessary and to my way of thinking this appears to be an absolute requirement. You can't separate the cells from their target with millipore membranes, even after PHA stimulation, without abolishing cytotoxicity. Indeed, you can't even interpose a thin layer of agar (0.5%), which is created by pouring it onto target cells, and immediately thereafter pour them out. Even this simple maneuver blocks cytotoxicity completely. Cytotoxicity can also be blocked by a layer of gammaglobulin molecules coated either on lymphocytes or on target cells. Lymphocytes or target cells coated with ALS are prevented from making the necessary contact; such lymphocytes although potentially toxic, can't express their cytotoxicity. In my view these findings obviously do not fit with the release of toxic factors.

What possibilities are there to explain this discrepancy? One possible explanation is contamination of lymphocyte populations with granulocytes; these cells release enzymes that detach the target cells from the glass. This looks exactly like cytotoxicity, but the cells are in fact not killed. I would predict that the results of Ruddle and Waksman, demonstrating toxic supernatants, is due to this kind of mechanism. If one counts only the number of living cells which remain on glass, it is impossible to distinguish between detachment and toxicity. We also know that lymphocytes release several factors which transform other lymphocytes do not release any factor which by itself is toxic, but rather an agent which is capable of transforming other lymphocytes into a toxic state. Not only granulocytes but also macrophages may release toxic factors. Dr. E. Möller has shown that mouse macrophages incubated with syngeneic or allogeneic erythrocytes release factors which lyse both murine and sheep erythrocytes but do not attack lymphocytes. These enzymic factors can be induced to be released and their effect is entirely nonspecific. Heparin and trypan-blue can suppress their effect. It therefore remains to be seen how we can equate our findings with those of Dr. Waksman.

DR. GRANGER: Dr. Möller has properly emphasized the very important issue of cell contact and its role in cytotoxicity. However, I would point out that in his experiments contact was invariably at the level of <u>initiating</u>

V. CYTOTOXICITY OR STIMULATION BY EFFECTOR MOLECULES

the reaction. Unless the cell can be initiated or triggered to undergo derepression, it is <u>obvious</u> one would not see any destruction. Thus separating target and aggressor cells by a cell impermeable millipore filter, effectively prohibits <u>initiation</u>; without induction there naturally would be no elaboration of effector molecules. Moreover, placing a millipore filter between PHA-treated lymphocytes and target cells introduces an additional complication for these filters are highly charged and would therefore impede free passage of LT.

In these systems the concentration of LT is very important, for when one activates only a small number of lymphocytes, the dilution effect in the culture medium is very great, except for what may briefly pertain immediately adjacent to the few producing cells. So the high local levels of LT immediately adjacent to the few triggered cells would be rapidly diluted out and therefore be undetectable in the medium. In contrast the triggering of large numbers of cells does effect the release of enough LT to be detectable.

Finally our own evidence of a requirement for aggressor cell protein synthesis for LT release would be consistent with the results of numerous investigators who have demonstrated a requirement of lymphocyte protein synthesis for target cell destruction. These results and those of Holm and Perlmann do not square with Dr. Möller's concept of antigenic recognition.

DR. MÖLLER: I think most other workers have initiated the lymphocytes beforehand. We have shown that lymphocytes stimulated for three days with PHA, so that they are strongly toxic, cannot express their effect on agar covered fibroblasts or on fibroblasts covered by ALS. It is obvious that contact is necessary for initiation, but in our experience <u>contact is also essential for expression</u>. The dilution argument does not impress me very much. Study of the reports of Ruddle and Waksman shows that they added lymphocytes to target cells and obtained a clear plaque at the site of addition. However, the supernatant of such cultures could be diluted ten times and when added to a new culture was capable of destroying the entire culture. Why didn't the supernatant destroy the initial culture, which was affected only at the site of addition of the cells?

351

DR. GRANGER: The objection you have raised is a very important one. I believe we have data that provide an explanation. We can protect cells from the effect of LT by coating their surface with antibodies. We can, moreover, also protect target cells by coating them with various polyanions. These protective effects are apparently due to blocking or altering target cell membrane receptors for LT. I emphasize again that one is introducing new and major complications by interposing materials that have charge effects or that restrict diffusion between cells. As a final bit of very important evidence, we recently reported that antibodies specific for mouse LT inhibit immune and PHA-induced normal mouse lymphocyte *in vitro* L cell destruction. Careful controls attested to the antibody being not reactive with either the aggressor or target cells, but rather blocking the effector molecule in the culture medium, i.e., LT.

DR. WAKSMAN: Dr. Möller has raised important and potentially disturbing problems about specific aspects of Dr. Ruddle's work (Ruddle and Waksman, J. Exp. Med. 128, 1237, 1968). I want to speak first of all to the basic question of whether she really observed killing or was merely dealing with detachment of cells from the plastic. We have checked this point rather carefully, counting cells in the supernatants of a fair number of cultures. In virtually every instance the fibroblasts in the supernatants were in fact dead cells. We satisfied ourselves that the number of surviving cells on the plastic was a valid representation of the number of surviving target cells in the culture. The question about the possible role of PMN cells or macrophages in the lymph node cell suspension is also quite to the point. I don't believe there were significant numbers of PMN in the suspensions we were using, but there undoubtedly were some macrophages. McLaughlin and Ruddle showed two years ago (this has not yet been published) the very situation that Dr. Möller described, i.e., that macrophages can be highly cytotoxic to fibroblast monolayers. Cytotoxicity was closely correlated with the degree of activation of the macrophages. Cells taken from the normal peritoneal cavity, i.e., small monocytic cells with a very low complement of lysosomal enzymes, had no effect on target cell monolayers. On the other hand, glycogen-induced exudate cells that are partly activated produced some degree

V. CYTOTOXICITY OR STIMULATION BY EFFECTOR MOLECULES

of cytotoxicity. Beef heart infusion broth gave rise to extremely active cells that destroyed the monolayer. This finding is already on the record in a sense. Dr. Zanvil Cohn and collaborators some time ago showed the release in macrophage cultures of certain lysosomal hydrolases, and Pincus had described target cell destruction by normal macrophages. The point is that in a recent experiment Dr. Ruddle has shown that column-purified lymphocytes produce cytotoxicity just as well as unpurified suspensions. This suggests to us that contamination with macrophages could not be responsible for the effect we reported.

DR. MÖLLER: Were you referring to toxic supernatants or toxic cells?

DR. WAKSMAN: I believe toxic cells.

DR. MÖLLER: But that is not the issue. The issue is whether the supernatant was also toxic for purified lymphocyte preparations.

DR. WAKSMAN: I don't know the answer. The next question concerned the effect of an agar or a gamma globulin monolayer on the surface of the target cells. My answer would be the same as Dr. Granger's: that this could very well cover up specific receptors for a cytotoxic molecule, one would therefore have operationally the same result. Finally we come to the question why, in a situation where one produces a plaque by putting a drop of lymphocyte suspension on the target cell monolayer, the whole monolayer is not killed. The issue here is probably the ratio of lymphocytes to target cells since in those cultures where more lymphocytes were used, the whole monolayer was killed.

DR. MÖLLER: There is an additional point I would make regarding procedures. I think the only reliable technique for cytotoxic studies is direct measurement of lysis, preferably by an isotope marker like chromium. All other methods are open to certain objections. If something makes the target cell detach from the glass they won't clone. Incorporation of amino acids may not be objectively accurate if the cells have to adhere to glass in order to grow well.

DR. GRANGER: Dr. Möller, your last objection is not relevant to our routine assay systems. In our C_{14} incorporation test, <u>suspension</u> cell cultures are used and therefore adherence to glass is in no way involved. In the matter of your previous concern about our direct cytotoxicity assays on monolayers, I would assure you that the cells are totally lysed and destroyed. As to the possibility of viable cells remaining in the medium in our cytotoxicity tests I would reply that by means of vital stains and the much more sensitive technique of radioactive isotope uptake, we have come to the conclusion that after appropriate exposure to LT there isn't a living cell in the medium, nor for that matter even fragments that can incorporate amino acids or nucleic acid precursors. I don't see how there can be any question regarding the free cells being dead. Indeed in many of these experiments we label every cell whether free or fixed to the glass.

DR. LAWRENCE: Since the discussion has taken this turn, I think it worth documenting that for the human system, very similar data have been reported by Dr. Lebowitz and myself (Lebowitz and Lawrence, Fed. Proc., <u>28</u>, 630, 1969) which affirms the work that Dr. Granger has presented. Our results have demonstrated the release of a soluble lymphotoxin from tuberculin-sensitive human blood lymphocytes incubated with tuberculin for 36 hours. Supernatants prepared in this manner are assayed for cytotoxic activity by their effect on the cloning efficiency of individual HeLa cells in culture. A representative experiment is given in Table 39, showing that the release of the toxin is antigen-specific, the material is inactivated by heating at $56°C$ for 30 minutes and is non-dialyzable. The concentration present in the flasks is considerably less than that achieved in Dr. Granger's system. Here, 0.75 to 1.0 ml of supernatant is added to the 3.5 ml of medium already present in the flasks. It may be that this relatively low concentration of LT would account for our disparate findings with regard to heat sensitivity and the lack of target cell cytolysis or detachment.

Seeking a clue to the mechanism of action of this material and some direct visual evidence of the type of damage inflicted on target cells by its presence, Dr. Lebowitz and I photographed the events in continuous time-lapse cinematography. The results of this approach are

V. CYTOTOXICITY OR STIMULATION BY EFFECTOR MOLECULES

TABLE 39

PERCENTAGE REDUCTION OF HELA CELL CLONES AS COMPARED WITH CONTROLS 10 DAYS AFTER ADDITION OF SUPERNATANTS *

Specific Additions to Medium	% Reduction of Clones
No addition	0
PPD alone	0
** SN of unstimulated sensitive lymphocytes	0
SN of PPD stimulated non-sensitive lymphs.	-5
SN of PPD stimulated sensitive lymphocytes	98
Heated SN of PPD stimulated sensitive lymphs. (56^0 x 1/2 hr.)	8
SN of PPD stimulated sensitive lymphocytes dialyzed	98
SN of PPD sensitive lymphs. incubated with histoplasmin	0

* 24 hr. old flasks containing 200 HeLa cells; each group contains 4 or 5 flasks.

** Supernatants (SN) from 36 hour cultures of 4×10^6 L/ml x 4 ml cultured with or without 2.5γ PPD/ml; PPD added to supernatant from unstimulated cultures.

documented in Fig. 45, a composite of sequential still photos taken from a time-lapse cinematography experiment illustrate the characteristic effects of human LT in our experiments. The main effects to be noted are rounding up of cells; the appearance of abnormal forms; the fusion of cells and finally the cessation of division after a variable number of cycles. We have not observed the occurrence of cytolysis or detachment of the target cells. This figure also illustrates the gross appearance of HeLa cell clones in flasks, comparing LT-treated cell populations with untreated controls. We have not yet secured definitive data on the nature of this material produced by human lymphocytes, as Dr. Granger has in the experimental animal models except, as we have indicated, human LT is inactivated by heating at $56^{\circ}C$ for 30 minutes and is non-dialyzable. It is appropriate in this context to recall our earlier discussion which emphasized the broad repertoire of sensitive lymphocytes as expressed by their production of a whole family of molecules simultaneously into the same supernatant following interaction with specific antigen (see Fig. 36). This recognition event results not only in the prompt liberation of preformed transfer factor within one hour in the human system, but also in the production of a heat-labile non-dialyzable LT just discussed; as well as a heat-labile, non-dialyzable material which in the presence of antigen causes normal lymphocytes to respond by transformation, repeated cell division and clonal proliferation; as well as MIF, which according to Dr. Thor is heat-stable in the human as well as the guinea pig models. The main point to be made is that Dr. Lebowitz and I can readily confirm Dr. Granger's observations on human LT in most essential details. The secondary and perhaps more important point to be made here is that since our laboratory is working mainly with human cell systems, we are constantly and acutely aware of the simultaneous presence of multiple biological activities (transfer factor, LT, lymphocyte transforming material and MIF) in each and every supernatant we prepare for assay.

DR. HIRSCHHORN: I think it is important to point out that these very elegant microphotographs look to me like cells that can still clone.

V. CYTOTOXICITY OR STIMULATION BY EFFECTOR MOLECULES

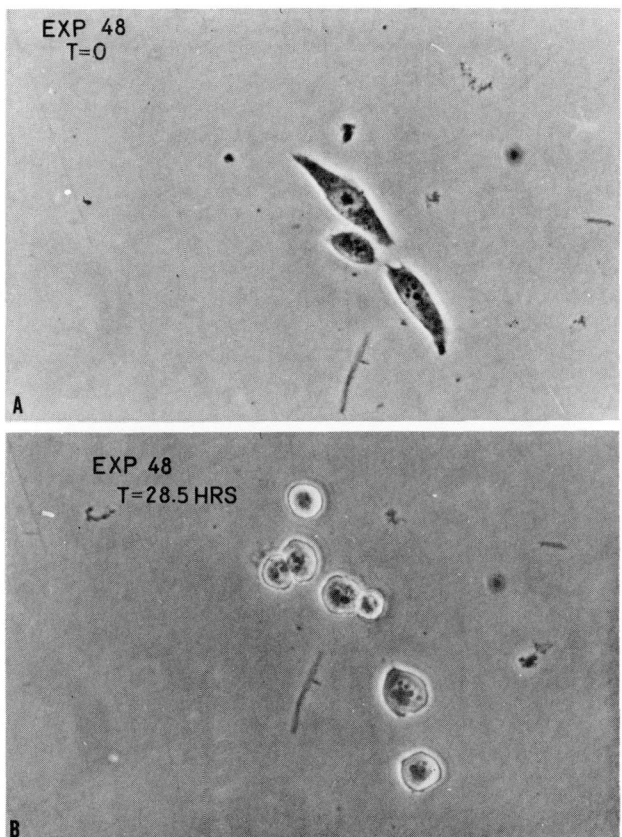

Fig. 45 Effect of human lymphotoxin (LT) produced by tuberculin-stimulated lymphocytes on HeLa cells in culture - time-lapse sequence of the same microscopic field.

A. appearance of HeLa cells at 0 time

B. same cells 28.5 hours after addition of LT

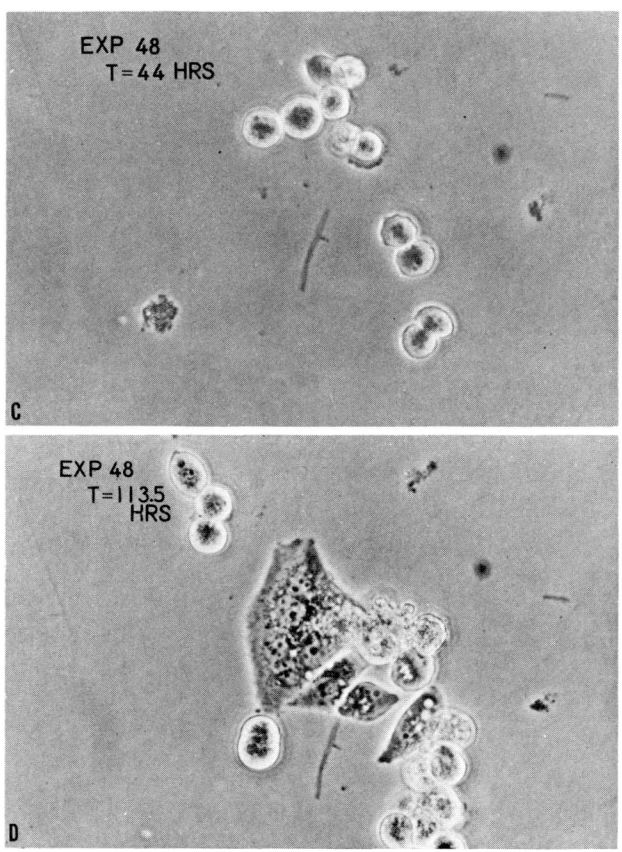

Fig. 45 (cont.)

C. same HeLa cells 44 hours after addition of LT

D. same HeLa cells 113.5 hours after addition of LT

V. CYTOTOXICITY OR STIMULATION BY EFFECTOR MOLECULES

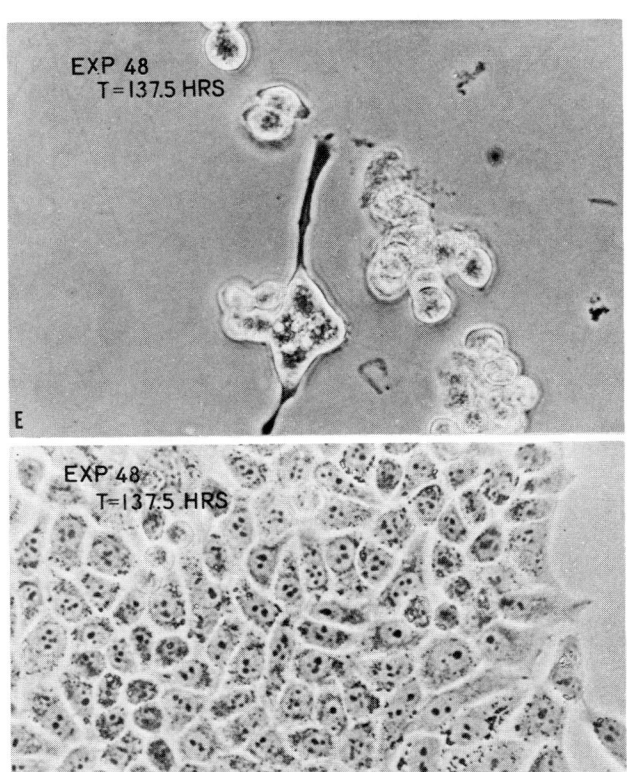

Fig. 45 (cont.)

E. same HeLa cells 6 days after addition of LT

F. appearance of HeLa cells in control flask cultured without LT at 6 days

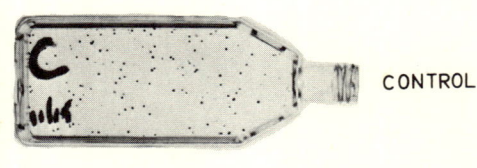 CONTROL

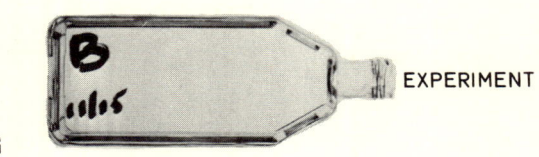 EXPERIMENT

G

Fig. 45 (cont.)

G. Gross appearance and numbers of HeLa cell clones in control flasks cultured without LT (above) compared to absence of clones in experimental flasks cultured with LT (below) after 12 days incubation.

DR. LAWRENCE: No, to the contrary, the HeLa cells seen attached on the falcon flask did nothing but sit there transfixed during a period of five additional days of observation with time-lapse cinematography - i.e. for a total period of 12 days in all (see Fig. 45). We have also done additional experimenta designed to answer this exact question. Culture media containing human LT were removed from HeLa cell cultures after four days exposure and replaced with fresh media. The HeLa cells were then incubated for an additional seven days. The reduction in clones observed in cultures treated in this fashion was the same as that observed in control flasks that had been cultured continuously in the presence of human LT.

DR. HIRSCHHORN: But do all the cells respond in this way or do some of them in fact come off the flask surface into the supernatant?

V. CYTOTOXICITY OR STIMULATION BY EFFECTOR MOLECULES

DR. LAWRENCE: No, that is another finding of interest, the cells remain adherent to the surface of the flask - all of them.

DR. HIRSCHHORN: Two points made by Dr. Granger relate to the problem of mechanism. One is the question of why some cells die while others get stimulated, in other words, the difference between the target cells and the lymphocytes which respond quite differently. I think that membrane phenomena must be involved and I would imagine that sodium pumps or lipid turnover in target cell membranes might be affected profoundly - also that lysosomal activation is involved. We have demonstrated that in the lymphocyte, lysosomal activation will in fact lead to stimulation of that cell. It is entirely feasible that in a dividing cell rather than a resting cell, lysosomal activation could lead to death. A macrophage is another type of resting cell, and in this cell lysosomal activation, induced by phagocytosis, would not necessarily lead to death.

Once again I would urge that we stop using the term "gene derepression." We have no evidence for gene derepression in the situations we have been discussing. The fact that actinomycin causes some diminution can reflect effects on ribosomal RNA synthesis and may have nothing to do with messenger. I think the point to be emphasized here is that these factors are produced in the absence of DNA synthesis. This event does occur very early; it is not completely inhibitable by actinomycin, and therefore we must search for a mechanism whereby pre-existing or constantly made messenger is transported out into the cytoplasm for the purpose of making a new substance on the newly made ribosomes in these stimulated cells.

DR. VALENTINE: I would like to comment on three of the questions posed by Dr. Möller, using information from the studies of Lebowitz and Lawrence which have been discussed earlier. In these studies blood lymphocyte populations of 95 percent purity were stimulated by PPD and produced supernatants with toxic activity. Thus, it is most likely that a soluble toxic material similar to LT comes from the lymphocyte. The second point is in regard to the assay of cell killing. We have seen that few clones remain. In fact also there are no unattached cells in the media of the HeLa cell cultures. We have no evidence to indicate that the absence of clones is the result of an interference with attachment. Thirdly, regarding the problem of contact being a requirement for the initiation of stimulation of the lymphocytes rather than a requirement for the killing mechanism, we find that lymphocytes preincubated with antigen for 36 hours and <u>then</u> placed on the HeLa target cells kill them in a much more efficient fashion. If the same number of lymphocytes are put on the HeLa cells directly and antigen added, killing is then very poor. We would interpret this as indicating that high density cell contact with antigen facilitates their interaction and indeed may be necessary for the immune cell to release this cytotoxic material.

DR. BACH: I mentioned previously that in MLC there is a factor present in the culture supernatant that is blastogenic. There is also a factor, and I mean to imply we know it to be a different factor, that is present in MLC and is cytotoxic, as Dr. Granger has pointed out. We find that the presence of the cytotoxic factor is dependent on cell concentration in the MLC producing the factor. High cell concentrations provide much inhibitory activity, so much indeed that blastogenic factor activity frequently cannot be detected. Inhibitory activity is assayed in terms of ability to inhibit another MLC reaction, or for its ability to destroy fibroblasts in a monolayer. In fact, if we take one person's cells alone, and test them at a high concentration (about six to ten-fold higher concentration than we generally use) such cells alone will release cytotoxic factor. In view of the findings of the Möllers on granulocyte toxicity, we have purified cells extensively and observe that preparations 98 to 99 percent pure produce just as much of this cytotoxic activity. This cell concentration effect is of particular concern to me, as we find that at low cell concentrations there is produced rather considerable amounts of blastogenic factor but no significant amount of inhibitory factor.

DR. BRAUN: I want to come back to the matter of target cell concentration. Dr. Granger, when you add your purified LT, is this to a constant or a variable number of target cells.

V. CYTOTOXICITY OR STIMULATION BY EFFECTOR MOLECULES

DR. GRANGER: We have examined the effects of target cell concentration on LT induced destruction. It was based on exploratory studies that we arrived at a standard number of 100,000-200,000 cells per tube in two ml medium as appropriate for our assay. These cells are in log phase growth during the 48-hour exposure to LT. We have noticed differences in sensitivity in old compared to young vigorous cultures and consequently have made efforts to standardize conditions to avoid these variables.

DR. VALENTINE: We have heard that supernatants of sensitive lymphocytes stimulated by antigen contain biologically active materials as determined by several different assay systems. The physical or chemical separation of a substance active in one system from materials active in a second system presumably would indicate that the biological activities were due to two different molecules. However, some of these biological effects may well be due to different concentrations of the same molecule or only _seem_ to differ because of the different ways we measure them. In studies comparing these systems I think we must be careful about the variables in the production and assay of active supernatants, the number of lymphocytes, the presence or absence of phagocytic cells, the dose and type of stimulant, the amount of supernatant used in the assay system, and the sensitivity of that system in reference to the number of activated lymphocytes producing the effect. On first thought one would assume that the _in vitro_ biological system that detects the smallest amount of supernatant activity, as related to the number of activated lymphocytes, might simulate most closely the events _in vivo_. However, the occurence of stimulatory effects at low concentrations of active supernatant and inhibitory effects at higher concentrations obviously suggests a possible control mechanism.

DR. HIRSCHHORN: I would be particularly interested in Dr. Granger's views on the relationship of LT, in partially purified form, to the other effector molecules that were discussed in the preceding session.

DR. GRANGER: We do not, at present, have any information on the relationship of human LT to chemotactic factor. However, as previously mentioned, sephadex and DEAE refined human LT does inhibit mouse or guinea pig macrophage migration from capillary tubes. Moreover LT and MIF derived from human, mouse, and guinea pig cells are both resistant to heating. While the information is still incomplete, it is entirely possible that they are the same; inhibition of migration may only reflect lower concentrations of the material, temporarily affecting macrophages, but not killing them. While we do not yet have sufficient data to verify an absolute relationship of LT to blastogenic factor, initial results suggest that MIF, LT and blastogenic factor may very well be the same material that at high concentrations is toxic, at intermediate levels temporarily incapacitates cells, and at low levels stimulates cells.

DR. VALENTINE: If the multiple biological activities measured in the supernatants of sensitive lymphocytes stimulated by antigen are due to different molecules then theoretically, one might postulate that each of these effector molecules was coming from a different lymphocyte. This theory must be plausible in the case of the nonspecific activation by PHA of a large proportion of the total lymphocytes. However, it would seem highly unlikely that there are different groups of lymphocytes, each of which is geared to the production of a particular factor and also capable of specific activation by a given antigen. It would seem more likely that multiple factors are produced by a single cell upon activation by specific antigen. There is, however, another slightly more complex view for which there is presently no evidence. A sensitive lymphocyte, upon activation by antigen, might release one product which in turn was capable of causing other types of lymphocytes, not themselves antigenically responsive, to elaborate the various effector molecules. This theory would allow for a specific immune initiation of events, a nonspecific intermediate product, and a variety of effector molecules dependent on what groups of cells were induced to respond. The fact is that such "cascade" mechanisms exist in other biological systems.

DR. LAWRENCE: Would Dr. Granger tell us whether LT binds to the target cells.

DR. GRANGER: A number of observations suggest that if LT does bind to target cells, the binding must either be weak or occur at low levels. We found that LT-induced target cell destruction, whether involving the products of human

V. CYTOTOXICITY OR STIMULATION BY EFFECTOR MOLECULES

or murine origin, could be reversed up to the point where the cells had rounded up and become vacuolated, provided the toxic medium were replaced with fresh medium. In the case of mouse LT, this can still be done many hours after initial exposure. Moreover, repeated absorption of toxic medium with large numbers of sensitive cells did not markedly reduce the level of toxicity. However, target cells are apparently able either to bind or to inactivate LT to some extent, for they do recover from exposure to medium containing low levels of LT.

DR. VALENTINE: I wonder if Dr. Granger has had information about the effects of a brief exposure of target cells to LT. Is there a sharp difference between the length of exposure causing a reversible inhibition of target cells and that causing irreversible damage? Also he mentioned that human LT requires certain co-factors. Could he elaborate on that?

DR. GRANGER: The effect of both human and mouse LT can be reversed up to a certain stage as mentioned previously in reply to Dr. Lawrence. This varies, of course, with the amount of LT present, the number of the particular target cells employed, and their physiologic state. The reversibility of this interaction is not sharply focused but rather is spread out over a period of time. For example, mouse LT cytotoxicity on L cells continues to be reversible for as long as 24 hours. However, during the next four hours it becomes irreversible.

As to your second question, I prefer not to elaborate in detail because the data are still of a preliminary kind. However, I can say that human LT requires divalent cations for its effects and that it may be inactivated by certain heavy metals. Moreover, its stability and effectiveness can be greatly enhanced by the presence of a critical amount of protein.

DR. LANDY: Dr. Granger, you have indicated that an extensive array of target cells are killed by LT. These represented both established cell lines and primary cultures from many animal species. Have your tests been conducted in such a way that you discerned either differences or similarities in their susceptibility to this cytotoxicity. My point is that widely divergent cell types would be expected to differ appreciably in the makeup and character of their membranes.

DR. GRANGER: It is clear that at high concentrations both human and mouse LT act in vitro in a nonspecific manner, suggesting that the LT-sensitive site must be a widely distributed common unit expressed on the membranes of many cell types. However, at lower concentrations of LT differences in the sensitivity of the same spectrum of cell types emerge, and we find that this same LT medium now can stimulate cellular protein synthesis. These diverse concentration-dependent effects could be attributed to the ability of different cell types to facilitate repair of small focal LT-induced lesions and the degree of expression (frequency) and accessibility of these sensitive membrane sites. Our studies suggest to us that both of these factors may operate to determine the effect of a given level of LT on a particular target cell.

DR. MÖLLER: Dr. Granger, in vitro situations are always difficult to translate into events that occur in the body. The release in vivo of highly toxic molecules would seem to be dangerous for the organism, unless they act over extremely short distances or are rapidly inactivated. How do you interpret your own findings with regard to function in vivo?

DR. GRANGER: It is, as Dr. Möller has already pointed out, difficult to propose direct correlations from in vitro situations, at least until we become more aware of the fundamental characteristics of these cellular immune reactions. However, I believe that for the present the answer to your question may lie in how the host controls these processes. Obviously in vitro systems operate independently of the elements of host control. One can visualize many steps where regulation would greatly influence the outcome with respect to effector molecules. For example: (a) activation – certainly the initiating agent would dictate which cells could be triggered and how many in a given population would respond, (b) cellular biosynthetic response – this would control the amount of the material actually fabricated and released, (c) a means of inactivating LT is presumed to exist, which would tend to keep the reaction localized and finally, (d) there must be some means of terminating the reaction when it is no longer necessary. By exercising control at one or more of these steps host lymphoid cells could induce specific destruction of adjacent foreign cells by the release of a nonspecific cell toxin,

V. CYTOTOXICITY OR STIMULATION BY EFFECTOR MOLECULES

such as LT. In pathologic situations, on the other hand, such as frequently characterize delayed hypersensitivity reactions and certain autoimmune disease states, the individual may in fact lack the capability to contain these reactions, with consequent generalized nonspecific tissue destruction.

DR. VALENTINE: As Dr. Granger has said, there must be some sort of control mechanism or limitation on the action of lymphotoxin. A very likely mechanism of limitation that has been mentioned is that lymphotoxin in amounts produced <u>in vivo</u> by a given focus of stimulated lymphocytes would be rapidly diluted below effective concentrations by diffusion away from the site of production. Additional mechanisms limiting the activity of this material might be that it is adsorbed and/or inactivated by non-lymphoid cells. A similar mechanism has been suggested to explain the greater yield of MIF activity from relatively pure lymphoid populations as compared with the total population of peritoneal exudate cells. More specific control mechanisms might include a circulating inhibitor molecule, or an immunologically specific mechanism which acted <u>in vivo</u> to keep antigen from triggering the lymphocyte and initiating lymphotoxin production; antibody would be an obvious candidate for this sort of regulation.

DR. LANDY: My comment is directed to Dr. Möller. I recall a series of papers some years ago by you and Dr. E. Möller, and also by Perlmann and Holm, that dealt with cytotoxicity of lymphocytes for target cells. The details of these reports escape me at the moment other than that the number of combinations of aggressor and target cells resulting in cell destruction of the latter were at that time difficult to assess in classical immunologic terms. The implications were that in these situations the recognition and destruction did not seem to depend on immunologic mechanisms. However, I would now be inclined to interpret that work in a quite different way, because in many, indeed the most interesting instances, the experiments involved inclusion of PHA in the lymphocyte-target cell interactions. You will recall from a number of our discussions in Stockholm and elsewhere, that at that time your view and that of Perlmann was that PHA was included as being helpful rather than necessary, in that it agglutinated the cells and served to bring them more closely into contact with target cells.

I would now view those published works as having really dealt with lymphocytes that were enormously activated by PHA; rather than resulting from cell-cell interactions that seemed to exclude conventional immunological considerations. We now appreciate, of course, that such powerfully activated lymphocytes would be elaborating effector molecules such as LT and be capable of destroying target cells quite independently of their particular immunological specificity.

DR. MÖLLER: Our original experiments were performed by adding normal human lymphocytes to allogeneic or to autologous fibroblasts in the presence or absence of PHA. The findings were as follows: in the absence of PHA there was no cytotoxic effect whatsoever, but in the presence of PHA the lymphocytes become strongly cytotoxic to both types of target cells. Cytotoxicity was, as Dr. Landy has said, due to stimulation of the lymphocytes by PHA rather than to the agglutination it produced. A similar stimulation of cytotoxicity could also be achieved with other non-agglutinating substances, such as streptolysin. However, close contact between lymphocytes and target cells was necessary and separation of the cells by a thin layer of agar or a layer of ALS molecules prevented the expression of cytotoxicity. Although PHA stimulated the lymphocytes to cytotoxicity this stimulation was not related to the increased RNA and DNA synthesis induced by PHA, since these synthetic processes could be suppressed without affecting cytotoxicity. Viable lymphocytes were essential however.

Lymphocytes from immunized individuals upon exposure to the corresponding antigen also transformed into a cytotoxic state active on fibroblasts. If the corresponding antigen were a histocompatibility antigen shared by the fibroblasts, cytotoxicity was specific for these target cells. However, if the lymphocytes were immunized against bacteria and added to target cells in the presence of bacteria, they also killed autologous target cells. Thus, in our experience the _inductive_ phase of cytotoxicity appeared to be specific but the _expression_ was nonspecific; as Dr. Landy has pointed out, our use of PHA resulted in the complete bypassing of the specific immunological recognition step.

DR. LANDY: Dr. Granger, it seems to me that in this fascinating area of lymphocyte aggressor capability against target cells, there has been reached a solid consensus that

V. CYTOTOXICITY OR STIMULATION BY EFFECTOR MOLECULES

lymphocytes can indeed directly express cytotoxicity against target cells; this involves direct contact. However, it appears to be quite another matter as regards the production by lymphocytes of a soluble toxin, such as LT, capable of acting on target cells in the absence of the producing cell. Apparently many workers have not succeeded in discerning this kind of activity under their particular experimental conditions. Having been able consistently to produce, and by various means assess LT as a potent toxin elaborated by lymphocytes, you surely must have given considerable thought to the reasons for your positive findings as opposed to the failure of others <u>apparently</u> working under similar conditions. Would you therefore summarize for us what you feel are the critical elements of your production and/or assay systems that could account for this dichotomy.

DR. GRANGER: These systems have been studied by many investigators using a variety of experimental conditions, animal species and techniques. It would, therefore, be well nigh impossible to assess independently or collectively the technical features operative in each instance. I have indeed asked myself why a soluble toxic factor has not been detected in some other systems. I believe the critical factors are most probably the following: The degree of lymphocyte stimulation achieved, inasmuch as the amount of LT released is directly related to this. In the experimental situations most widely employed the actual number of responding immune aggressor cells in the population is rather low. In these instances LT levels in the immediate vicinity of the secreting cells might be considerable but the overall level in the medium would be low and, in the absence of concentration, perhaps even be imperceptible. A similar situation also applies to normal lymphocytes stimulated by mitogens. At optimal dosage of mitogen the levels of LT developed are high, whereas with limiting amounts of mitogen the concentration of LT is greatly reduced. The nature of the assay for cellular destruction is critical. With high levels of LT total destruction of monolayers can be obtained and the results would be apparent to anyone. However, relatively low concentrations require more sensitive techniques and here parameters of number, type, physiologic state of the target cells and the tissue culture medium employed become highly critical. Finally, I believe that the culture medium used in these systems is of particular importance. It determines and in some ways controls

the magnitude and duration of the lymphocyte response within
the limits imposed by the stimulant; moreover it affects
the stability of LT and to some degree its effectiveness on
target cells.

CHAIRMAN SILVERSTEIN: From this point on I believe we
should move on to deal with three other areas. One is the
relationship of the macrophage and all that it implies, in
the process of delayed hypersensitivity and in tissue damage.
Secondly, we might look at several models for the involvement of delayed hypersensitivity in damage to host tissues
and to homografts. Thirdly, I think it would be desirable
to consider the role of delayed hypersensitivity in the
grand scheme of defense and immunity, particularly with
respect to some of the more compelling problems of disease.

I would call on Dr. Mackaness to begin the discussion of
the macrophage as part of the effector mechanism in cell-
mediated immunity.

DR. MACKANESS: We have heard a great deal about mediators
of cellular immunity, but there are circumstances in which
it is difficult to invoke such a concept in the ultimate
mediation of immunity. The most obvious example is in
defense against infectious disease. Earlier in this
session the question was raised whether LT had bacterio-
static or bactericidal properties. In the absence of knowledge on this point, we must still ask how it is that the
host defends himself against an infectious disease in which
humoral antibody does not contribute significantly to protection. This situation obtains in some, if not all, intracellular microbial infections, and notably in tuberculosis
and related diseases. It is obvious that if delayed-type
hypersensitivity has a part to play in defense against
microbial invasion, some form of cooperation would be
needed on the part of phagocytic cells, since I think there
is no obvious way in which lymphocytes, being non-phagocytic,
can interact effectively with the parasite. To highlight
the contribution made by the phagocytic components of the
reticulo-endothelial system in defense against intracellular
bacterial parasites, I would like to consider a familiar
model. In the course of an intravenously initiated infection
with BCG the organism multiplies for 12-14 days in all of
the organs into which it is seeded. Despite continuing

V. CYTOTOXICITY OR STIMULATION BY EFFECTOR MOLECULES

multiplication of BCG in the liver and spleen, changes develop in the fixed phagocytic cells of these organs. These changes can be closely monitored by challenging representative animals at frequent intervals with heterologous organisms. Listeria monocytogenes is a good organism for this purpose; it survives and multiplies in normal macrophages, but is effectively killed by fully activated macrophages. If one challenges BCG infected animals with L. monocytogenes, the degree to which they multiply or die in the spleens and livers varies according to the stage of the BCG infection. The rise and fall in the antimicrobial status of the reticulo-endothelial system is described by the observations recorded in Fig. 46. Anti-Listeria resistance reaches a peak on the 12th-14th day. This happens to coincide with the inflection in the growth curve of BCG itself. Another feature of the host response, namely, the development of delayed hypersensitivity, initially manifest on about day nine and is unequivocally in evidence by the 12th day; it increases beyond this time to reach a well sustained peak after about 21 days.

It is reasonable to ask why the reticulo-endothelial function should diminish so abruptly after reaching peak activity at the end of the second week of infection. One of the most likely explanations is that the metabolic activity of BCG is sharply depressed at about this time, as evidenced by its growth curve in spleen and liver. Suffice it to say that Blanden et al. (J. Exp. Med. 129, 1079, 1969) have shown that isoniazid treatment of BCG infected mice effectively interferes with the development of enhanced microbial activity in cells of the reticulo-endothelial system. This implies that it is occasioned by the metabolic activity of the parasite which induces the change.

If one looks at a representative sample of the cells of the reticulo-endothelial system at intervals during the course of a heavy BCG infection, one finds a period of about three days on either side of the time of peak resistance when the macrophages of the peritoneal cavity are grossly and dramatically altered. The activated macrophage has enhanced microbial ability, and it is to this property that the BCG-infected animal owes its resistance to infections. Dead BCG or drug-inhibited BCG do not increase host resistance; this involves a host response dependent on continuing metabolic activity of the parasite.

CELLULAR IMMUNITY

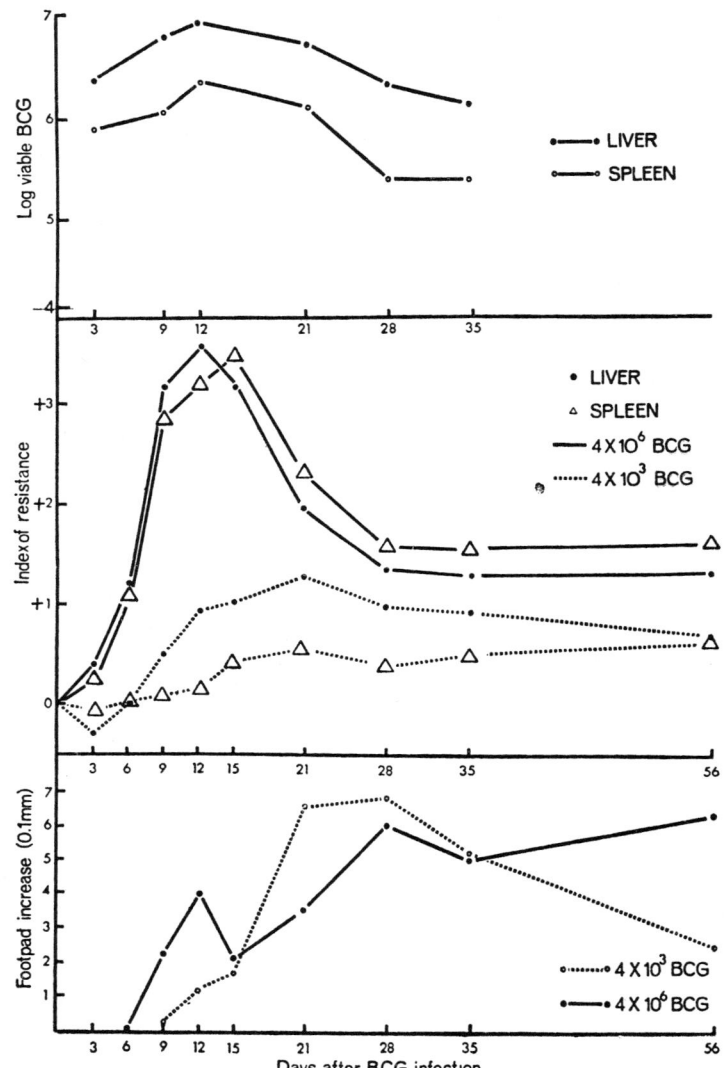

Fig. 46 Growth and survival of BCG <u>in vivo</u> following intravenous inoculation of 4 x 10^6 viable units.

Middle: Change in antimicrobial activity of reticuloendothelial cells of mice infected intravenously with

V. CYTOTOXICITY OR STIMULATION BY EFFECTOR MOLECULES

BCG. Index of resistance is difference, after 24 hours, in viable counts of Listeria, in control and BCG infected animals.

Bottom: Levels of tuberculin sensitivity in BCG infected mice.

(Reproduced with permission of Journal of Exp. Medicine)

Because events move too slowly in BCG-infected mice for a clear demonstration of the time-course of the changes leading to acquired resistance we turned to a simpler model. L. monocytogenes produces a more rapidly moving intracellular infection in mice and the same clearcut changes in host macrophages as occur in BCG-infected mice. Fig. 47 depicts the growth curve of Listeria in the spleens of normal mice.

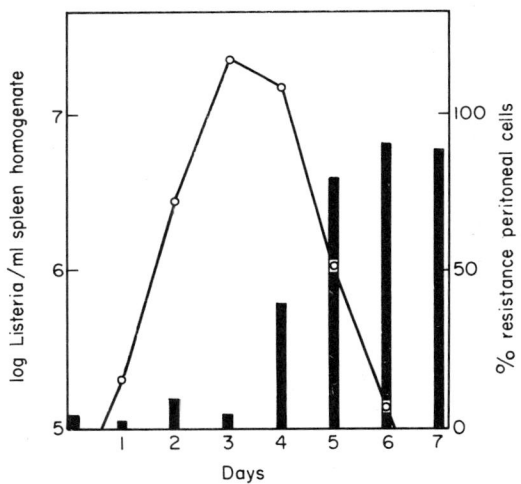

Fig. 47 The development of Listeria resistant macrophages in the peritoneal cavity (histogram) in relation to the onset of immunity as revealed by the growth curve of L. monocytogenes in the spleen during a primary infection in mice.

(Reproduced with permission of Journal of Exp. Medicine)

CELLULAR IMMUNITY

It is obvious that a conspicuous change occurs on or about the third day of infection. From this time on, the further proliferation of the organism ceases and bacterial inactivation ensues. The microbicidal potential of the cells in the peritoneal cavity changes significantly on day four of the infection. For the next few days the percentage of macrophages that have learned to inactivate Listeria increases to involve virtually all cells in the peritoneum. Their enhanced microbicidal activity is apparently intrinsic, because the activated macrophage can handle organisms which are quite unrelated to those used to induce this general state of cellular immunity.

The cells of the peritoneal cavity of animals which have survived a 50 percent lethal dose of Listeria, retain this highly activated state for about two weeks. During this time the convalescent animal is completely resistant to challenge as shown by the bacterial survival curves of Fig. 48. From the second week onwards, however, the

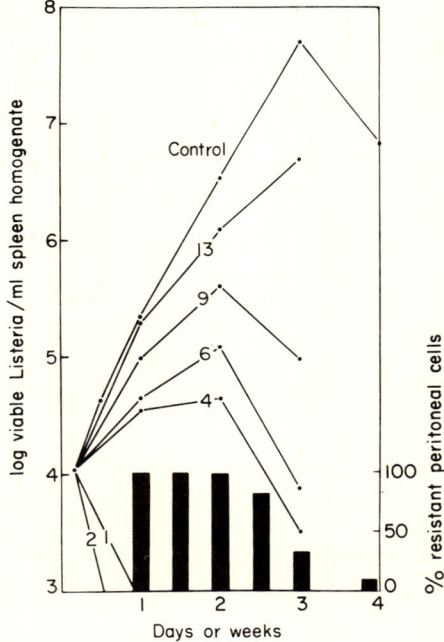

Fig. 48 A family of curves depicting the three-day growth of L. monocytogenes in the spleens of mice challenged,

V. CYTOTOXICITY OR STIMULATION BY EFFECTOR MOLECULES

as numbered, 1 to 13 weeks after a primary Listeria infection. Histogram shows percentage of Listeria-resistant macrophages measured in the peritoneal cavity on the first through the fourth week of convalescence.

(Reproduced with permission of Journal of Exp. Medicine)

percentage of activated cells diminishes, becoming virtually normal by the third week of convalescence. By the fourth week of convalescence, when few activated macrophages persist, the quality of the host's immunity changes. Only a memory of the previous infection remains; but with it the host can recall a microbicidal mechanism very promptly. With the passage of time, even this property is lost, so that the 13th week of convalescence finds the animal substantially normal in his response to re-infection.

What is the nature of the immunological process responsible for this memory of past infection, and the means by which it affords protection against infection? The first important point is that the serum of animals which have recovered from a Listeria infection contains no humoral factor that will make recipient mice behave like convalescent mice. The second significant finding is that mice develop, in the course of infection, a delayed type hypersensitivity to Listeria antigens. It is apparent from Fig. 49 that Listeria-infected mice do not react to culture filtrate during the first three days of infection. From the fourth day onward, however, they become progressively more reactive to Listeria antigens. The first appearance of this altered state of reactivities coincides with a break in the growth curve of Listeria in the spleen. This suggests a causal relationship between the development of delayed reactivity to Listeria antigens and ability to control the growth of the organism. If so, it would be possible to confer protection passive with the lymphoid cells of convalescent animals.

The experiment recorded in Fig. 50 shows that animals can be adoptively immunized with immunologically committed lymphoid cells. The left-hand panel depicts the growth curves of L. monocytogenes in the spleens and livers of animals which received filtered spleen cells from normal

CELLULAR IMMUNITY

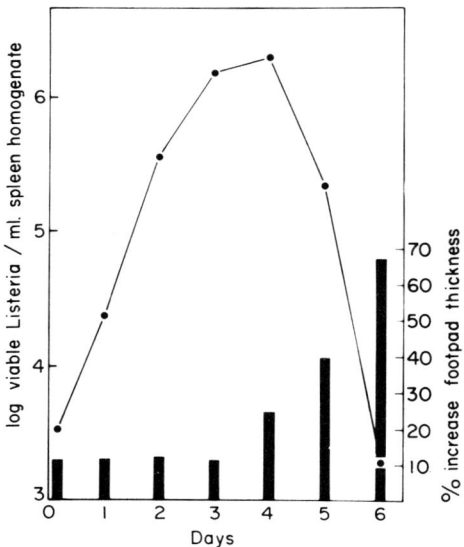

Fig. 49 Mean spleen counts of four normal mice on successive days after infection with a sublethal dose of L. monocytogenes. Histogram shows the corresponding percentage increase in footpad thickness produced by Listeria culture filtrate injected 24 hours previously.

(Reproduced with permission of Journal of Exp. Medicine)

or seven day infected donors. The growth of the challenge organism in animals protected with 2×10^8 immune spleen cells (one spleen equivalent), shows that protection was conferred immediately upon the spleen, but was delayed for 24 hours in the liver. Dr. Sutton and I have evidence to suggest that this difference may be due to the tendency of lymphoid cells to home in on lymphoid organs preferentially. In contrast to the conspicuous protective protective effect of immune spleen cells, the serum of the cell donors was quite inert as shown in the center panel of Fig. 50. Moreover, the third panel reveals that the cells must be alive in order to confer protection on a recipient. In this part of the experiment the inoculum of bacteria was incubated with the immune or normal lymphoid cells. The latter was

V. CYTOTOXICITY OR STIMULATION BY EFFECTOR MOLECULES

then killed by ultrasound before injecting them into recipients. No antibacterial antibody was secreted by the immune lymphoid cells; the lymphoid cells must be alive in order to confer protection.

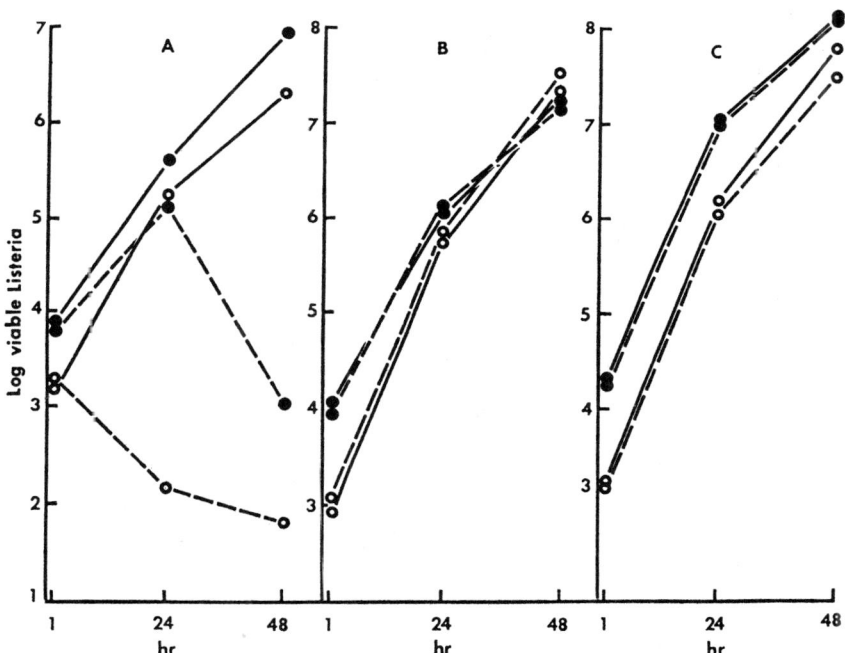

Fig. 50 A. Comparative growth curves of a Listera challenge in the livers (●) and spleens (o) of mice injected with 2×10^8 spleen cells from normal (—) or 7-day immune donors (------). B. Growth curves of L. monocytogenes in animals that received only serum from the normal and immune donors described in A. The organisms were incubated with the sera before injection. Groups as designated in A. C. Growth curves obtained with inocula of Listeria that had been incubated in the presence of the normal or immune spleen cells used in A. The cells were disrupted by untrasound prior to injection.

(Reproduced with permission of Journal of Exp. Medicine)

The development of the cell population that possesses this protective property is illustrated in Fig. 51, which

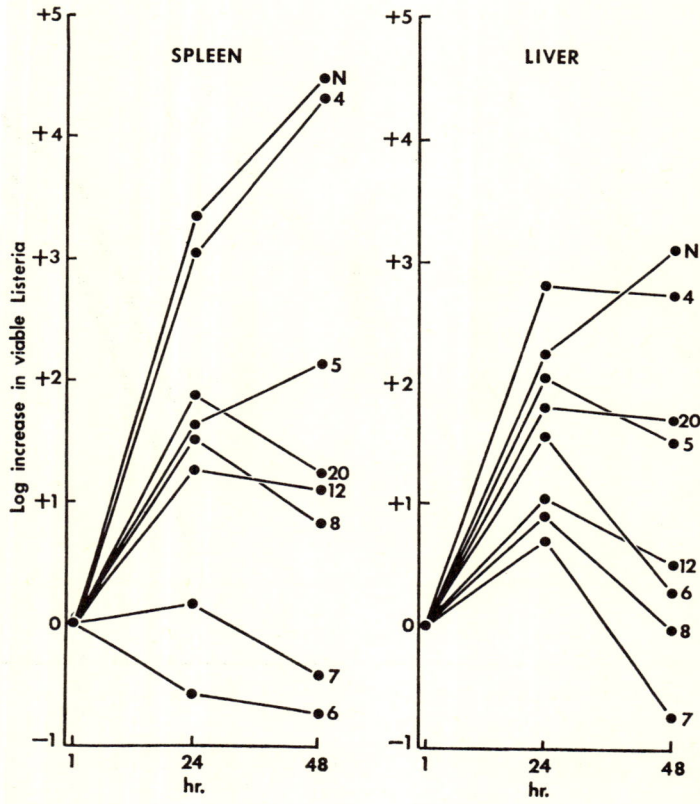

Fig. 51 Inhibition of Listeria challenge in the liver and spleen of mice protected with 10^8 lymphoid cells from the spleens of immunized donors. Numbers indicate day of immunizing infection upon which cell transfer was made.

(Reproduced with permission of Journal of Exp. Medicine)

depicts the growth curves of challenge organisms in mice that had received 10^8 spleen cells harvested at successive stages of an immunizing infection. Cells harvested on day four were almost inactive; but those obtained on the fifth,

V. CYTOTOXICITY OR STIMULATION BY EFFECTOR MOLECULES

sixth and seventh days were very effective. Thereafter the efficiency of protective transfer diminished.

The next study (Fig. 52) illustrates a feature central to the whole problem. Days five to seven of an immunizing

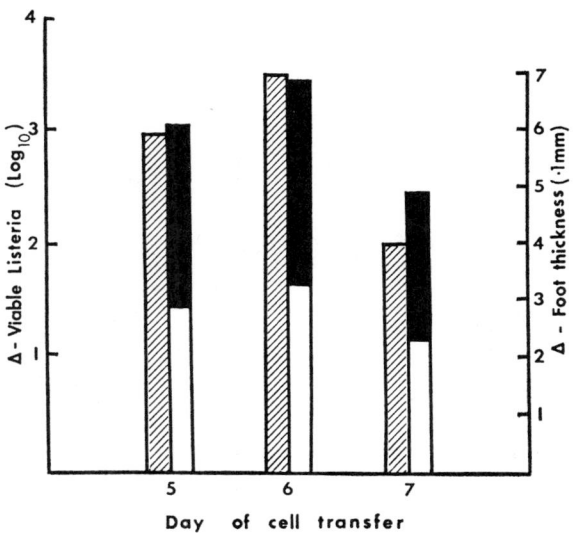

Fig. 52 Comparison between protection (hatched) and level of hypersensitivity (white) conferred with 10^8 spleen cells from 5, 6 or 7 day-immune mice. The level of hypersensitivity in the donors is shown in black. Protection is expressed as the difference between log of the viable count in the spleens of normal and immune cell recipients. Recipients of normal cells gave no measurable reaction to Listeria antigens.

(Reproduced with permission of Journal of Exp. Medicine).

infection showed the sharpest differences in the efficiency of the spleen cell population in terms of protective capacity. Do similar differences occur in the levels of hypersensitivity which could be transferred with cells harvested at these times? The observation recorded in this Figure

CELLULAR IMMUNITY

shows a significant parallel between the levels of delayed hypersensitivity prevailing in donors at different stages of infection, and the levels of sensitivity and protection conferred on normal recipients with a standard number of spleen cells. In view of this parallel, it is significant that ALS deletes the protective capacity of the immune lymphoid cells (Fig. 53). It is immunosuppressive

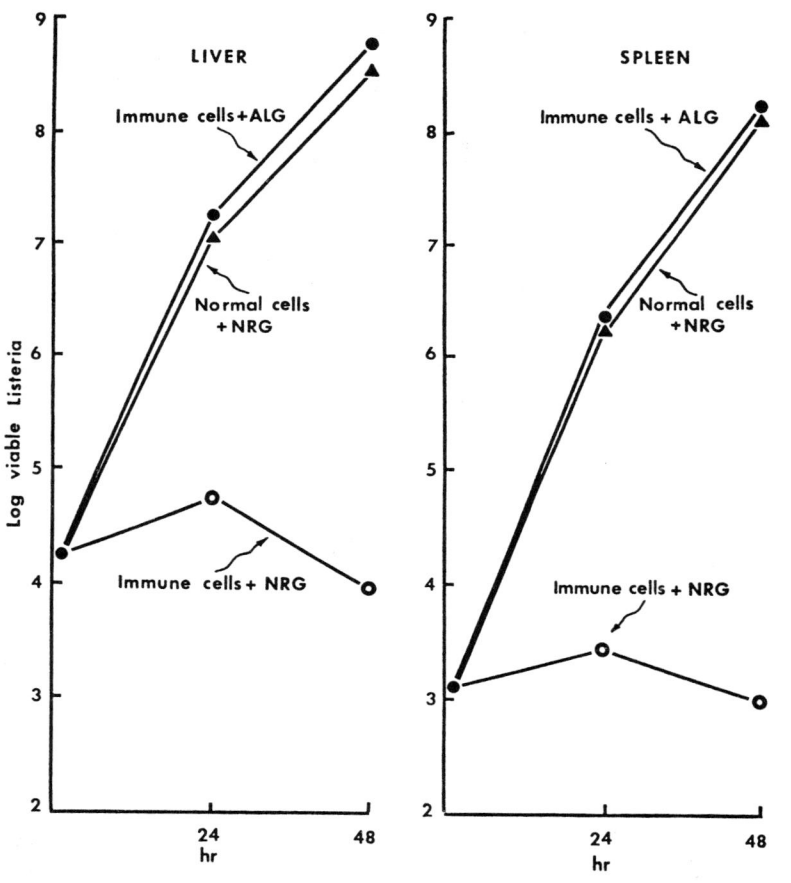

Fig. 53 Growth curves of L. monocytogenes in liver and spleen of mice that were protected passively with normal

V. CYTOTOXICITY OR STIMULATION BY EFFECTOR MOLECULES

or Listeria-immune spleen cell suspensions. The cells were treated with ALG or normal rabbit globulin immediately prior to transfer.

(Reproduced with permission of Journal of Exp. Medicine)

---

when given either before, with or soon after the cells; and blocks the transfer of hypersensitivity in the same unequivocal manner. Since ALS had no detectable effect on mouse macrophages, it seems that the protection and hypersensitivity conferred in this way is vested in vells of the lymphoid series.

The question of specificity in the transfer of cell-mediated immunity is of special interest. As indicated earlier, the BCG-infected mouse becomes highly resistant to heterologous organisms because of the non-specific microbicidal activity of its macrophages. Can the Listeria resistance of BCG-infected mice be transferred to normal recipients? The results shown in Fig. 54 indicate that spleen cells from BCG-infected mice could confer none of the Listeria resistance present in the cell donors.

However, in one experimental group, group B. a significant degree of resistance to Listeria was found. These animals received not only the cells of tuberculin sensitive donors, but an eliciting dose of BCG as well which was mixed with the cells before injection. The dose of BCG used to achieve this effect was not large enough to influence host resistance in recipients of normal cells. Apparently the level of host resistance is not raised by the immune lymphoid cells alone: it takes, in addition, the organism to which the lymphoid cells are specifically sensitive.

We can now consider briefly the basic change in the reticulo-endothelial cells which makes a specific immune reaction into a powerful but nonspecific antibacterial defense mechanism. When the macrophages of the peritoneal cavity were examined in animals which had received normal or immune lymphoid cells obtained from BCG-infected mice, no changes occurred in them unless the passively sensitized animals were also injected intravenously with an eliciting dose of BCG. Within 48 hours the macrophages in animals so treated became functionally and morphologically altered. Since in this and other similar experiments, the sensitized cells and BCG were injected intravenously, and the latter could be recovered almost quantitatively from spleen and liver, it follows that the cells of the peritoneal cavity become changed by an agent that circulates systemically. During the elicitation of a delayed-type hypersensitivity

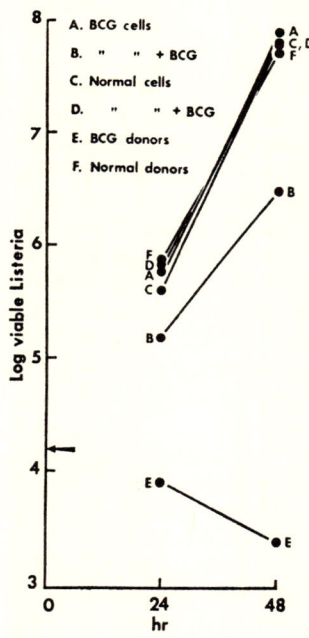

Fig. 54 The behaviour of a population of L. monocytogenes in the spleen of mice that had received 10^8 normal (C and D) or BCG-immunized spleen cells (A and B); and in the spleens of the normal (F) or immune (E) donors. Half of the recipients of normal (D) and immune (B) cells were also injected with a small dose of BCG at the same time.

(Reproduced with permission of Journal of Exp. Medicine)

V. CYTOTOXICITY OR STIMULATION BY EFFECTOR MOLECULES

reaction in an animal, whether actively immunized or passively sensitized with immune lymphoid cells, a systemic change occurs even in secluded anatomical compartments such as the peritoneal cavity. This could mean that systemic effects are produced by something liberated from lymphoid cells when they react with the antigens to which they are specifically sensitive. Substances with the properties of the effector molecules such as MIF or LT could very well be responsible. For this reason it was particularly interesting to learn from Dr. Granger that LT in low concentration stimulates macrophages *in vitro* and produces in them the morphological changes that I consider characteristic of the activated macrophages of infected animals.

CHAIRMAN SILVERSTEIN: It is interesting that over sixty years ago, the stimulation of the phagocytes and their subsequent activity was so popular a topic in society that even Bernard Shaw in his Doctor's Dilemma dealt with it at length. Somewhere up in a Franco-Russian heaven, Ilya Metchnikoff must be smiling with pleasure now.

DR. OPPENHEIM: Dr. Mackaness, can you rule out the possibility that lymphoid cells may be making cytophilic antibodies that are coating the macrophages and in this fashion promote opsonization, and also that this is all secondary to humoral rather than delayed hypersensitivity mechanisms?

DR. MACKANESS: I happen to favor the view that cytophilic antibody is involved in cellular immunity. It seems to me likely that circulating antigen encounters macrophages that have been sensitized by cytophilic antibody, and that their interaction at the cell surface provides the stimulation of membrane activity needed for macrophage activation. For this reason I believe that at least some aspects of delayed hypersensitivity is explicable in terms of cytophilic antibody, but I know that in this respect I am very much in the minority.

DR. BRANDRISS: Can you elicit the type of macrophage change you just described by giving a non-bacterial antigen along with the corresponding specifically sensitized lymphocyte?

DR. MACKANESS: The answer is yes. Macrophages can be modified by the injection of any protein antigen provided that the animal is rendered sensitive to it in the delayed sense.

DR. BRANDRISS: Will culture supernatants prepared by lymphocyte-antigen interaction give any demonstrable effect on macrophage morphology or phagocytic function?

DR. MACKANESS: Those who are enthusiastic about a role for MIF may be disappointed to learn that I have been quite unable to protect animals with lymphocyte culture supernatants, which I assume contain MIF; nor have I been able to induce *in vitro* the morphologic changes in macrophages, that I associate with their enhanced microbicidal activity, with such supernatants. I should point out however that the actual presence of effector molecules in the supernatants was not verified.

DR. BRANDRISS: I believe you stated that four weeks after infection with Listeria the state of resistance to another infection had declined but that "memory" persisted in that the animal could respond more quickly to challenge than normals. However, this accelerated response was gone by the 13th weeks. Is this not quite short-lived compared to the usual duration we associate with immunologic memory?

DR. MACKANESS: Yes, but only because of pre-conceptions on the part of immunologists. I think it is now possible to say that animals that remain tuberculin-sensitive do so because they are constantly stimulated antigenically. The evidence for this is quite substantial. In humans when recent tuberculin conversions are treated with isoniazid, a high proportion of patients lose their sensitivity; mice also do so under the same experimental conditions. This adds significantly to the concept that constant antigenic stimulation is needed to sustain the state of delayed hypersensitivity. In Listeria an effective immune mechanism develops, so that the parasite, and hence the antigenic stimulus, is eliminated. What we see then is the natural decay of the cell population which mediates delayed hypersensitivity in the mouse.

V. CYTOTOXICITY OR STIMULATION BY EFFECTOR MOLECULES

DR. LAWRENCE: In earlier experiments that Drs. David, Thomas and I did in an attempt to relate the in vitro inhibition of macrophage migration to in vivo reality, we found that peritoneal exudate cells from tuberculin sensitive guinea pigs transferred not only cutaneous tuberculin sensitivity but also in turn conferred on the peritoneal exudate cells of the recipient the capacity to be inhibited in their migration by tuberculin (J. Exp. Med. 120, 1189, 1964). This finding should have a bearing on some of Dr. Mackaness' observations. I would therefore suggest that the capacity to make MIF is also being transferred to his recipient animals. Would you agree to that conclusion Dr. Mackaness?

DR. MACKANESS: I guess so.

DR. BRAUN: I wonder, Dr. Mackaness if your observations might not be related to a finding we described a few years ago. I refer to the release in vitro by spleen cells of sensitized animals of a 260 OD absorbing factor when these spleen cells are exposed in vitro to the original immunizing antigen, which in this case was sRBC. The resulting supernatant factor was capable of stimulating all sorts of humoral responses to antigens of an entirely different sort. Since then we have found that the very same materials also stimulate macrophages as measured by carbon clearance. Inasmuch as we know that all of these effects are being inhibited by kinetin ribosides, one would like to know whether the sort of measurements you made in your studies with Listeria might also be inhibited by kinetin riboside.

DR. MACKANESS: I think your observations are highly pertinent. I would like to make it clear that my inability to induce macrophage changes in vivo with preparations expected to contain MIF, does not rule out the possibility that these effector molecules do operate in vivo. My tests thus far may very well have been inadequate in terms of dosage and timing. I think it is entirely possible that your explanation of what happens to clearance rates is analogous to the phenomena I described in relation to host resistance.

DR. SMITH: Dr. Mackaness' finding that six days is the optimal time for transfer of cell mediated resistance to Listeria differs from our in vitro observations on antigen stimulated lymphocyte activation of cells obtained from

BCG-infected mice. At one week there is practically no lymphocyte activation detectable in the presence of tuberculin, whereas this response is maximal at three weeks and has almost disappeared by the eighth to ninth week.

DR. MACKANESS: This seeming discrepancy is easily explained. The development of delayed sensitivity in the Listeria system is rather rapid whereas that for BCG is found to be much slower to evolve. What we have is two events of a quite different tempo which undoubtedly reflect the metabolic habits of the two organisms; one microbe has a generation time of about 35 minutes while the other has a generation time of 24 hours or more. No doubt their respective metabolic rates differ accordingly. Since we know, in the case of intravenously infected animals, that BCG must be alive and metabolically active to induce changes in host resistance, it follows that metabolic rate would be a determining factor in establishing the time at which cells would acquire sensitivity to antigen stimulation *in vitro*.

DR. SMITH: Would you predict, then, that the Listeria sensitivity *in vitro* would occur much earlier than we have observed using BCG?

DR. MACKANESS: Yes, I would expect it earlier, since evidence of immunity can be found within 48 hours of infection in the Listeria system.

DR. GOOD: I am really impressed by these beautiful studies, and I think one can dissect them a bit further with respect to the kind of lymphocytes that are involved in this process. When Dr. Salvin was in our laboratory, he and Dr. Peterson did experiments with another pathogen, Candida, in which they could transform mice essentially into a tissue culture equivalent by means of neonatal thymectomy and eliminating the thymus-dependent system, leaving intact the thymus-independent lymphocyte population.

I think it would be illuminating to know what you can achieve in your system with respect to macrophage activation. Can you use a soluble antigen when the animals are sensitive and do your macrophages have anything on their surface that will combine with that antigen? I think the

V. CYTOTOXICITY OR STIMULATION BY EFFECTOR MOLECULES

question of cytophilic antibody may be crucial. I look upon these angry macrophages as an amplification system for the cell-mediated immunity and not as cells themselves involved via a specific receptor.

DR. LANDY: The implications of data that Dr. Mackaness has presented are broadened further by some rather remarkable work of Howard (Brit. J. Exp. Path., $\underline{42}$, 1961). He found that GVH disease induced in adult F_1 hybrid mice by intravenous injection of parental strain spleen cells enhanced greatly the phagocytic action of the RES as determined by clearance of intravenously injected colloidal carbon. He showed that the markedly proliferating cells in spleen and liver were largely histiocytes similar to those seen following injection of bacterial endotoxin. I believe that this was paralleled by a greatly enhanced resistance to challenge with <u>Salmonella</u> typhimurium Dr. Howard's findings tell us that allogeneic interactions can also activate histiocytes and that while destructive in one sense, can nonetheless effect an enhanced nonspecific host resistance.

DR. THOMAS: Can you produce anything analogous to enhancement in homograft systems if you superimpose in the system very high levels of circulating antibody by passive transfer? Can you ablate this defense mechanism?

DR. MACKANESS: Yes, we can do so under certain conditions. As you probably know, delayed sensitivity to protein antigens can be induced in mice by means of Freund's incomplete adjuvant. In unpublished observations, Blanden immunized animals with soluble hemocyanin and subsequently with hemocyanin incorporated in Freund's incomplete adjuvant. These animals did not develop the minor increase in resistance to a Listeria challenge which was found in animals immunized only with hemocyanin in adjuvant, a regimen which induced delayed sensitivity to hemocyanin. I therefore suspect that antibody to the antigen interferes with the induction of the altered macrophage activity which is a feature of delayed hypersensitivity. Blanden was unable to obtain convincing evidence of the same phenomenon using Listeria antigens instead of this somewhat bizarre system. He attributed his difficulties to the multiplicity of antigens in <u>L. monocytogenes</u>, and lack of information on which are the important ones for host resistance.

CELLULAR IMMUNITY

CHAIRMAN SILVERSTEIN: I think we come away from this aspect of the discussion with the conclusion that the macrophage is one of the primary nonspecific elements which the system of cellular immunity brings into play. We have identified in several models the involvement of macrophages and sensitized lymphocytes for tissue destruction. One of these is the allograft rejection reaction, in which there is obviously a participation of these cellular elements in various combinations and permutations in the destruction of the allografted tissue. I would now ask Dr. Billingham to open the discussion on the manner in which a skin allograft is rejected, and what the specific and nonspecific events might be.

DR. BILLINGHAM: There are several fellow tissue transplanters present, and I am sure we have all listened with great interest to the preceding and present discussions and tried to revise our opinions as to how the familiar mononuclear cell infiltrates found in allografts procure their rejection. I think that so far as most solid tissue and organ grafts are concerned humoral isoantibodies can be excluded as playing any significant role in the rejection process. There are probably two separate effector mechanisms underlying the homograft reaction: first, there is the "kiss of death" resulting from specific contact of a host effector or specifically activated cell with a foreign cell in the graft. This phenomenon was discovered from *in vitro* studies by Rosenau and Moon, Wilson and others. However from *in vitro* and other findings it seems obvious that there are probably too few specifically "armed" lymphocytic effector cells to account for the death of the entire cell population in a graft in this way. Mediators of the type we have been discussing here, must in some way or another be involved and probably account for the major part of the tissue destruction observed. Furthermore, it seems necessary to postulate that agents like MIF must play an important recruiting and indoctrinating role coercing non-specific mononuclear cells, probably of bone-marrow origin, to join forces in procuring the death of the homograft.

I suppose a crude analogy of my interpretation of the events is as follows. You might have a small group of "specific" communist agitators demonstrating against the British Government in Trafalgar Square whose activities

V. CYTOTOXICITY OR STIMULATION BY EFFECTOR MOLECULES

attract a large crowd of politically uncommitted listeners. The latter may become emotionally roused and a hell of a lot of windows and heads may be broken largely as a result of a nonspecific process. This is a very crude analogy, but I think reflects the present status of our knowledge.

There are one or two observations we must not forget however, when we are tempted to argue that presumably diffusible non-specific agents are the ultimate effectors of graft rejection. In the first place as Medawar pointed out a long time ago, when a homograft is destroyed the infiltrating cell population of host origin always dies with it. This may not be entirely the result of vascular deprivation. It could reflect the non-discriminatory action of diffusible, biologically active substances such as LT.

However, if one postulates that the mononuclear cell infiltrate in an allograft undergoing rejection, is liberating a variety of effector reagents which diffuse through the graft's parenchyma, there are one or two observations which are difficult to reconcile with this interpretation. Medawar has shown that if you inlay small skin autografts into much larger skin allografts in rabbits, destruction of the compatible grafts does not accompany that of the incompatible grafts. This was a crude experiment in terms of the size of central, potentially compatible graft. However, even when refinements were introduced similar results were obtained - the rejection process seemed to be highly specific. Revesz and Klein have mixed very small numbers of compatible tumor cells with very large numbers of incompatible tumor cells and inoculated the mixture into mice. In nearly every case the small minority of compatible tumor cells succeeded in generating tumors, implying that whatever was responsible for the destruction of the massive preponderance of incompatible cells, did not harm the intimately mixed minority of compatible cells.

Dr. Silvers and I have carried out essentially analagous experiments in guinea pigs with similar results. Using appropriately designed experiments it is possible to get pigment cells from a strain 13 guinea pig to grow in the superficial epidermis in an initially white skin area of a strain 2 guinea pig. Secondarily, blackened epidermis of the latter therefore contains strain 2 malpighian cells with a small minority of pigment cells of strain 13 origin. If such epidermis is transferred to a strain 13 guinea pig sensitized against strain 2 tissues the melanocytes will survive despite the destruction of the neighboring strain 2 malpighian cells. Thus there is no evidence of any non-specific destruction of the minority cells. Furthermore in rabbits, if you mix epidermal cell suspensions from two animals, A and B, and "seed" them over a large, full-thickness bed prepared in the integument of B, a large sheet of epidermis of composite origin will be generated. Despite the presumed destruction of B's cells, the wound remains fully epithelialized.

There is one experimental observation, however, which points in the opposite direction. Drs. Elkins and Guttman have recently been doing experiments involving the ortho-topic transplantation of renal grafts in rats. They are using (Lewis x BN) F_1 hybrid rats as hosts into which Lewis strain donor kidneys are transplanted and which are of course accepted. If suspensions of Lewis strain lymphocytes were injected beneath the capsules of these Lewis kidneys in the hybrid hosts, local graft-versus-host-type reactions developed which destroyed significant amounts of the renal tissue. Clearly the reacting cells were Lewis lymphoid cells confronted and stimulated by F_1 mononuclear cells circulating in the blood of the transplanted kidneys. The damage inflicted upon the latter therefore must necessarily have been non-specific damage. Drs. Wilson and Elkins have suggested that the lesions in these kidneys were essentially one-way mixed lymphocyte interactions. However, one cannot escape the conclusion that some kind of non-specific agent was responsible for the destruction of the Lewis renal tissue.

CHAIRMAN SILVERSTEIN: Dr. Billingham has highlighted in a clear and concise fashion the most important point that we are dealing with in this part of the present session. That is whether there is any significant amount of non-specific damage in the vicinity of a specific delayed hypersensitivity reaction.

DR. BACH: I think another point of particular interest might now be added. Studies demonstrating non-specificity are largely derived from _in vitro_ tests. If you sensitize animals _in vivo_, and then test for the capabilities of

V. CYTOTOXICITY OR STIMULATION BY EFFECTOR MOLECULES

killing cells in vitro, you do get specificity in the killing. Here you can establish contact between the sensitized cells and cells other than those to which they have been sensitized - such cells they will not kill. There thus seems to be specificity.

DR. GOOD: Dr. Billingham has made a very able summary of the issues. There is however one that we might focus on a little more and perhaps derive an experiment that will give us an important answer, I am thinking of the GVH reaction. There is no question that initiation of the GVH reaction is a highly specific immunological event. There is also no question however, that there are delayed events in the GVH reaction. The extensions are not immunological, and if you look at the lesions in man, you can see very clearly that at the sites where the destruction of tissue is taking place, there are precious few lymphocytes; often it is hard to find any lymphocytes, yet the destruction goes on. I would attribute such damage to angry activated macrophages. The kind of experiment I would like to suggest is that the GVH reaction might provide an extraordinary way of sensitizing mice to kill infectious agents such as Listeria.

DR. MACKANESS: I have a specific answer to that proposal. Dr. Blanden, induced GVH reactions in A/J x C57B1 hybrids. Despite a severe ongoing GVH reaction the animals were able to survive many lethal doses of Listeria (Transplantation - in the press 1969). The peritoneal cavities of the grafted mice contained the "angriest" macrophages we have seen except perhaps for those which appear in brucella-infected animals. Blanden and I, among others, have already suggested that the GVH reaction is a generalized delayed hypersensitivity reaction.

DR. LANDY: Dr. Billingham, your vivid delineation of the complex process involved in the rejection of a skin graft and the associated tissue damage, reminds me of a very interesting paper by Steinmuller, given at the recent International Congress of the Transplantation Society (Trans. Proc. 1, 593, 1969). As I recall he demonstrated most convincingly that skin allografts that had been largely freed of passenger lymphocytes survived much longer on the host. Wouldn't you consider this important and relevant to our understanding of this process?

DR. BILLINGHAM: I am glad you brought this point up, Dr. Landy. There is increasing evidence from Dr. Good's laboratory; from the work of Guttman and Elkins, parts of which I cited; from Dr. Merrill's group; and, of course from Dr. Steinmuller, that the principal inciters of immunity against tissue and organ allografts are not necessarily the indigenous population of cells in those grafts. A very significant contribution to the incitement of host resistance may be made by "passenger" cells, donor leucocytes of some kind either present in the vasculature or actually in the parenchyma of the donor graft.

However, I think that even if we could clean out <u>all</u> the postulated passenger cells from a graft, although we would probably get prolongation of survival, rejection would ultimately occur.

DR. HIRSCHHORN: The question of specific versus non-specific reactions reminds me of two experiments, one an early one from our own laboratory which is not as discriminating as the second one which I will mention in a moment. Our experiment consisted of cultivating lymphocytes from one individual on fibroblasts of another without the presence of PHA. If these were left on the monolayer for eight days, they did eventually cause tissue damage. If they were transferred at this time to fresh fibroblasts prepared from the initial fibroblast donor, they were now much more rapidly effective in their destructive ability. This response had not been observed on autologous fibroblasts. The reaction was accelerated similarly by PHA.

This was much more clearly demonstrated by Ginsberg in his experiment involving rat lymphocytes on mouse fibroblasts in which cytotoxicity after transfer was H-2 specific, in causing rapid destruction following sensitization of the lymph node cells by the fibroblasts upon which they were initially cultured.

CHAIRMAN SILVERSTEIN: I too have a contribution to the question of the role of non-specific elements in tissue damage. Following Billingham and co-workers, we have done some work on the heterotopic transplantation of corneal epithelium onto a prepared skin site. This is very useful model in which one can look through this

V. CYTOTOXICITY OR STIMULATION BY EFFECTOR MOLECULES

transparent layer of corneal epithelial cells with a microscope, to see what is going on underneath. It is also a model in which there is no involvement of donor vascular endothelium, since no donor vessels are transplanted.

It is usually suggested in the literature that the first target of specific graft rejection is the donor endothelial cells. In this model, which has no donor endothelium one typically sees the first sign of involvement between the host and the graft in the recipient's capillaries under the epithelium. These vessels, it should be noted, do not even penetrate up into the donor epithelium. Yet, one sees the same sequence of disturbance of the recipients endothelial cells and vessels, which start to leak and often thrombose. Cells come out of these vessels and then invade and actively destroy this avascular epithelial graft.

I think it is quite clear now that we are faced with an interesting problem in view of the data that Dr. Billingham has presented on the lack of damage to "host" cells in the presence of a violent delayed hypersensitivity reaction in the immediate vicinity. There are other situations that we are all aware of, in which this type of damage to neighboring, naive onlooker cells does take place, and it might be worth a moment to explore this.

DR. BILLINGHAM: Over the last few years, Dr. Möller and his wife and his colleagues, the Hellstroms, have reported on two interesting and potentially important phenomena, those of "allogenic inhibition" or syngeneic preference and that of "contact-mediated cytolysis." According to them, to inhibit the activities of target cells or to kill them does not necessarily require mediation by immunocompetent cells. They instead result from intimate or very close contact of cells having different surface configurations.

Much, but not all, of their work has been done with _in vitro_ systems, and from their findings they have made certain predictions about possible surveillance mechanisms operative _in vivo_. Over the last year or two, several different _in vivo_ phenomena, such as the production of allophenic mice and the long-term survival of heterografts in ALS-treated animals have been described which are inconsistent with these postulated phenomena. This is a good opportunity to ask Dr. Möller his present feelings about contact mediated cytolysis and allogenic inhibition.

DR. MÖLLER: I think we have to distinguish two reactions-- allogeneic inhibition, which I will define as growth inhibition by a non-immunological mechanism when histoincompatible cells are confronted with each other and the cytotoxic effects which you see with activated lymphocytes. In the human system which I have talked about, we have no evidence at all for allogeneic inhibition and target-cell killing by lymphocytes requires metabolically active and living lymphocytes. So that is a clear case of an aggressive lymphocyte killing.

In the mouse system, though, this is not the case. There we have both in vitro and in vivo models. In vitro we can show that mouse lymphocytes in the presence of PHA will kill allogeneic target cells to a larger extent than syngeneic cells. This differential effect is quite different than in the human system. In the mouse system, F_1 hybrid cells will kill parental target cells. Therefore, we have a process which shows immunogenic specificity, but does not obey immunogenetic rules. It is obviously not an immunological process, because tolerant lymphocytes can kill cells of the tolerated genotype.

In order to explain these data we used the concept of allogeneic inhibition, developed by Hellström in another context. I think one should remember that allogeneic inhibition is basically an in vivo concept revealed as inhibition of tumor growth in F_1 hybrids, in the absence detectable immune reactions. When you mix two tumor cells of different genotypes in the presence of PHA and inoculate this mixture into an irradiated host, tumor growth is inhibited as compared to syngeneic mixtures. It is an old observation initially described by Snell, that tumor cells of lymphoid or fibroblastic origin as well as normal bone marrow cells and normal lymphocytes, are inhibited in F_1 hybrid hosts in the absence of any immune reaction. All these in vivo phenomena have been used to interpret the in vitro findings: the interpretation being that we are dealing with a surface to surface interaction between two cells which are incompatible with regard to the structure of their histocompatibility antigens. Somehow the target cell

V. CYTOTOXICITY OR STIMULATION BY EFFECTOR MOLECULES

detects these differences and this leads to growth inhibition or direct kill. Now you can bring up new data that is apparently in contradiction to this concept; the allophenic mice being the example that this situation could be predicted from allogeneic concept. Of course there is no direct answer to this. There is some way out of it however. Hellström has demonstrated that repeated passages of the tumors in a foreign environment makes it specifically resistant to allogeneic inhibition in their particular genotype, but not in another. Thus, one could postulate that there is a mechanism for induction of, let's call it tolerance to this surface recognition phenomenon. If this is so, the allophenic mice may have developed such tolerance. Allogeneic inhibition is thus a weak but definite reaction.

CHAIRMAN SILVERSTEIN: I would now ask Dr. Waksman to introduce the question of the delayed hypersensitivity reactions in which there is distinct damage to host cells uninvolved, as far as we know, with the antigen itself.

DR. WAKSMAN: First I have a comment on what has been said so far. This session makes it clear that specifically or nonspecifically activated lymphocytes can produce a cytopathogenic effect on target cells, either by direct contact with them or by way of a mediator. It is also clear, from what was said before, that macrophages can produce non-specific damage of certain types of target cells. By suitable labeling techniques, it has been shown, in most types of cell-mediated reactions, that both specifically sensitized lymphocytes and bone marrow-derived cells (monocytes or histiocytes), are present in each type of lesion. The question to address ourselves to is: which produces the damage and why:

The experiment that Dr. Billingham quoted has always seemed totally inconsistent with the idea that target cell damage mediated by soluble factor(s) or by histiocyte or macrophage enzymes, could be responsible in a situation where only the correct one of two intimately mixed tumor cells is rejected. Two recent findings appear relevant. Dr. Lubaroff, now in Dr. Billingham's laboratory, has apparently been able to show that skin homograft rejection occurs whether or not bone marrow-derived macrophages are present to participate in the lesion. The other study was carried out last year in our laboratory by Dr. Nomoto. In rejection of a hamster lymphoma, the presence of marrow-derived macrophages were found to play no role. In the absence of macrophages, he observed as rapid and intense destruction of the tumor by sensitized lymphocytes as that seen in the presence of macrophages. In the former case there was no delayed reaction, and in the latter there was quite a conspicuous reaction at the site of transfer. It is clear, then, that in these tumor and graft situations, lymphocytes alone account for the cytotoxic effect one sees. The simplest reason one could advance to explain this, since histiocytes are present in these lesions under ordinary circumstances, is that the target cell is in some degree resistant to macrophage enzymes in low concentration. In GVH lesions, on the other hand, one has extremely large epithelioid cells. These were shown by Dvorak a number of years ago to be the same type of cells, hematogenous and certainly bone marrow-derived as we deal with in ordinary delayed lesions. However, in these situations they are highly activated cells with an enormous content of lysosomes and thus quite different from the histiocytes in ordinary delayed reactions. In the GVH lesion, there is total destruction in the area of the infiltrate, as also was shown in Dvorak's studies. In the experimental autoallergies, like autoallergic encephalomyelitis, one has a puzzling situation. There is clearcut destruction of certain tissue elements but not others in the zone of cell infiltration. Myelin, for example, breaks down while the axis cylinder is preserved, even in zones of dense cell infiltration involving again both lymphocytes and histiocytes.

CHAIRMAN SILVERSTEIN: I would like to pose the following question: Let us grant, in the situation that Dr. Billingham posed, that there does not seem to be any involvement of the intimately associated host cells in the neighborhood of a violent delayed type sensitivity reaction. Can we gather from this that the destruction of host tissue observed in certain types of delayed hypersensitivity reactions, may be because the host cells have become "contaminated" by the antigens involved in the more specific aspects of the destruction, and that this may be responsible for much of the damage that we see? Does this provoke anyone to reply?

V. CYTOTOXICITY OR STIMULATION BY EFFECTOR MOLECULES

DR. CHASE: I believe we are dealing here with a dependence on local concentration which can be of great importance. In the immediate neighborhood of producing cells, mediators or effector molecules may be present in sufficient concentration to produce their effects and yet be too dilute to do so even a short distance away.

DR. GRANGER: We suggest that the destructive effect of the lymphocyte is intimately associated with what we refer to as a microenvironment. This would be defined as that area adjacent to an activated cell. This microenvironment would lead to a nidus of total cellular destruction and as materials begin to diffuse away and become diluted there may be differential cytolysis based on the metabolic state of the cells in the adjacent area. In addition, we should consider the total concentration and location of activated cells.

DR. GOOD: I too think the microenvironment is critical. I think if we are to take examples from the way nature does handle this kind of a complicated and potentially extraordinary threatening mechanisms, that organisms use in their bodily defense, there must be modulators, homeostatic controls and inhibitors. If you look at the complement system, the other well established biological amplification system there are at least three specific inhibitors operating at specific points along the chain of events leading to cell destruction and other biological actions. One sees also the rheumatoid factor that can exert a modulating effect, conglutinin is another such component and there may be still others. We have just now begun to appreciate homeostatic and regulatory mechanisms in the microenvironment.

DR. LANDY: We have had presented much evidence based on both MIF and LT assays showing that once lymphocytes are triggered, whether by antigen or by mitogen, they go on to produce effector molecules as long as they can be maintained in a viable state. This continued production can be for at least a week under conditions of tissue culture where homeostatic control mechanisms, such as we expect are provided by the host, are absent. It seems to me virtually mandatory that we envision the host as possessing tissue components capable of counteracting or blocking the action of these effector molecules. Otherwise their continued elaboration and their persisting actions would go on in an uninterrupted fashion and the ensuing tissue destruction would be massive and infinite. Since we know, however, that this does not occur in vivo, I would venture the prediction that host components capable of blocking, counteracting or inactivating these effector molecules will soon be demonstrated. It seems to me these inhibitors must prove to be at least as important as the effector molecules themselves for our understanding of the overall process. The bioassay of such hypothetical components should be straight-forward and indeed is presently manageable.

DR. BARAM: I would like to suggest the possibility that we already have the necessary information to construct a model in which modulation or feedback control does exist to prevent excessive destruction of tissue in vivo (Fig. 55).

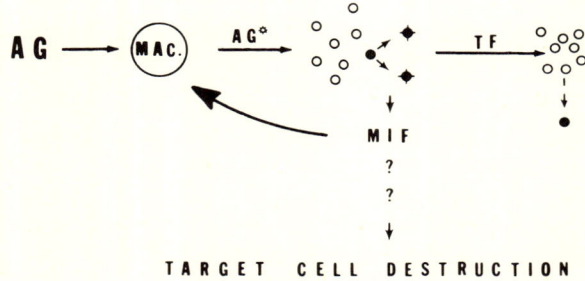

TARGET CELL DESTRUCTION

Fig. 55 Modulation of the hypersensitivity reaction. Mac=macrophages, small open circles=nonsensitive lymphocytes, closed circles=sensitive lymphocytes, closed starred circles=cell division, TF=transfer factor, MIF=macrophage inhibitory factor.

In most cases antigens are processed by the macrophage and are only then capable of stimulating hypersensitive lymphocytes. This is made apparent by the fact that one cannot stimulate hypersensitive lymphocytes in vitro by the addition of specific antigen if almost all of the

V. CYTOTOXICITY OR STIMULATION BY EFFECTOR MOLECULES

macrophages have been removed. However, if macrophages are added to these lymphocytes plus the antigen, then stimulation will occur. It is likely then that only macrophage-processed antigen is capable of stimulating the specifically sensitized lymphocytes. These cells release at least one factor (MIF) which, in low concentration, stimulates the macrophages so that they are capable of processing and degrading still more foreign antigens. In addition, cells adjacent to the lymphocytes are destroyed by factors released from the stimulated lymphocytes (LT). As additional antigen is processed through the macrophages, the intensity of the lymphocyte response increases. The hyper-sensitivity of the lymphocyte response increases. The hypersensitive lymphocytes upon contact with the processed antigen also release specific transfer factor which causes sensitization of a small number of additional lymphocytes capable of being sensitized by the specific transfer factor. As cell division continues and the MIF and/or LT accumulate, increased cell death occurs in the area of the reaction.

As the concentration of MIF increases, it becomes inhibitory to the macrophages. Antigen processing either decreases, or stops if macrophage sickness or death occurs. As the processed antigen is utilized by the lymphocytes or diluted in body fluids, the lymphocyte stimulation ceases. Cell division returns to normal levels; MIF and cytotoxic factors are no longer produced and tissue destruction ceases. When the concentration of MIF has been reduced in the area, then the macrophages are again capable of processing additional antigen, if any remains. The stimulation of macrophages is nonspecific and the cells are capable of processing all foreign antigens present. But the hypersensitive lymphocytes can, of course, be stimulated only by the processed antigens to which they are sensitive.

Since every hypersensitivity reaction of lymphocytes with processed antigen does not result in the host becoming increasingly more sensitive, it is possible that those lymphocytes that are stimulated during the processed antigen-lymphocyte interaction may die. The host sensitivity may be maintained partially by those cells receiving transfer factor late in the reaction but at a time when there is not sufficient processed antigen to stimulate them.

DR. MÖLLER: I think everyone agrees the initial step in the discussion of the homograft reactions or in delayed hypersensitivity, is the specificity of the attachment. The question is, if the cell transformed becomes non-specifically cytotoxic, it is possible that it does create a microenvironment, but it is also necessary to take into account differences in the target cells. It has already been pointed out that lymphocytes don't seem to destroy themselves. Yet, in GVH reactions, that is just what is happening. One rather puzzling thing which has not been mentioned is the immunoselection you can accomplish with tumor cells. If you passage a tumor in a foreign environment, it will be rejected. However, under appropriate circumstances, a tumor cell line will emerge which is not rejected, and will grow progressively in foreign strains. These tumor cells still have their original antigenic determinants, but in lower concentration. I think this an extremely interesting situation, since we are here dealing with cells that have the required determinants; lymphocytes should attach and then transform and thus result in rejection of the tumor. We have yet to account for the manner of this kind of "escape."

DR. HIRSCHHORN: There has been rather frequent reference to lymphocyte derepression. I would like to stress the point that in mammalian systems, there is at this time little if any evidence for the derepression of a specific gene rather than the simplification of a message. In fact, there is good evidence against specific derepression in the bacterial sense, at least without the occurrence of cell division.

Since most of the molecules that we have been discussing during this conference are produced before cell division it would be highly unlikely that a gene is being turned on by the stimuli. This fact indicates that we should rather be searching for a specific transport mechanism that can transport from the nucleus, messengers that are constantly being made and move them into the cytoplasm where they can be read and expressed.

DR. UHR: Dr. Hirschhorn is correct about the lack of formal proof that a small lymphocyte encountering antigen and becoming a plasma cell is derepressed. There certainly is no argument that this change represents a differentiation

V. CYTOTOXICITY OR STIMULATION BY EFFECTOR MOLECULES

process. I think it would be very uneconomical for the long lived small lymphocyte to synthesize all the messenger RNA's that are needed for the formation of the complicated plasma cell, and then simply destroy the messages. I think it is far more likely that stimulation represents derepression.

DR. HIRSCHHORN: There is now good evidence from the recent work of Cooper that in the resting lymphocyte a great deal of nuclear polydispersed RNA is constantly being made and degraded and never leaves the nucleus. We don't know what this is, but perhaps it is a complex of messengers of all kinds. Before small lymphocytes change into plasma cells I am sure that division must occur. I insist that without such division there is really no good evidence that there can be a real turning on of genes, because these events are not completely actinomycin repressible.

CHAIRMAN SILVERSTEIN: There is one other issue we would be remiss not to discuss in this session. This concerns the importance of the delayed hypersensitivity mechanism in defense of the host against infection and in surveillance against somatic mutation. I would ask Dr. Good to discuss the participation of delayed hypersensitivity in viral and other chronic infectious diseases, and how he views the various mechanisms to operate against the pathogen.

DR. GOOD: We have already discussed a number of possible mechanisms that could explain a variety of possible disease states both from our experimental work and from the clinic. I will therefore just summarize some of the issues that have been placed clearly in focus by some of the clinical observations.

When Bruton in 1952 opened Pandora's box by discovering agammaglobulinemia, many questions arose. One of the most pertinent was why are these individuals selectively susceptible to the infections of the virulent encapsulated pyogenic pathogens; and while they are unable to make antibody, how is it that they effectively resist many kinds of virus infections? It was subsequently established that these patients do not lack cellular immunity, their deficiency is restricted to antibody production. These deficits in immunoglobulin formation were so great that in selected patients among this group, it seemed impossible to explain this resistance to viral infection on the basis of the very limited production of immunoglobulin they could effect. It is a fact that patients with Bruton's type of agammaglobulinemia have few difficulties in handling most virus infections; they are however extraordinarily susceptible to the hepatitis virus. So in these patients we have evidence of a major bulwark of the bodily defense against certain organisms based on criteria of how the host resists, rather than on classifications of microbial virulence.

At the other end of the immune deficiency spectrum are the patients with the DiGeorge syndrome who are born without a thymus, unable to reject skin homografts and incapable of mounting cell-mediated immunity of any sort. These patients cannot survive because in our particular ecological niche, although there are innumerable viruses, fungi and bacteria for which they are capable of making antibody efficiently. Although antibody is not effective against intracellular microbes of this type, it is effective against encapsulated pathogens. The DiGeorge patients do not tend to be particularly vulnerable to the virulent encapsulated pyogenic pathogens. In considering the DiGeorge type patient with lymphopenic agammaglobulinemia, smallpox vaccination does not protect them and indeed usually gives rise to a progressive, fulminating, destructive vaccinia reaction.

However, such patients in which marked deficiencies of both immune systems occur in variable degree, generally have an early demise caused by either virus or fungus or indolent pyogenic infection.

What I seek to bring out here is that there is clear evidence from the clinical observations made on patients with cellular immune deficiency states that are now corroborated in the laboraotry; the experimental models include agammaglobulinemic chickens on one hand, the athymic chickens on the other and the irradiated thymectomized rodent all providing very clear models of this type of cellular immunity.

These patients even the ones with the lymphopenic agammaglobulinemia, make interferons in response to infections, just as well as normal individuals. They can be induced to make interferon and yet they can't resist viral infection. Therefore, we have sought to link up their ability to resist these infections with their deficiency

V. CYTOTOXICITY OR STIMULATION BY EFFECTOR MOLECULES

in cellular immunity. A critical test of this conclusion is afforded by our ability to reconstitute these cellular deficiencies and restore their capacity to respond. These recent results would seem to exclude other possible immunological interpretations.

DR. UHR: I want to ask Dr. Good why he thinks it has been so difficult to get experimental data to support the evidence that in agammaglobulinemia in humans, delayed hypersensitivity is an important factor in resistance to viral agents. I am thinking of the work of Baron and Friedman at the NIH, in which they failed to demonstrate such a role for delayed hypersensitivity in their extensive studies of vaccinia infection in guinea pigs.

DR. GOOD: I really think that the laboratory models that have thus far been used leave a great deal to be desired. I think the only critical model is the ablation of one of the distinct immunologic systems, which they have not thus far done. When the system for cellular immunity is eliminated then you have marked evidence in support of this concept. The study of virus infection such as vaccinia in newly thymectomized animals, yield results more closely reflecting what we have described in patients of the DiGeorge type.

DR. LAWRENCE: I would make two additional points in support of Dr. Good's statement: First, the inability to grow lepra bacilli in experimental animals has recently been overcome by Gaugas et al. (Nature $\underline{221}$, 1033, 1969) by means of combined thymectomy and administration of ALS. Thus in animals with impaired or abrogated cellular immune mechanisms, lepra lacilla grow freely. These findings are also germane to the concept of immunological surveillance, since a high proportion of these animals developed spontaneous tumors. Secondly, the successful use of transfer factor for the immunologic reconstitution of cellular immune deficiency in patients suffering from generalized vaccinia (Kempe, Pediatrics $\underline{26}$, 176, 1960, O'Connell, et al. Ann. Int. Med. $\underline{60}$, 282, 1964) or disseminated moniliasis (Buckley et al. Clin. Exp. Immunol. $\underline{3}$, 153, 1968) that I alluded to in our earlier discussion has resulted in prompt recovery from infection coincident with the acquisition of transferred delayed cutaneous reactivity in these anergic patients (see Session II).

CELLULAR IMMUNITY

The conclusion that transfer factor induced a reconstitution of their cellular immune mechanisms and resulted in the recovery of each of these patients is strongly suggested by the temoral sequence of events viewed against the uniformly bleak and often fatal outcome of such infections in this setting. Moreover, the detection of high titer circulating antibody in each patient and the failure of repeated administration of high titer anti-vaccinial or anti-monilial gamma globulin to eradicate the specific infection in the control period before cellular transfer was undertaken, provides compelling evidence for this conclusion.

CHAIRMAN SILVERSTEIN: Would anyone like to address the question of the situation in which the delayed hypersensitivity reactions to an apparent pathogen is in fact a disease itself? I am thinking now of lymphocytic choriomeningitis as an example of this state.

DR. DIXON: There is little evidence that all the specificity involved in the LCM disease cannot be explained by serum antibody. That includes the perivascular mononuclear infiltration and the so-called viral nephritis. The effector cells are undoubtedly lymphoid but in most situations it appears that serum antibody can direct these cells.

CHAIRMAN SILVERSTEIN: I have interpreted your data as indicating that LCM is really two diseases, both of them primarily host mediated. I have assumed that the inflammatory disease is essentially via a mechanism of delayed hypersensitivity such as we have been discussing, and that the glomerulonephritis is, as you have often pointed out, an antibody mediated immune complex type of disease.

DR. DIXON: The immune complex disease is clearly and obviously caused by complexes of serum antibody and viral antigen. The other lesions - cell death and mononuclear cell infiltration may well also result from anti-viral antibody reacting with virus in cells.

CHAIRMAN SILVERSTEIN: That may be, but do you know of any other situation where it is possible to mediate this type of chronic inflammatory response with an antibody of any variety.

V. CYTOTOXICITY OR STIMULATION BY EFFECTOR MOLECULES

DR. DIXON: No, but I have never made the attempt.

DR. GOOD: I really think that one can make a case for the possibility that the animal congenitally infected with LCM is indeed unresponsive with regard to cell-mediated immunity. I think the one critical issue in these animals is whether they are tolerant with respect to cell-mediated immunity. Obviously they can make antibody and get lesions attributable to the antibody-antigen combination. But why does the virus persist in their bodies? Where studies have been made with respect to some cellular immune functions they have been found to be defective in this regard.

VI

SPECULATIONS ON THE NATURE OF ANTIGEN RECOGNITION BY THYMIC LYMPHOCYTES AND ITS CONSEQUENCES

Concept of delayed hypersensitive cell with non-secretable antibody as postulated receptor site for antigen — Thymus-dependent cells predestined to function in cellular immune responses — Questionable relevance of cell-associated immunoglobulins to cellular immune responses — Expression of cellular immunity in situations where immunoglobulin is blocked or absent — Inhibition by anti-light chain antibody of MLC and antigen-induced lymphocyte transformation — Recognized classes of immunoglobulin uninvolved in antigen-recognition — All antigens could involve "thymus-dependent" lymphocytes; differences may be quantitative rather than qualitative — Evolution of cellular immunity to recognize and destroy mutant cells — Massive immunosuppression and consequent development of neoplasia and disseminated microbial infection — Environmental alteration of histocompatibility antigens; the self + X hypothesis of cellular immunity.

VI. MODELS FOR RECEPTOR SITES ON THYMIC LYMPHOCYTES

CHAIRMAN THOMAS: Ten years ago or for that matter as recently as five years ago, conferences on delayed hypersensitivity tended toward nearly general agreement that the phenomenon was terribly interesting but basically a simple and rather primitive one. Diagrams were regularly and easily drawn to display the two or three chief cellular participants, and there were always scenarios describing what they did to each other. My own impression, as this conference draws to a close, is that the field has now become extremely disorderly, even violent in spots, and the nice sense of vague neatness has vanished. It may even be that at long last the figure of Metchnikoff is no longer quite the domineering contemporary that he has always seemed until just recently. Mind you, he still dominates, but one senses that the field is at last in active movement. Soon he will be far enough behind so as to be waved at respectfully, instead of, as usually happens, our finding him greeting us as we come up the road.

I think we can agree that there is no longer any center of the problem of delayed hypersensitivity, which I personally take to be a piece of good news. There are now instead several centers, depending upon the point of view of the particular investigator and his laboratory. Even the lymphocyte now seems to be in danger of being replaced by its products. We are perhaps already in some danger of being swept away by the array of mediators elaborated by this cell. I suspect that we are only at the beginning of this fascinating state of affairs and I suspect that we will experience complications before a process of simplification emerges.

DR. UHR: The information we have received in the course of the five preceding sessions suggests that the effector mechanisms of delayed hypersensitivity are being rapidly elucidated, whereas the mechanisms of induction and specificity of delayed hypersensitivity remain less clearly defined. Undoubtedly the situation is caused in part by the increasing number of different in vitro assays which measure the events that follow interaction of specific antigen and delayed hypersensitive cells. A general picture has emerged in which a small population of sensitive cells encounters antigen and is then stimulated to synthesize and release one or more factors which eventually involve a large number of cells that are not sensitive. We have heard about lymphotoxic (LT) chemotactic, mitogenic and macrophage immobilizing (MIF) factors. It is clear that there has been progress in sorting out these factors. In a relatively short period of time we should know the structure, indeed the amino acid sequence, of each of these effector molecules and presumably their biological function.

I think one of the problems involved in progress in this area will be methodology. I would like to comment on several aspects of it. We still have to deal with the fact that delayed hypersensitivity in vivo, usually means a red spot, and microscopically, perivascular lymphocytes. Dr. Dixon mentioned experiments which suggest that serum antibody interacting with LCM virus in specifically tolerant mice can cause perivascular infiltrates. It is possible therefore that such infiltrates are not necessarily an anatomical hallmark of delayed hypersensitivity, and they may be no more helpful than edema or fibrinoid as markers of particular pathogenic events. Tests for resistance to intracellular infective agents as a manifestation of delayed hypersensitivity based on the elegant experiments of Dr. Mackaness will not be useful as general practical methods for analyzing delayed hypersensitivity. Thus, our in vivo assays continue to be unsatisfactory.

We are left therefore with a number of in vitro tests each of which measures a particular aspect of the in vivo event. The first point to be made is that the in vitro assays may not all be measuring the same thing, therefore, at suitable times, they will have to be compared to each other. Further, at some point the in vitro assays have to be related to the events in vivo. This is a critical point; factors elicited from lymphocytes in vitro may not be those primarily concerned with the pathogenic mechanisms that underlie delayed hypersensitivity responses in vivo. I suppose the simplest approach is to use serum antibody specific to a particular mediator and by immunofluorescent

VI. MODELS FOR RECEPTOR SITES ON THYMIC LYMPHOCYTES

or radio-autographic techniques search for the presence of the mediator in delayed hypersensitivity lesions. Also, the capacity of such specific antiserum to block lesions can be studied. Drs. Möller and Granger have already alluded to preliminary evidence about this important type of experiment which offers the possibility to link the in vitro to the in vivo phenomenon. The final point I want to make concerning methodology is that attempts should be made to develop methods for measurement of macrophage function other than their mobility and their morphologic appearance. Since the macrophage is intimately concerned with the development of the delayed inflammatory lesion, this cell deserves a radioactive assay analogous to thymidine incorporation in lymphocytes, if this is possible. In this regard, Elsbach (J. Clin. Inv. 47, 2217, 1968) has found that the rate of membrane synthesis increases in macrophages that are actively phagocytizing and the change can be detected by determining rates of P_{32}-lysolecithin incorporation into lecithin. It is possible that such a technique might be useful for measuring changes in macrophage function induced by various mediators. So much for methodology.

Despite recent progress, there clearly remain significant gaps in our knowledge of the effector events. First of all, the site of interaction of antigen and the delayed hypersensitive cell is still not known. The site could be the endothelium of the post-capillary venules or it could be extravascular such as the surface of macrophages or it could be free in the loose connective tissue. It is not clear whether a single factor only is secreted by stimulated hypersensitive cells. The data presented by Granger suggests a single factor whereas the presented by Bloom and by David is indicative of more than one. Personally, I would be surprised if we were dealing with only one molecule with many biologic functions. Reasoning by analogy with what is known of mediators in antigen-antibody induced tissue damage, one would expect an analogous complexity in delayed hypersensitivity. If there is more than one type of molecule mediating tissue damage in delayed hypersensitivity, the question arises as to whether one call forms one type of molecule only or whether one cell can make all the mediators.

The problem of whether synthesis of the mediators is entirely de novo is not settled. The puromycin experiment in the MIF-system as presented by David and Bloom suggests that this mediator must be synthesized de novo in order to produce the in vitro phenomenon. On the other hand, Hill's experiments (J. Exp. Med. 129, 363, 1969) have shown an accelerated and magnified delayed hypersensitivity lesion after skin testing animals at the site of a saline injection done 24 hours previously. There was considerable macroscopic inflammation in the skin within an hour or two after injection of antigen, and 70-80 percent of the maximal inflammation by three or four hours. This observation suggests the possibility that there are preformed mediators already present.

Indeed, the situation may be somewhat analogous to the cellular events in an animal "primed" for antibody formation. Such an animal may have two cell types: a memory line waiting to be stimulated and to give massive antibody synthesis, and a small number of plasma cell constantly arising from the memory line either stimulated by antigen or arising randomly and accounting for a plateau level of serum antibody. Similar events could occur in delayed hypersensitivity. There may be a small number of stimulated cells constantly arising that can be mustered at the site of local antigen injection and "dump" their ammunition there. At the same time, resting small lymphocytes enter the lesion, are stimulated, and synthesize large amounts of the mediators.

The problem of cell division and its relationship to delayed hypersensitive lesions is also not clear. It has been demonstrated that the in vitro synthesis of mediators occurs well before cell replication. However, this does not exclude the necessity of cell replication for the development of the full inflammatory response in vivo. Certainly, cell replication is a prominent feature of the skin lesion. It is also not known whether the replicating cells in the skin lesion are derived directly from the bone-marrow or are the thymus-dependent cells.

Another problem that was brought out clearly in earlier discussions is the possibility that cell contact may be necessary for producing cell damage in certain delayed

VI. MODELS FOR RECEPTOR SITES ON THYMIC LYMPHOCYTES

hypersensitivity models. I think a helpful experiment would be to determine the effect of antibodies to LT on in vitro cell systems in which contact appears to be necessary for cytolysis. If antibody to LT can prevent this type of cytolysis, it would be a formidable argument that it is mediated by a soluble product of cells rather than by intimate contact between cells.†

The final point I want to make regarding gaps in our understanding of the effector mechanism, is that the relationship to the effector mechanisms of antibody-induced tissue damage is not known, in particular, the relationship to the complement and kinin system. Recent studies of Perlmann et al. (Science 163, 937, 1969) which suggest that lymphocytes can contribute a C'8-like activity to a reaction mixture adds particular impetus to relate the mediators in the two kinds of immune systems.

I would summarize the effector aspect by saying that it is a very important area in delayed hypersensitivity with immense practical implications for human transplantation, for immunity to certain microbial pathogens and also for the important possibility that this type of immunity may represent a surveillance mechanism for somatic mutations. I think the road ahead looks clear. What is needed is good chemistry, some imagination, and the answers should be forthcoming in a relatively short period of time.

In contrast, I think understanding of the induction of delayed hypersensitivity and the nature of its specificity is still not clear. In the past, many exotic mechanisms have been postulated. I would like to approach the problem of induction by asking if we can design the development of a delayed hypersensitive cell with appropriate specificity for antigen without resorting to unusual mechanisms, but simply by borrowing current concepts of antibody formation and cell biology.

---

†Editors Footnote: Such experiments have in fact already been carried out (see Session V). Rabbit anti-mouse LT blocked the direct cytotoxic action of either immune or of PHA-activated mouse lymphocytes on target L cells.

CELLULAR IMMUNITY

The following model which I present to you encompasses a series of events, many of which have been described for the plasma cell, which it seems to me can now satisfactorily explain the development of the delayed hypersensitive cell.

1. The precursor of the delayed hypersensitive cell is a thymus-dependent lymphocyte or lymphoblast which synthesizes one type of H and one type of L chain.

2. The precursor cell contains the same cytoplasmic equipment as a plasma cell but in small amounts. Thus, it has polyribosomes, endoplasmic reticulum and a Golgi complex. L and H chains are synthesized on polyribosomes of the rough endoplasmic reticulum, are assembled into immunoglobulin (IG) and transported through the cisternae to the Golgi complex.

3. In the Golgi vesicles, the IG becomes bound to a site on the membrane either through the H or L chain. The Golgi vesicle containing IG is transported across the cytoplasmic matrix to the plasma membrane.

4. At the plasma membrane, reverse pinocytosis takes place but the IG remains attached to the membrane (rather than being detached, as in the plasma cell).

5. For stimulation of the cell, specific antigen interacting with surface IG must induce conformational changes in the plasma membrane to produce a signal for stimulation.

6. Multiplication and differentiation then occur: (a) production of more hypersensitive cells (memory); (b) synthesis and secretion of effector molecules such as chemotactic factor, MIF, LT, etc.

7. These effector molecules produce local tissue damage and recruit nonsensitive cells from the circulation into the local inflammatory lesion.

As regards the antigen-specific receptor, it is for me unthinkable that nature would have in the course of eons evolved the beautiful and magnificently functional IG molecule and then proceed to abandon it and substitute another type of macromolecule which provides, in general, a similar

VI. MODELS FOR RECEPTOR SITES ON THYMIC LYMPHOCYTES

range and degree of specificity. For this reason, I think that the receptor must contain an L and H chain probably in the usual tetrameric form. There is no impetus for suggesting a new H chain, but this is not critical to the argument.

The next point is whether the precursor of the delayed hypersensitive cell has the equipment necessary to make and assemble L and H chains and to transport the molecule to the plasma membrane. The precursor of the delayed hypersensitive cell is not known but it may be a lymphoblast. I want to emphasize however that even small resting lymphocytes may have all the necessary equipment. Dr. Zucker-Franklin (Seminars in Hematology 6, 4, 1969) has observed that these cells frequently possess polyribosomes, a small Golgi complex and an occasional bit of endoplasmic reticulum. I would postulate that in the precursor cells the same initial events take place as in the plasma cell (Fig. 56). In the plasma cell, we have evidence to support this scheme of assembly and transport to the Golgi complex (Zagury et al., C. R. Acad Sci., Paris 268, 1664, 1969) but the events thereafter have not been proven. A key point is that after crossing the rough endoplasmic reticulum, the IG is enclosed in membranes during the remainder of its intracellular life, and after reaching the Golgi complex, it is bound to the membrane. The IG molecule eventually reaches the outside of the plasma membrane, but, in contrast to the plasma cell in which secretion takes place, the IG molecule is not cleaved from the plasma membrane of the hypersensitive cell.

The simplest possible binding is attachment by the Fc fragment with the two antigen binding sites available to the outside to act as receptors. Another possibility is binding by one of the L chains, with at least one, and perhaps both of the antigen binding sites available to the outside.

There is nothing mysterious about this pathway. It has been described for secretory molecules that are stored, such as zymogen granules in the pancreas. Moreover, as already mentioned, data on mouse myeloma cells provide evidence for similar events in the plasma cell. The only novel points are the postulations that molecules destined to act as surface receptors bind to the Golgi membrane and go through the same events as secretory molecules right up to the crucial point of cleavage from the plasma membrane.

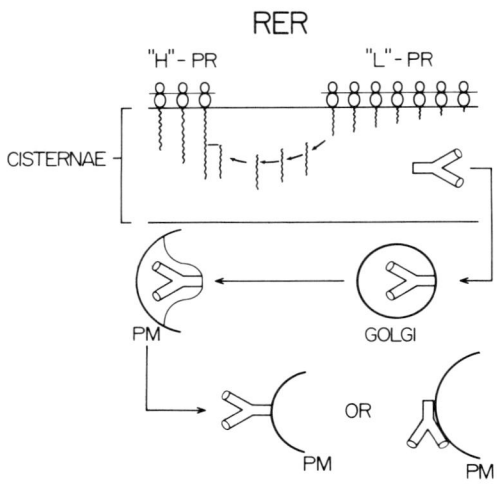

Fig. 56 Synthesis and transport of antibody-receptor in precursor of delayed hypersensitive cell.

The problem of stimulation of cells is a critical one. The first point to be made is that the requirements for stimulation of delayed hypersensitive cells and antibody forming cells may be similar. Dr. Schlossman has obtained evidence which suggests that elicitation of a delayed hypersensitive response requires an immunogenic molecule. Thus, the role of carrier protein may be important in distinguishing the difference between immunogenicity and antigenicity (combining with antibody) rather than between delayed hypersensitivity and antibody formation. The unstimulated delayed hypersensitivity cell may therefore be strictly analogous to the memory cell for antibody formation except that the former is programmed to synthesize mediators after encounter with antigen, whereas the latter

VI. MODELS FOR RECEPTOR SITES ON THYMIC LYMPHOCYTES

is destined to secrete antibody in massive amounts.

Another implication of Dr. Schlossman's findings is that there are similarities between the events in the skin during elicitation of delayed hypersensitivity and those in the regional lymphoid organ when delayed hypersensitivity is induced. Thus, mediators may be released in the lymph node during sensitization and account for some of the nonspecific stimulation which occurs.

The key point in stimulation of immune cells is that antigen must do something "extra" to antibody receptors other than to combine with them with sufficient energy of interaction. I suggest that this "extra" is a change in the conformation of the plasma membrane resulting from the binding of antibody receptors by antigen in a particular manner. This need for delivery of antigen in a special way may explain the requirement for macrophages or other cell-to-cell interactions in certain models, the role of carrier protein or even the role sometimes played by small amounts of antibodies. For example, it may be necessary for antigen to bridge two or more antibody molecules on the immune cell in order to produce this conformational change in the membrane (Fig. 57); "bridging" has been suggested as a mechanism for eliciting anaphylaxis (Levine, J. Immunol. $\underline{94}$, 121, 1965). This bridging may require the surface of macrophages in order to "stack" antigen molecules and this in turn may be accomplished by "natural" antibody (Jerne, PNAS $\underline{41}$, 849, 1955) binding to antigen and directing it to appropriate sites on the macrophage that bind IG. Conformational changes in the antibody molecule as suggested by Bretscher and Cohn (Nature $\underline{220}$, 444, 1968) may occur but are not essential to produce changes in the membrane. There are a variety of other models that could be suggested. The common denominator is the need to do something special to the membrane of the precursor cell.

There is no impetus in this hypothesis to consider passive sensitization of lymphocytes. If a cell can generate its own IgG receptor, it seems unnecessary to have an additional mechanism to obtain antibody receptors on sensitive lymphocytes particularly since these cells have nonspecific mechanisms for magnifying their response to antigen.

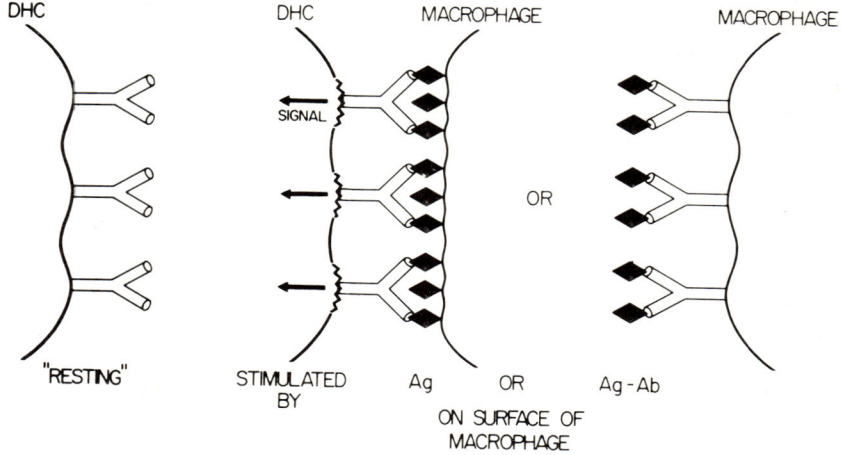

Fig. 57 Stimulation of delayed hypersensitive cell by antigen.

I would like to say one word about transfer factor and RNA-rich extracts. I suggested during an earlier session that transfer factor and indeed the extracts described by Thor and Schlossman, might contain superimmunogens. By that term I meant a fragment of antigen still retaining its tertiary structure attached to another molecule, which is particularly effective at performing that something "extra" necessary for stimulation of cells, e.g., the superimmunogen may have a much higher ratio of successful collisions (causing stimulation) to unsuccessful collision with precursor cells. I want to re-emphasize that this is a possibility suggested mainly by exclusion; it does not easily explain all the findings. On the contrary, a number of very pertinent objections have been raised to this possibility. We simply need more information about transfer factor before it can be properly integrated into a general theory of delayed hypersensitivity. Such information will come rapidly now that a number of laboratories are working on different facets of the problem. The chemistry of transfer factor undoubtedly will give considerable

VI MODELS FOR RECEPTOR SITES ON THYMIC LYMPHOCYTES

information about its possible biologic functions. Further testing of specificity of transfer factor, including the in vitro model, will be crucial in evaluating its nature. Finally, it should be possible to find out if antigenic determinants are actually present in transfer factor, and several possible experiments were suggested in previous discussions.

In summary, the essential message I would leave with you is that it is possible to explain the development of a delayed hypersensitive cell with antigen-specificity in terms that puts delayed hypersensitivity in the mainstream of immunology and cell biology without resorting to exotic mechanisms. The hypothesis can be tested.

DR. MITCHISON: I would ask Dr. Uhr for some clarification: when you talk about thymus-derived cells, is it your idea that there is another line of cells that goes ahead to antibody-synthesis, or is there something which enables a thymus-derived cell at the time of stimulation to make a choice between the delayed type sensitivity pathway or the antibody synthesis pathway?

DR. UHR: The assumption is that the choice has already been made; i.e., the thymus-dependent cell is destined to function as a delayed hypersensitive cell.

DR. EISEN: I think that Dr. Uhr has done a superb job of sketching a model which many of us find, and have found, to be attractive and reasonable. His last statement was that one of the main attractions of the model is that "it is easily tested". Since this model has been present more or less conspicuously in front of us for a number of years, and has not yet been tested adequately, I wonder what Dr. Uhr had in mind saying that it could be tested easily.

DR. UHR: One example that I had in mind is the experiment of Greaves et al. (Nature 222, 885, 1969) referred to by Dr. Möller, in which the lymphocyte receptor site for cell-mediated immunity, could be blocked by anti-light chain antibody or by its Fab monomer. I think experiments can be designed along this line, that would indicate whether or not immunoglobulin molecules are in fact present on the cell surface and are associated with the receptors that bind antigen specifically.

In addition, the receptor can be approached from the biosynthetic viewpoint. Studies can be done of macromolecular synthesis and transport in stimulated lymphocytes similar to what we have done in plasma cells using radioautography of electron micrographs. These approaches should give information that would have a direct bearing on the model.

DR. GELL: I would like to suggest that it is possible to do a formal test of Dr. Uhr's model with anti-allotype antisera - that is to say the model of determinants on the surface. By using antisera against these postulated IgG-like molecules on the surface of the cell, it can be shown that a specific proliferation stimulus occurs.

Now it may be that this is a model of proliferation stimulus produced by antigen, but there is no formal proof of this. As regards the distortion of the surface which you suggest as the trigger for proliferation, Dr. Sell and I have a certain amount of evidence indicating that at least two, possibly contiguous, hits on the cell are needed to produce lymphoblasts: there is also the evidence I mentioned previously; that if you bind onto the cell any allotypic antibody and then pile on top of it an antibody directed against that antibody; i.e., producing a larger lump of material and presumably producing greater surface distortion, there results a large number of cells going into cycle. So it seems to me the formal proof of gamma globulin determinants on the surface of the cell is there if you accept our demonstration that they are produced by that cell. There is also strongly suggestive evidence that surface distortions are involved in the proliferative stimulus. But there is not, I agree, in this system any formal indication that what we are doing is analogous to what antigen is doing under the same circumstances, something that is of course essential to your model.

VI. MODELS FOR RECEPTOR SITES ON THYMIC LYMPHOCYTES

DR. UHR: The "piggyback" experiment is nicely explained by the concept of a conformational change of antibody on cell surfaces.

DR. SILVERSTEIN: Dr. Gell's demonstration suggests that there is immunoglobulin on the surface, but it does not tell us anything concerning the importance of that immunoglobulin to the question at hand. To illustrate the complexity of the problem of the recognition immunoglobulin being on the cell surface, I want to mention some experiments on graft rejection in the presence of heterologous anti-host-immunoglobulins (Silverstein and Kraner, Transplantation 3, 535, 1965). These experiments could uniquely be done in vivo in the agammaglobulinemic fetal ungulate. Orthotopic skin allograft rejection by the competent fetus proceeded unhindered despite the fact that the fetus was overloaded with rabbit anti-sheep immunoglobulin chains, both light and heavy. Yet this treatment, involving a persisting excess of anti-immunoglobulins in the fetal circulation, did not seem to interfere with the graft rejection reaction. Were a conventional immunoglobulin recognition molecule to exist on the surface of the sensitized lymphocyte, it should have been neutralized under the conditions of this experiment.

DR. GOOD: The experiments that Dr. Gell referred to have, since they were published, been a source of great concern and some distress to me. I think that although they formally demonstrate that many lymphocytes may have an antibody receptor on their surface, there is a very real question as to whether this has anything at all to do with cell-mediated immunity.

Dr. Alm has done a critical experiment in which he has first of all established for the chicken, in confirmation of Ivanyi, that the Sell and Gell phenomenon works in this species. He introduced antibody against almost any immunoglobulin component to lymphocytes and, as in the rodent system, he observed blast transformation of many of the lymphocytes. However, if he did this in chickens that have an intact cell-mediated immunity and a normal thymus-dependent system, but who were irradiated and bursectomized so that they lacked the capacity to produce antibody, their lymphocytes did not transform. This work has been published recently (Alm and Peterson, J. Exp. Med. 129, 1247, 1969); the data are absolutely convincing.

DR. EISEN: I am also troubled by the demonstration of immunoglobulin molecules, or parts of them, on cell membranes, because the question always comes up to what extent these molecules are picked up from serum. How can one be certain that these are formed by the cell in question, and attached to its membrane in some very significant way, relevant for delayed type hypersensitivity. Perhaps the ideal material to use in the search for lymphocyte-attached immunoglobulins would be cells from persons with agammaglobulinemia, who have little or no circulating gammaglobulin, but who have delayed type hypersensitivity. Can one demonstrate immunoglobulin light chains or heavy chains on the lymphocyte membranes of such individuals?

DR. UHR: The experiment of Alm and Peterson that Dr. Good described is in essence a negative one. It may be a quantitative problem. If one succeeded in stimulating these cells by the maneuvers described by Dr. Gell, the interpretation would be just the opposite.

DR. GOCD: I think so; I think what I am objecting to is the interpretation of Dr. Gell's experiment as a positive demonstration. I think there is clear evidence that that is not the case. We still have no evidence that there is any antibody of this sort on or in the lymphocytes involved in the process we are discussing.

In chickens that have been previously bursectomized and irradiated, and by this maneuver have been made agamaglobulinemic or markedly hypogammaglobulinemic, their lymphoid cells could not be induced to undergo blast transformation after treatment with anti-gamma globulin antisera.

DR. GELL: The point I wish to emphasize is that in the chicken, bursectomy apparently abolishes antibody-mediated

VI. MODELS FOR RECEPTOR SITES ON THYMIC LYMPHOCYTES

blast transformation, but leaves intact antigen-mediated blast transformation. The implication of this is either that the antigen-receptor is in the latter case not an immunoglobulin, or that the effect is quantitative - that cells from a bursaless chicken have too few receptors to respond to anti-IgG antigen, but perhaps there are some. I should like to suggest that Dr. Good might do an experiment along the lines I quoted earlier, using an antibody in a second stage against the first anti-IgG antibody; this might magnify any response, as it does with rabbit cells.

In reply to Dr. Eisen's concern that the presence of immunoglobulin on cell membranes might reflect what was picked up from serum, I would assure him that Sell and I were award of such a possibility and endeavored to control it by means of a genetic experiment (Sell and Gell, J. Exp. Med. 122, 823, 1964). This indicated that the determinants demonstrated on cells were indeed products of the cell itself, and were not merely taken up from the serum.

DR. GOOD: During our previous discussions there has arisen confusion concerning the precise designation of immunocompetent cells in relation to their point of origin. I personally object to the use of the terms "bone-marrow-derived" cells and "thymus-derived" cells. To me it is absolutely clear that thymus-derived cells are also cells derived from bone-marrow. I think that we are contributing to confusion if we talk about thymus-derived versus marrow-derived cells. Clearly there are many marrow-derived cells which differentiate to completely distinct lines of cells. The marrow-derived cells which come under thymus influence represent one example. These then are thymus-dependent lymphoid cells. The bone-marrow cells that come under another influence, the equivalent of the influence of the bursa of Fabricius, in birds, represent another but separate bone-marrow-derived cell line. This line in the chicken can be considered bursa-dependent. It could be thought of as representative of the immunoglobulin-producing system in man and mammals, since we do not yet know what the equivalent of the bursa might be. Another example of a marrow-derived cell is the monocyte line. This line must be induced to achieve its final differentiation at some site which has not yet been defined, but which may reside in marrow itself. It should be thought of as a phagocytic line or a monocytic line, not a marrow-derived line of cells.

I think we will avoid much semantic confusion if we are clear on these concepts and stop using these confusing terms that seem to be gaining current popularity. It is now clear from work on in vitro systems such as antibody production to sRBC, that this is a function of cells that are not derived from thymus, but rather are thymus-independent immunoglobulin producing cells. This important conclusion can be derived from the recent contributions by Davies and by Mitchell and Miller. What I think is unclear right now is how certain immune responses resulting in antibody synthesis are also thymus dependent. I cannot take very seriously, at this juncture, the view that there occurs an exchange of information from cell to cell in the lymphoid system. To me it is unnecessarily cumbersome to think of the thymus-dependent system operating any way except by making, through its known function in cellular immunity, a more efficient delivery of antigen to the surface of antigen-sensitive cells of the thymic-dependent system.

DR. MÖLLER: I want to restate some of Dr. Greaves' findings since they are of decisive importance to Dr. Uhr's proposition. Anti-light chain antibody either as intact antibody or as the Fab monomer inhibited mixed lymphocyte cultures, inhibited stimulation of lymphocytes by PPD and prevented inhibition of migration by antigen. Furthermore, Dr. Greaves in collaboration with Dr. E. Möller showed that thymocytes from animals immunized with sRBC had the ability to combine with sRBC and form rosettes, despite the apparent absence of antibody production by the thymus cells.

Furthermore, Drs. R. and J. Falk demonstrated that in rats immunized with sRBC, the first cells to react specifically with the antigen in the migration inhibition tests were thymus cells. Later on antibody-forming cells appeared in the spleen and these cells were also inhibited in migration. Obviously, the first event in triggering lymphocytes must be the antigen interaction with the antibody receptor. However my guess is that something more is

VI. MODELS FOR RECEPTOR SITES ON THYMIC LYMPHOCYTES

needed, probably some extra factors, that are necessary for the secondary events.

I would like also to report some experiments concerned with antigenic competition. Animals subjected to GVH disease, which have been immunized with hRBC, do not produce antibody to sRBC - a clear case of antigenic competition. However, when these animals are irradiated and subsequently transfused with cells hyperimmune to sRBC, mixed with this antigen, the cells do not produce antibody in this environment. This can be interpreted in many ways. A simple interpretation would be that a vigorous active immune response has removed something from the environment which is necessary for the secondary triggering events leading to cell division, because if the cells are removed all the antigen-sensitive cells can be detected in another environment.

DR. GOOD: I hope you understood, Dr. Möller, that the cells in the thymus are not necessarily the cells first stimulated and that they are not required in some way to initiate an immune response. I say this because it is very clear from study of patients with the DiGeorge syndrome, who never had a thymus, that antibody production can be initiated to many antigens and can be essentially normal. This is also the case with respect to neonatally thymectomized and irradiated mice. With appropriate antigenic models such animals can make really good antibody responses despite an absence of cell-mediated immunity. Such animals, now entirely lacking a thymus, can be immunologically reconstituted with peripheral lymphoid cells from lymph node or spleen, resulting in immune responses (including their response to sRBC) being restored to normal. They still have no thymus. Thus, a view that an essential step in immune reaction involves direct stimulation within the thymus seems to me untenable.

DR. MÖLLER: I don't contest your point. I would remind you that in employing RBC as the antigenic model we were of course dealing with a thymus-dependent antigen.

CELLULAR IMMUNITY

DR. GOOD: True, but what I am saying includes responses to sRBC. You do not have to have the thymus as such to produce a good antibody response to this very antigen. Indeed one can initiate the response to sRBC in neonatally thymectomized or neonatally thymectomized and irradiated animals, by giving them sufficient supply of differentiated peripheral lymphoid cells from spleen or lymph nodes or other peripheral lymphoid tissue.

DR. UHR: I think the remarks that have been made in this last interchange are relevant to evaluating the evidence that might be interpreted as supporting the model. As I see it, no evidence has thus far been given that excludes it. The only possible exception is Dr. Silverstein's finding that antiglobulin does not block the cellular immune reactivity of the fetal lamb. His experiment does not rule out the possibility that immunoglobulin antibody is present on delayed hypersensitive cells. First, I don't believe there was evidence obtained that the rabbit anti-sheep IG was in excess at the time that the grafts were rejected. Second, even the presence of excess anti-sheep IG does not exclude interaction between IG receptors on sensitive lymphocytes and specific antigen. After all, enormous excess of serum antibody does not prevent a minute dose of antigen from stimulating memory cells to give a secondary antibody response. In some way, not yet clear, antigen supposedly fully coated with antibody contacts receptors on these cells. The thermodynamics of such interactions *in vivo* including those of Dr. Silverstein's experiment, are complex and not yet understood.

DR. SCHLOSSMAN: The mechanism of antigen recognition by the sensitized lymphoid or processing cell, while still poorly defined, is crucial to our understanding of the cellular immune responses. The production of an observable delayed skin reaction, the anamnestic response and the biologic mediators associated with these responses are direct consequences of antigen-induced cellular proliferation and/or biosynthesis. Clearly, the expression of the cellular immune response involves an exquisitely specific receptor system for antigen. It is precisely the same physicochemical requirements for antigen that are requisite for

VI. MODELS FOR RECEPTOR SITES ON THYMIC LYMPHOCYTES

triggering the sensitized cell that are also obligatory for the induction of the immune response in the virgin animal. These observations suggest that studies of the specificity of the established immune response may yield clues to the mechanism by which the immune response is initiated. Thus, the cellular receptor plays a key role in both the induction and the elicitation of the cellular immune response. If one assumes, as Dr. Uhr has, that the only mechanism available for antigen recognition is antibody, he would then have to agree that the antigen receptor on the sensitized lymphoid cell possesses a binding site, and L and H chains, similar to those found on gamma globulin. Unfortunately, the available experimental data do not support this conclusion: there is neither direct evidence to show that antibody is in fact the receptor for antigen, nor do the available immunochemical studies comparing cellular specificity with antibody specificity, (i.e., binding site size, affinity etc.) support the conclusion that the receptors are identical in these two situations. One is required to postulate that "cell associated antibody-antigen interactions" require something above and beyond the mere interaction of antibody with its ligand. It is precisely this "something extra" that leads me to the conclusion that for now it is premature to assume that the mechanism for antigen recognition by the sensitized cells proceeds through an antibody-binding step. Moreover, the critical experimental findings described for us by Drs. Good and Silverstein show that the cellular immune response proceeds in the absence of detectable gamma globulin on the cell surface or even in the presence of antibody to gamma globulin, an interaction that clearly should inhibit the cellular response. Thus, there would seem to be provided tangible support for the view that conventional antibody is not involved in antigen recognition by the sensitized cells. However, in view of the present imperfect state of our knowledge in this area, one should not rule out the participation either of an unique form of antibody, or conventional antibody that undergoes a highly specific change as a consequence of antigen interaction, or finally the participation of an as yet undefined molecule or "exotic mechanism" for antigen recognition.

DR. TURK: The model Dr. Uhr has developed takes a lot for

granted and in my opinion leans too heavily on analogy with humoral antibody formation. Moreover the analogy is with a special type of antibody production - that exemplified by the production of antibody to sRBC in the mouse. In contrast, there is no evidence in the mouse for a two-cell system in antibody production to pneumococcal polysaccharides or to flagellin. Thus, the two-cell system is far from being a universal phenomenon, even in antibody production.

I would like to make my points within the context that all immunological responses involve several separate stages; (a) recognition of foreignness; (b) proliferation of cells; (c) rejection of that which is foreign and the possible involvement of pharmacological agents. As Dr. Medawar has suggested the main differences between humoral antibody production and cell-mediated immunity is that in the latter, recognition takes place in the periphery. In humoral antibody production, antigen has been shown to drain down to the macrophages in close relation to the plasma cell precursors at the cortico-medullary junction or in the medullary cords. In cell-mediated immunity, on the other hand, initial contact with the potentially immunologically responsive cell appears to take place in the periphery. The next event that can be observed is the proliferation of lymphocytes in the paracortical area of lymph nodes or the equivalent area of the spleen. The significance of this as a site of proliferation is that under normal conditions this is a place where the mobile pool of small lymphocytes are passing through continuously. The lymphocytes that are traversing it are those dependent on thymus integrity in neonatal life and while in the periphery are susceptible to the action of ALS. During the development of a cell-mediated immune response the passage of these cells out of the lymph node is temporarily stopped. Lymphocytes accumulate in the lymph node and proliferate. This phase of proliferation of lymphocytes could be likened to the action of an electrical transformer, as a result of which the immune response is magnified. We have no evidence as yet from *in vivo* studies that, when lymphocytes are released from the lymph node after the first proliferation phase, these are either the effector cells or even precursors of the effector cells. However, similar proliferation of lymphocytes has been shown by Dr. Ginsburg to

VI. MODELS FOR RECEPTOR SITES ON THYMIC LYMPHOCYTES

occur in culture leading to the production of effector cells that in turn can kill the target cells that had stimulated their proliferation. In Ginsburg's cinematography of this kind of interaction one can actually see normal lymphocytes proliferating in contact with foreign cells and following these effector lymphocytes after division as they make direct contact with and kill the target cells.

Despite Dr. Uhr's contention I know of no evidence that the effector lymphocytes in cell-mediated immune reactions have sufficient polyribosomes, a Golgi apparatus or endoplasmic reticulum to produce peptide chains analogous to those produced by plasma cells. I fear that we are all wishing so much that these cells would produce a counterpart to the immunoglobulin molecules that we are beginning to take it for granted that they do. All these essential elements are present in the blast cells during lymphocyte division. However, most small lymphocytes are surprisingly free of these subcellular elements. The blast cells formed during the proliferation of lymphocytes may be likened to the erythroblast as viewed by electron microscopy, but this would hardly lead one to suggest that erythrocytes manufacture hemoglobulin.

From this point onwards, it seems to me important to examine the relationship between the so-called "in vitro" correlates and cell-mediated immunity "in vivo". As of now none of the in vitro correlates, correlate completely. Coombs and his group have shown that inhibition of macrophage migration in vitro can be mimicked under certain circumstances by means of cytophilic antibody. Transformation in vitro can be detected in rabbit lymphocytes under conditions where antibody production exists without delayed hypersensitivity. Pokeweed mitogen stimulates the transformation of small lymphocytes into cells that display an endoplasmic reticulum and the characteristics of antibody-producing cells. But even if one accepts that the in vitro correlates are in fact relevant to the cell-mediated immune reaction as we see it in vivo, what is their relationship to the actual mechanisms by which these reactions are produced?

Dr. Uhr has stated that cell replication is a prominent feature of the lesion in delayed hypersensitivity. I would immediately take issue with this. In my view there is no evidence for cell-replication occurring within the lesion itself. Mononuclear cells infiltrating the lesion may have been derived from bone-marrow lymphocytes that have been replicating within the previous 24 hours, and thus may be labeled with H_3-thymidine injected at this time. However, mitoses are not seen within the infiltrating cells in the dermis. The only increase in cell replication that occurs in delayed hypersensitivity does so in the epidermal cells of the skin, and increased cell turnover in the epidermis also occurs with any inflammation in the underlying dermis.

Now what about the most intensively studied _in vitro_ correlate - the inhibition of macrophage migration. Can we in any way fit this into the picture of delayed hypersensitivity as we see it _in vivo_? No evidence has yet been provided indicating that aggregation of macrophages leads to any of the observed _in vivo_ effects. Mononuclear cells do accumulate in delayed hypersensitivity lesions, notably the tuberculin reaction in the guinea pig and the rat. However, there is no evidence that there is a specific aggregation _in vivo_. Spector has suggested that the infiltrate in a delayed hypersensitivity reaction is typical of normal inflammation and it is known that PMN migrate from such lesions more rapidly than mononuclear cells. It is well documented that at 48 hours one cannot distinguish between Arthus reactions and delayed hypersensitivity reactions by just looking at the cellular infiltrate. Moreover, in the mouse the infiltrate remains mainly PMN as late as 24 hours. The infiltrate in a delayed hypersensitivity reaction, if it is mononuclear, probably consists mainly of bone-marrow-derived cells, whether these show at the particular time phagocytic features such as the ability to ingest carbon particles or the presence of lysosomes or for that matter give the superficial appearance of small lymphocytes. The number of thymus-influenced lymphocytes in a particular lesion at any time is not known.

The production of an inflammatory lesion with erythema and induration (swelling of collagen) as a result of the injection of protein fractions derived from the incubation of "sensitized lymphocytes" with antigen is the only indication that MIF or a similar substance might be related to a factor produced _in vivo_ during the development of a

VI. MODELS FOR RECEPTOR SITES ON THYMIC LYMPHOCYTES

delayed hypersensitivity lesion. The nature of the inflammatory infiltrate, whether mainly PMN or mainly mononuclear, as I have mentioned is not related to the <u>form</u> of the lesion but more to the <u>time</u> the lesion takes to develop, the degree of necrosis and species in which the reaction takes place.

There is no doubt in my mind that we and others, as reported in preceding sessions of this conference, have isolated a true pharmacological agent involved in delayed hypersensitivity. However, its action <u>in</u> <u>vivo</u> may not be limited to macrophages but it may produce membrane changes similar to those which Dr. Diengdoh and I described in cells other than the macrophages. Another group of pharmacological agents that may contribute to inflammation are the components of complement. I do not suggest that these act in the same way in delayed hypersensitivity as in erythrocyte lysis, yet delayed hypersensitivity can be inhibited by a number of systems which reduce the level of one or more complement components <u>in</u> <u>vivo</u>. These include anti-complement serum, ALS and antigen-antibody precipitates. However, pure C'6 deficiency alone does not inhibit the development of these reactions. Then too there is a hint of other pharmacological agents being involved, as delayed hypersensitivity reactions can be inhibited by a serum directed against membrane free extracts of lymph nodes which do not drop complement levels. I myself do not believe in a "lymph node permeability factor" as a mediator of delayed hypersensitivity and I have identified the reasons elsewhere. However the serum produced by such an extract does have remarkably specific anti-inflammatory effects on delayed hypersensitivity reactions while not affecting nonspecific reactions induced by turpentine.

Thus defects in our knowledge occur at all levels in our understanding of the mechanism of cell-mediated immune responses. The ones I have mentioned can be charted along the afferent arc of sensitization through the lymph node and down the efferent arc to the final manifestation of the reaction in the periphery. I would agree with Dr. Uhr that one of the most vital points is to clarify the chemical nature of the "recognition factor" in cell-mediated immunity. However, even when this is accomplished the battle will be far from over. There are so many differences between "cell-mediated immunity" and "antibody immunity" during the recognition stage and the cell proliferative stage of the development of the reaction that we are all likely to be occupied for a long time afterwards. However even more challenging will be the elucidation of the pharmacological events which produce the various manifestations of cell-mediated immunity, such as the tuberculin reaction, homograft rejection and of course, the defense of the body against bacterial pathogens, and viruses. Many of these problems cannot yet be effectively approached with the type of *in vitro* models that have been developed thus far.

DR. UHR: I have two general comments in reply to Drs. Schlossman and Turk. They have cited no evidence that would exclude any important features of the model, nor have they spelled out any alternatives. Thus, if IG is not the receptor for antigen, what other types of molecules are being considered as candidates? If the sensitive cell does not synthesize its own receptor, where does the receptor originate? In considering alternatives for the receptor, it is clear that for potential antibody-secreting cells the receptor must have the same specificity in general as the product in order for antigenic stimulation to result in specific antibody formation. This argument supersedes the objection that there can be apparent discrepancies between the specificity or binding affinity of serum antibody versus cell-associated antibody for specific antigen. I have several additional points to make concerning Dr. Turk's discussion. His description of the differences between humoral antibody formation and delayed hypersensitivity as regard fate of antigen and the cellular events in the responding lymphoid organ, is not helpful in evaluating theories of delayed hypersensitivity, since most of us now accept that there are two different cell populations involved. Moreover, the differences he described are not convincing, because there is no method as yet for distinguishing irrelevant antigen from immunogen. Also, since there is no suitable criterion for identification of a specific immune cell other than an antibody-secreting cell, the *specific* cellular events underlying the early phase of antibody formation or any phase of delayed hypersensitivity cannot presently be characterized in a definitive manner. I am also puzzled by Dr. Turk's statement that there are so

VI. MODELS FOR RECEPTOR SITES ON THYMIC LYMPHOCYTES

many differences between cell-mediated immunity and antibody formation in the recognition stage. I think that in general the two immune responses show a similar range and degree of specificity.

Debate on whether or not small lymphocytes have the cytoplasmic equipment for making IG is beside the point since lymphoblasts actively synthesize protein and could have synthesized IG before giving rise to small lymphocytes.

I agree with Dr. Turk that there are considerable numbers of unsolved problems regarding the skin lesion, but I think he has overemphasized the methodological difficulties of determining mechanisms of inflammation in delayed hypersensitivity. Not only are there a variety of *in vitro* models for obtaining information about the biology and chemistry of potential mediators, but antibody to these mediators provides an exceedingly powerful tool for determining their importance in the *in vivo* lesion.

DR. CHASE: As our chairman has pointed out, there is no single "center" to the problem of delayed type hypersensitivity, but "several centers", depending upon the point of view of the particular investigator and his laboratory. One can choose either to study in detail single aspects of the phenomenon, or to range widely over multiple examples of delayed hypersensitivity in a search for divergencies or common factors in manifestations of the delayed reaction. While all information secured in the several areas enriches and leads to new experiments, to confine one's attention exclusively to single segments of the problem may prove insufficient for total understanding. Thus, cell-to-cell contact triggers reactions which properly constitute part of the mechanisms of delayed hypersensitivity; yet other examples, equally applicable, scarcely support cell-to-cell contact as a necessary generalization.

Hypersensitivity to tuberculin, once studied exclusively in tuberculous animals, is now largely determined in animals sensitized by injection of relatively large antigenic amounts of mycobacterial cells administered in paraffin oil. The manner of reaction to tuberculin differs in the two cases; yet few are those who now make parallel studies of the two systems. Both the character and temporal sequences of the cellular infiltrate are unlike in these systems. In the artificial sensitization represented by the Coulaud-Saenz-Freund phenomenon, large amounts of circulating antibody, nearly wholly anti-carbyhydrate, are present. How much the co-existing antibody system contributes to the greater speed and early necrosis when tests are made with "tuberculin" cannot yet be judged. (Favour has found total globulins in animals so sensitized to be present in abnormally large amounts). The form of tuberculin called "PPD" contains more than one protein, at least tuberculocarbohydrate, and some nucleic acid. Can safe generalization be made if this antibody is ignored?

Yet other problems of interpretation can arise when sensitization is induced to proteins, hapten-protein complexes, or hapten-polylysine complexes, providing studies are made after the participation of circulating antibody becomes a possible factor. All who have worked in this area are aware of the difficulties in the sure recording of so-called "mixed reactions", in which early type reactions occur but are succeeded in the same intradermal site by "delayed" reactions.

Contact hypersensitivity with simple chemical allergens appears also, at times, to exhibit an antibody component. Recent studies from our laboratory (Maguire and Chase, J. Invest. Dermatol. 49, 460, 1967) and unpublished experiments have indicated ways to establish and study delayed-type, contact hypersensitivity of an exquisite degree of sensitivity in the essential absence of PCA and other types of circulating antibody. A wide experience with the various forms of delayed hypersensitivity in vivo is needed, even in order to interpret the bearing of in vitro studies.

DR. GOOD: In the course of our discussions there have been repeated references to Experiments of Nature. Dr. Silverstein has tried to persuade us that Experiments of Nature are poor experiments and that we might be better off had we done them in our laboratories. I disagree vigorously with his obviously biased view. My position is that Experiments

VI. MODELS FOR RECEPTOR SITES ON THYMIC LYMPHOCYTES

of Nature must be recognized and properly interpreted to have maximal meaning. Simply to equate empirical clinical observations with interpretation of Experiments of Nature is incorrect. Such an approach yields nothing but gross empiricism and, more often than not, is incorrect. It is those instances where Nature's Experiments ask a critical question which we cannot think of from the restricted point of view of our current hypotheses where I believe the natural experiments are the most useful. The usefulness of the question and the establishment of the credibility of a relationship often supported by most critical laboratory analysis. None the less the laboratory analysis will be carried out in the new perspective provided by the insight or creative impulse which has been contributed by the natural experiment.

Jenner's concern for the shiny-faced milkmaids in the presence of the disfiguring pox could have been entirely wrong but that one insight, and Jenner's initial observations concerning it, gave us the first real studies of immunity; the first evidence of hypersensitivity or allergy; the first use of an attenuated virus vaccine; and the first glimpse of interferon. That is quite a contribution from which we are still deriving direction.

This is but one of the numerous examples I could cite in which interpretation of natural experiments has played the crucial role in guiding progress in medical science. Knowledge is not a succession of answers, but a succession of questions, and it is in that succession of questions to which the Experiments of Nature provide an extraordinary usefulness.

DR. GELL: I am deeply concerned about the situation where some antigens seem to be "thymus-dependent" while others are not. I should like to keep open the possibility that all antigens are in fact really thymus-dependent, and that the differences observed are essentially of a quantitative nature. Thymus-derived cells are to me a perfectly simple concept, meaning cells that are the product of division in the thymus, and exposed there to thymic influence, whatever that may be. These cells are, I suppose, being seeded out into the peripheral tissues from the very earliest embryonal stage of thymic development. Consequently neonatally thymectomized (or bursectomized) animals will prenatally have recorded some thymus-derived cells in its immature lymphoid tissues: the ablation of this organ merely prevents its getting any more. Accordingly non-thymus dependent antigens will be those that are easily recognized because there is, in that species, a high probability of a randomly produced IG molecule "fitting" them and therefore there is likely to be potential antibody to them despite a residue of only a small population of thymus-derived cells: in such a situation it would obviously be difficult and perhaps even impossible for thymus-dependent antigens to be recognized.

There are two sorts of objections to this hypothesis: first, though the evidence from neonatal thymectomy and other experimental procedures can perhaps be brushed off on the interpretation that a few surviving thymic cells can do the job; the findings on individuals with the DiGeorge syndrome really seem to reflect a total congenital thymectomy. This, together with the lack of effect by anti-sheep immunoglobulin on cellular immune responses in the immunologically virgin fetal lamb constitutes a formidable objection. The other is, if one argues that "just a few cells, somewhere or other" can account for the experimental results, this then became a very hard hypothesis to test. This of course doesn't mean that it may not be true - nature is constantly playing this sort of low trick on us. But it seems to me an entirely reasonable expectation that antibodies arising from a very small initial cell population should be demonstrably different from those derived from a large population, e.g., they should be of low binding affinity and high homogeneity. I do not believe that thymus-independent antibodies, in thymectomized animals, have yet been looked at from this point of view.

A nice tidy theory of this sort could be a useful step in delineating the difference between delayed hypersensitivity and antibody production at the stage of cell interaction, whatever this process may actually be. The "delayed-sensitive" cell would be one which has not interacted with a potential antibody-producing cell; we instead make it react in vitro with antigen to produce the effector molecules we have been discussing. Were it normally to

VI. MODELS FOR RECEPTOR SITES ON THYMIC LYMPHOCYTES

interact by way of an antigen-bridge, as suggested by Dr. Mitchison, there would then be an obvious and very important function for some of these effector molecules in enlarging the subsequent clone. The state of pure delayed hypersensitivity would then be envisioned as one in which such interaction has been discouraged either by our experimental procedures or by the nature of the antigen.

CHAIRMAN THOMAS: I would now like to see us move from the general discussion of Dr. Uhr's concept of cellular immunity and begin to complete our assignment. To this end I have asked the Chairmen and Discussion Initiators to summarize what they view as significant and noteworthy in each of the preceding sessions.

DR. MÖLLER: We sought in Session I to delineate the processes leading to activation of lymphocytes in delayed hypersensitivity states and to differentiate between triggering events in humoral antibody synthesis and in cell-mediated immunity. Lymphocytes can be activated by an array of nonspecific substances as well as by specific antigens. In both situations the initial interaction seems to occur at the surface of the lymphocytes between the inducing substance and membrane receptors. The nature of these receptors is unknown for nonspecific inducers such as PHA, ALS, and various bacterial products. Antigen-antibody complexes, which appear to be nonspecific triggers in lymphocytes, may stimulate the cells in the same way as antigen itself. Alternatively the complex may merely make more efficient the interaction of antigen with lymphocytes and thereby magnify the response. Activation of lymphocytes by antibodies to allotypes of gamma globulin involves receptors that appear to be at least part of the immunoglobulin molecules normally present on cell membranes. Immunoglobulins may also be the receptors for antigens in situations where antigens stimulate sensitized lymphocytes. Because of notable differences in the specificity requirements between humoral antibodies and lymphocyte receptors, the antigen receptors on lymphocyte surfaces are viewed as different from humoral antibodies.

Although induction of DNA synthesis has been most commonly used as an indicator of lymphocyte activation, this is now recognized as representing a late stage that may, moreover, occur only in a small proportion of the cells initially triggered. A considerable number of events are now known to occur well within one hour after triggering; indeed pronounced changes affecting the DNA-histone complex can be detected within five minutes. Changes of membrane permeability as well as alterations of lysosomes also occur very early. The initial change involving the synthetic processes appears to affect the RNA metabolism. In a general biological sense, these early events also occur in other activated diploid cells, and seem in no way peculiar to lymphocytes. Activation can be reversed early after triggering but becomes irreversible later on. Most of these data have been obtained either with anti-allotype antibody or PHA and provide important analogies to the *in vivo* situation in humoral antibody synthesis, where antigen appears to drive the cells involved during the early events and removal of antigen prevents the subsequent steps leading to antibody synthesis.

The mechanism of triggering remains obscure, involving definite threshhold events by nonspecific as well as specific agents. Neither PHA nor ALS stimulates lymphocytes in low concentrations despite the fact that a significant number of molecules have reacted with the cells. An increase in number of molecules results in activation, and a further increase in lack of stimulation. The number of antigen molecules needed to trigger sensitized cells remains unknown and it is still uncertain whether triggering represents a "hit-and-run" process or is determined by the number of receptors triggered.

A major problem emerges from the discrepancy between the high frequency of 1-2% of initially reactive cells in cell-mediated immunity, as opposed to values of only 0.0001-.01% for cells engaged in humoral antibody synthesis. In terms of a strict clonal selection approach implying a one cell-one recognition unit concept, these findings create difficulties, since they imply that cell-mediated immunity would be restricted to a limited number of perhaps 100 antigenic determinants. However, the high values for antigen-reactive cells have been derived from systems where multiple

VI. MODELS FOR RECEPTOR SITES ON THYMIC LYMPHOCYTES

antigenic specificities were involved. It is noteworthy that the estimates of the frequencies of reactive cells in these two systems is not directly comparable, since humoral antibody synthesis is carried out by cells derived from bone-marrow whereas cell-mediated immunity involves thymus-derived cells.

Assuming that only a few determinants are involved in these experimental situations, the major alternative explanations that emerge are: (1) clonal selection is not valid and lymphocytes are actually pleuripotential; (2) clonal selection is indeed operative and the results are attributable to: (a) nonspecific recruitment of innocent "bystander" cells; (b) specific recruitment or spread of information from a few specific cells to many others; (c) histocompatibility antigens are distinctive in the sense that many antigen-sensitive cells carry receptors for them; (d) in transplantation systems the lymphocytes have always been exposed to antigens previously, i.e., their high frequency is a consequence of specific selection by immunization; (e) in cell-mediated immunity the antigen-capturing receptors express a wide cross-reactivity, possibly because of low affinity; (f) non-immunological recognition may operate in histocompatibility systems.

DR. WAKSMAN: In Session II we sought to identify the controlling factors that make for cellular immunity as opposed to antibody production. Although there is now good evidence for two and three cell systems in immunology, the relative roles of thymus-derived cells, bone-marrow derived cells, and macrophages are still poorly defined. These experiments are current, and we have no established body of knowledge as yet. At the rate that new data are being accumulated, within a year or certainly two at the most, we will have a fairly precise definition of the systems discussed in the preceding sessions.

We have not managed to come to grips with the issue of whether the specificity determinants (combining sites) of thymus-derived cells, on the one hand and bone-marrow derived cells on the other, act in relation to what we know as the carrier specificity and determinant specificity of the antigenic molecule, respectively. Dr. Mitchison advanced evidence that a thymus-derived cell could help another thymus-derived cell, in other words, respond to the carrier function while the other responds to the determinant function of the antigens. Here again, our knowledge is too fragmentary to permit a really valid synthesis.

Dr. Mitchison has formulated the distinctions between thymus-derived and bone-marrow derived cells as we know them at the moment. The issue of recirculation of thymus-derived cells as against bone-marrow-derived cells, for example, is a very weak point. While this in no way negates the value of his overall scheme, a great deal of new information based on this scheme must now be obtained.

There is preliminary evidence that in delayed sensitivity, the sensitized cell is a thymus-derived cell. It seemed to me that we left at least two questions quite unanswered. We do not know the role of the macrophage, or of a reticular type of cell, in relation to immunization for the delayed type of immune phenomenon. Secondly, we do not really yet know the relationship of the thymus-derived "sensitized cell" of delayed hypersensitivity and the thymus-derived cell engaged in antibody synthesis; and their possible relation, in turn, to what has been called a "memory cell".

A subject not touched on at all, which is also extremely important, concerns the relationship between the immunizing event, involving a particular antigen and these two or three cell types, and the events which result in immunologic tolerance. Tolerance must also involve some of the same cells and presumably the very same antigen.

We explored the contributions made by the "Experiments of Nature" and artificial experiments which might permit one to separate delayed hypersensitivity events and immunoglobulin events, or perhaps I should say humoral antibody events. The main impression left by that discussion was that many of the "Experiments of Nature" have not proved very definitive. The only case that seems wholly clearcut is the DiGeorge syndrome, where we are dealing with a key organ such as the thymus. Here at least one can say that whatever develops does not involve thymus-dependent cells.

VI. MODELS FOR RECEPTOR SITES ON THYMIC LYMPHOCYTES

The largest specter looming behind all our discussions, one which never even rose to the level of question or answer, is how is the specificity of these cells generated, and what happens within an organ like the thymus. The possibility that these cells maturing within the thymus may carry immunoglobulin is, I think, extremely important. We have no evidence at present that the cells that enter the thymus from the bone-marrow and differentiate there have any type of immunocompetence or immunoglobulin on the surface. This problem has been referred to as the problem of the generator of diversity. We have a long way indeed to go before we have anything really substantive to consider in this area.

DR. LAWRENCE: In the general consideration of transfer factor in Session III, the overriding issue that generated recurring discussion concerned Dr. Uhr's view of transfer factor as an immunogen. He carefully alluded to certain data which his interpretation must temporarily ignore. I too am puzzled about the behavior of an immunogen that is not immunogenic in rabbit or in man. Indeed, this finding was a disappointment to us since an antibody to transfer factor would provide such a useful reagent; we are seeking to render dialysable transfer factor immunogenic by coupling it to methylated serum albumin. I am also puzzled about the idea that transfer factor may represent a cell-bound immunogen ("superantigen") with the unusual properties we have detected, namely that of interacting with antigen in a stereospecific fashion, being liberated into the supernatant and the cell from which it originates being desensitized in the process. This could perhaps be explained if transfer factor had an immunogenic configuration at one end of the molecule and some other stereospecific configuration at the other end.

Dr. Uhr's suggestion of interacting transfer factor with high-affinity immunoglobulin prepared against the antigen to which reactivity is specifically transferred is a very good one and should be pursued. We have not tried this approach, although Baram and Mosko have (Immunology $\underline{8}$, 461, 1965). They used rabbit antiserum to BCG and were unable to detect mycobacterial antigens in dialysable transfer factor either by immunodiffusion in agar gel or by the much more sensitive technique of equilibrium dialysis. Mixing the rabbit antiserum with transfer factor also failed to block transfer factor activity.

Another broad issue raised in our discussion concerned the specificity of transfer factor. Specificity has been repeatedly documented in vivo starting with viable cells, cell extracts, antigen-liberated supernatant transfer factor and finally dialysable transfer factor. The low molecular weight of dialysable transfer factor calls for additional and broader studies of specificity to reinforce this conclusion. Nevertheless where multiple sensitivities have been transferred in vivo as well as in vitro using dialysable transfer factor, the correlation has been exact and precise. However, the range and variety of specific combinations can and should be enlarged.

A final issue was the consideration of serial transfer from individual A to B to C. It is of course possible that an immunogen could be carried over by A's leucocyte extract to B, but it is more difficult to postulate such carriage from B to C. So the question remains what kind of an immunogen, other than a virus or living microbe, is capable of making more of itself in the process of inducing sensitivity?

DR. GOOD: Dr. Lawrence has already given us an authoritative summary of the issues concerning transfer factor. Our discussions in Session III, resulted in a consensus that whatever transfer factor is, the system for its demonstration is consistent and reproducible, as demonstrated with a variety of antigens of bacterial, viral and fungal nature. We have reached agreement that it is especially crucial to exclude antigenicity or an immunogenic nature of transfer factor. Dr. Lawrence has persuasively presented arguments from serial transfer studies that if transfer factor is an immunogen, it must be a very special replicating immunogen. Others, still skeptical, argue that his serial transfer studies are not absolutely conclusive because antigenic stimulation might have been introduced by the testing used after each successive transfer.

We have also considered the more recent adaption of in

VI. MODELS FOR RECEPTOR SITES ON THYMIC LYMPHOCYTES

<u>vivo</u> models to the study of the properties and mechanism of action of transfer factor. Here, however, one of the factors liberated by antigen from sensitive lymphocytes <u>in vitro</u> has characteristics somewhat different from those established for the dialysable transfer factor that induces the systemic transfer of delayed allergic reactions <u>in vivo</u>. It is going to be important, I think, to elucidate these differences.

We are still faced with the overwhelming fact of the human-animal paradox: why is it that one can readily demonstrate transfer factor in man but not in experimental animals? I think this problem remains as a challenge, although perhaps some inroads have been made from our recent findings that similar activity can be liberated into plasma <u>in vivo</u>, and from the studies on <u>in vitro</u> models described at this conference. It is obvious that if transfer factor is not acting as an immunogen, it is acting as some sort of a specific derepressor. However, it is difficult to conceive of a specific mechanism of derepression other than that mediated by antigen. This may be a direction into which further thought and work should go. At any rate, there is much work yet to be done with the challenge that is posed by transfer factor.

DR. BLOOM: Our discussion on effector molecules in Session IV, centered on the distinctive factors released by sensitized cells under the influence of antigen. A major issue that emerged was whether the same factor or putative effector molecules were released from sensitized cells by antigen stimulation as were found after stimulation with various mitogens. The answer is not easily provided at the moment, but the activities and factors are there to be tested, and I think that this part of the scheme developed by Dr. Uhr is easily tested and will be known shortly.

What we now have is a series of activities <u>in vitro</u>, about seven at the moment, produced by supernatants of activated lymphocyte cultures, and surely more to come. In a sense, these activities, such as migration inhibition, cytotoxicity, mitogenicity, etc., represent only a first step towards determining the actual effector molecules of delayed-type hypersensitivity, and we should not let their newness and variety confuse us. It seems to me an entirely reasonable expectation that the question of which molecules are responsible for the individual *in vitro* activities can and will be answered satisfactorily rather soon. However, I am not so sanguine as Dr. Uhr in the belief that it is going to be easy, even with fluorescent antibodies to the factors, to demonstrate the presence of these effector molecules in delayed-type reactions *in vivo*. I would hold that this criterion, namely the demonstration of the putative effector molecule at the site of an active reaction is, however, a *sine qua non* for establishing the role of any given factor in the reaction.

While the multiplicity of factors and activities is presently the source of some confusion, I would suggest that the concept that there exists *the* delayed-type hypersensitivity reaction *in vivo*, to which each of the *in vitro* activities is compared, may indeed be deceptively simplistic. On the formal level, one wonders whether all activated cells make all effectors, and whether all effectors are produced in all types of delayed-type hypersensitivity reactions. Further, how can we compare the microbial model of cellular immunity, in which there is a specific release of a component with nonspecific effects on macrophages, with the cell cytotoxicity reactions that seem to involve specificity in the killing of target cells in the homotransplantation model. Then too, there is the possibility that delayed-type reactions in different parts of the body may be directed against different antigens and display separate and distinctive histology as emphasized by Dr. Dixon.

The possibility is thus recognized that under different circumstances, in different environments and milieu, the same factors may in fact have rather different effects. In some cases factors released from sensitized lymphocytes may affect primarily macrophages; in other situations they may act on target cells, endothelial cells or even other lymphocytes. Additionally there has evolved at this conference the realization that the same molecule might have very different effects depending on local concentrations. What has emerged from our discussions is the awareness that the study of *in vitro* models for delayed-type hypersensitivity reactions is quite a new and exciting area,

VI. MODELS FOR RECEPTOR SITES ON THYMIC LYMPHOCYTES

but really has only just begun. It now seems clear that each of the present models and in vitro systems has serious limitations and drawbacks, viz, in terms of sensitivity, the time and effort required, and above all else uncertainty of its real relevance to the events in vivo. Clearly still other models are required that are maximally discriminating and analytically objective. There is little reason to doubt that such tools will be forthcoming.†

DR. SILVERSTEIN: In Session V, we devoted considerable time to what one might call the more biological and medical questions of the effector limb of the delayed hypersensitivity reaction. One might almost subtitle it delayed hypersensitivity in health and disease. I don't know that we came to substantive conclusions as a result of our discussions. Perhaps we are historically not ready to do so.

---

†Editors Footnote: Even before this conference, the Allergy and Immunology Branch of the NIAID had given consideration to the desirability of organizing a series of workshops on in vitro models of cellular immunity, patterned after the successful workshops on Histocompatibility Testing. The present conference, which itself had been stimulated by rapid pace of developments in cellular immunity, served further to crystallize the need for such a workshop. As a direct consequence of this conference, the planning and organization of the first of a series of such workshops was effected and is scheduled for an entire week in November, 1969.

It is anticipated that the principal in vitro techniques now in use will be standardized, and various preparations of effector molecules will be assayed by all of the principal procedures. There will be an associated conference devoted to the theoretical base for present methodology and oriented especially towards the development of new techniques.

CELLULAR IMMUNITY

It is of interest that a very strange quirk of history permitted the circulating antibody to be the first discovered of the immunologic manifestations, in all of its protective aspects. Only some twenty odd years later was it found that it could do some harm to the host, so that the concept of humoral immunity preceded that of hypersensitivity. Delayed hypersensitivity (note the very name we use for it) was on the other hand discovered in the context of disease and damage to the host. It has only been in recent times that we have had any notions that it might be concerned with protection against infection, and might have immunologic implications in the purest sense.

It might be appropriate to return to the biologic problem of why we have delayed hypersensitivity, or if you would prefer, cellular immunity. The suggestion made originally by Dr. Thomas and subsequently taken up by Burnet, was that this is a surveillance mechanism to control somatic mutations. I think that proposal is a fascinating one and we are destined to hear a great deal more about it. Yet, I want to bring up for your consideration a critical experiment in the literature that argues against the surveillance hypothesis. Most of us would, I think, agree that for this kind of duty, a very sensitive surveillance mechanism would be required to pick up the mutational event early, well before the mutant cells get out of hand. The system must be able, in fact, to recognize the existance of but one or at most a few cells. It is very significant, in my view, that Billingham and others working with histocompatibility antigens, that if anything are stronger than tumor antigens, demonstrated that a sprinkling of allogeneic cells implanted in a recipient can go unrecognized for very long periods of time, if not indefinitely. This is, I believe, a very significant observation. I would submit that the putative mechanism for surveillance, if such indeed exists, is falling down on the job in this instance. If this is indeed so important a mechanism, I don't think we can afford such a lapse. The point I want to make is that there is thus far only an imperfect case for the prime function of the cellular immune apparatus being the detection and destruction of naturally arising mutant cells.

I do however feel strongly that there is a great point

VI. MODELS FOR RECEPTOR SITES ON THYMIC LYMPHOCYTES

to be made for the involvement of the cellular immune mechanisms in the mobilization of predominantly nonspecific factors for the defense of the host via the inflammatory reaction. Many have been perplexed by the local plasmacytosis and antibody formation found in association with delayed-type inflammatory reactions. We have here a very good example of the efficacy of the cellular immune mechanisms in its mobilization of the mononuclear cell inflammatory reaction in its broadest context. In point of fact, we see mobilized not only lymphocytes and macrophages, but also the very cells (which may not be different) that produce antibody at a local site where it is most needed. This is the picture we see consistently in chronic inflammation, in the type of defense mechanism that I would identify with cellular immunity in its broadest sense.

CHAIRMAN THOMAS: Dr. Silverstein's point is well taken, but we should not scrap the whole idea of immunological surveillance because it happened to fail in one specific experimental situation. Unhappily this is the precise point of my postulate: surveillance does not invariably function with the efficiency that Dr. Silverstein demands, and as a result a high percentage of individuals eventually succumb to cancer.

The suggestion we made some years ago (Thomas, in Cellular and Humoral Aspects of Hypersensitive States, Ed. Lawrence, Hoeber, 1959) has cropped up repeatedly in these discussions, namely that cellular immunity evolved in multicellular organisms as a protective device designed to recognize mutant cells as foreign and reject them forthwith. This postulated immunological defense against neoplasia has been subsequently termed "immunological surveillance" (Burnet, Lancet $\underline{1}$, 1171, 1967). Neoplastic cells, antigenically foreign and recognizable, are continually appearing in many tissues, in the same way that they regularly appear, sooner or later, when normal cells are placed in tissue culture. It would seem essential to have at hand a mechanism constantly alerted to recognize the new cells and then to destroy them. The issue of survival would be determined by the foreignness of the cells, the sensitivity of the recognition process, and by the efficiency of the immunologic mechanism involved in their destruction.

CELLULAR IMMUNITY

This, I would like to think, is the purpose of the reaction we have been considering. It is fortunate that the same device appears useful in preventing and eradicating viral infections as well as certain intracellular microbial infections. Of further interest is the participation of the same central mechanism in the tissue damage encountered in certain human and experimental animal diseases. The transplantation biologists are fortunate indeed to have been provided with such a fascinating puzzle for their entertainment. But the real business of delayed hypersensitivity or cellular immunity is, I submit, to keep the animal kingdom from being overrun by cancer.†

DR. LAWRENCE: It is noteworthy that observations made in the decade following Thomas's original formulation of an immunological surveillance mechanism, have in large measure tended to substantiate the validity of his idea. The increased incidence of tumors in a host with depressed or ablated cellular immunity is now an increasingly recognized hazard of interference with this central recognition event. Examples of this correlation are now being observed and documented with increasing frequency in recipients of transplants receiving immunosuppressive therapy (Lancet $\underline{I}$, 505, 1969) as well as in experimental animals subjected to total immunosuppression by means of thymectomy + ALS (Gaugas et al., Nature $\underline{221}$, 1033, 1969).

---

†Editors Footnote: Information relevant to immunological surveillance has now been augmented considerably, notably as regards lymphocyte products with the capacity to eliminate target cells. The reader will find marshalled in these pages the basic data and points of view that has led to the selection of Immunological Surveillance as the focus of the next conference in this series. Indeed it should be apparent that a considerable portion of the groundwork for this topic has already emerged in these discussions.

VI. MODELS FOR RECEPTOR SITES ON THYMIC LYMPHOCYTES

As a result of the idea proposed by Dr. Thomas, we were stimulated to formulate the self + X hypothesis which virtually identified all delayed type responses as homograft reactions. (Lawrence, Physiol. Rev. 39, 811, 1959). Mitchison was the first to call direct attention to this possibility when he pointed out the similarity to a haptene-altered protein complex and an iso antigen and suggested an analogy between homograft sensitivity and sensitivity to simple chemicals (Proc. Roy. Soc., Ser. B. 142, 72, 1954).

The factual basis of the self + X hypothesis may help resolve some of the conflicts that have arisen in our discussions whenever the realities of delayed sensitivity collide with immunologic theory. The facts are quite simple: the most intense and durable states of delayed reactivity result from an inductive phase characterized by prolonged, intimate association between the inducing agent (bacterium, fungus, virus or simple chemical) and the intracellular microenvironment of the host's phagocytic mononuclear cells. Classical examples of this situation are afforded by infections caused by preferential (e.g., Mycobacteria, Salmonella, Brucella) as well as obligatory (e.g., viruses) intracellular microbial parasites (Mackaness and Blanden, Progr. Allergy 11, 89, 1967).

We made the prediction that such prolonged intracellular residence of microbe or virion (X) could alter host histocompatibility antigens (self), resulting in the formation of a self + X complex and thereby create, in effect, a new histocompatibility antigen. Considering the tubercle bacillus as the prototype, the conditions favorable for such an outcome are met - namely a relatively amicable intracellular residence of bacilli in host macrophages without necessarily killing such cells on the one hand, nor being autolyzed and digested on the other. Upon phagocytosis by other reticuloendothelial cells, such effete macrophages possessing the self + X marker would be recognized as foreign in the sense of having acquired a minor histocompatibility difference. This recognition event would in turn result in sensitization of immunocompetent cells (presumably small lymphocytes) with the induction of a transfer factor to the new antigenic determinant and thus acquisition of a highly reactive site in or at such cell

CELLULAR IMMUNITY

surfaces directed at all other cells bearing the self + X marker. This view of the induction of delayed type hypersensitivity is diagrammed in Fig. 58.

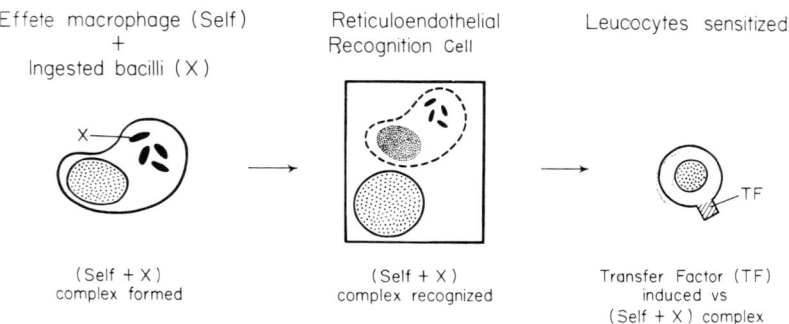

|Effete macrophage (Self) + Ingested bacilli (X) | Reticuloendothelial Recognition Cell | Leucocytes sensitized |

(Self + X) complex formed ⟶ (Self + X) complex recognized ⟶ Transfer Factor (TF) induced vs (Self + X) complex

Fig. 58 Induction of tuberculin type hypersensitivity in the context of the self + X hypothesis.

(Reproduced with permission of Physiological Reviews)

Ordinarily, in the absence of antigen, the tissues of tuberculin-sensitive individuals do not undergo inflammation or necrosis. When tuberculin does coat such host cells, in skin or lung, a brisk inflammatory response ensues which may progress to cell death. We view this expression of tuberculin sensitivity as a special type of homograft response undertaken by the host against his own tissues. This outcome is illustrated in Fig. 59, where the intradermal injection of antigen is shown bound to host epidermal cells converting them from cells recognized as self to a population of cells recognized as self + X. The latter attract and interact with sensitized leucocytes bearing transfer factor specifically directed as the self + X marker. Mild reactions result in the usual red, indurated lesion; severe reactions result in blister and eschar.

450

VI. MODELS FOR RECEPTOR SITES ON THYMIC LYMPHOCYTES

formation. The fully developed necrotic eschar is indistinguishable from that of a rejected skin allograft. Thus, recognition of only slightly foreign cells may evoke a response unique to itself (tuberculin sensitivity), or may vary only in intensity from reactions invoked by allografts expressing major histocompatibility differences (homograft sensitivity). From this vantage point, the similarity to homograft rejection is unmistakable in the tissue necrosis of the Koch phenomenon expressed by tuberculous guinea pigs and its human counterpart observed in caseating, cavitary pulmonary tuberculosis; both are triggered by antigen and sensitized lymphocytes bearing a specific transfer factor elaborated by the host. These situations illuminate most clearly the nature of the host's predicament: in attempting to reject the tubercle bacillus he cannot dissociate bacillary antigens from histocompatibility antigens and in effect inadvertently reacts to his own tissues as well.

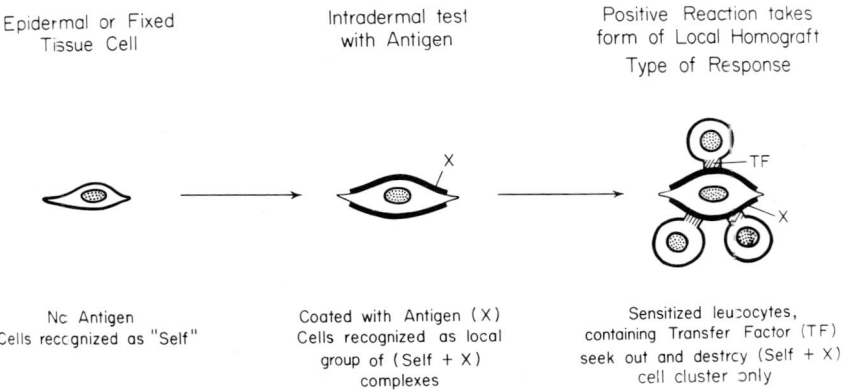

Fig. 59 Manifestations of tuberculin type hypersensitivity in the context of the self + X hypothesis.

(Reproduced with permission of Physiological Reviews)

CELLULAR IMMUNITY

In relation to Dr. Uhr's view of transfer factor as an immunogen, it is of interest that we had considered this possibility and indeed actually proposed a mechanism whereby transfer factor, not immunogenic by itself, might acquire the properties of an immunogen as diagrammed in Fig. 60. We suggested then that the early appearance of sensitivity following transfer (i.e., a "passive" phase), could result from the prompt engagement of host leucocytes by transfer factor which then interact with antigen-coated epidermal cells (a suggestion which has subsequently received experimental support from our recent <u>in vitro-in vivo</u> observations with dialysable transfer factor). The

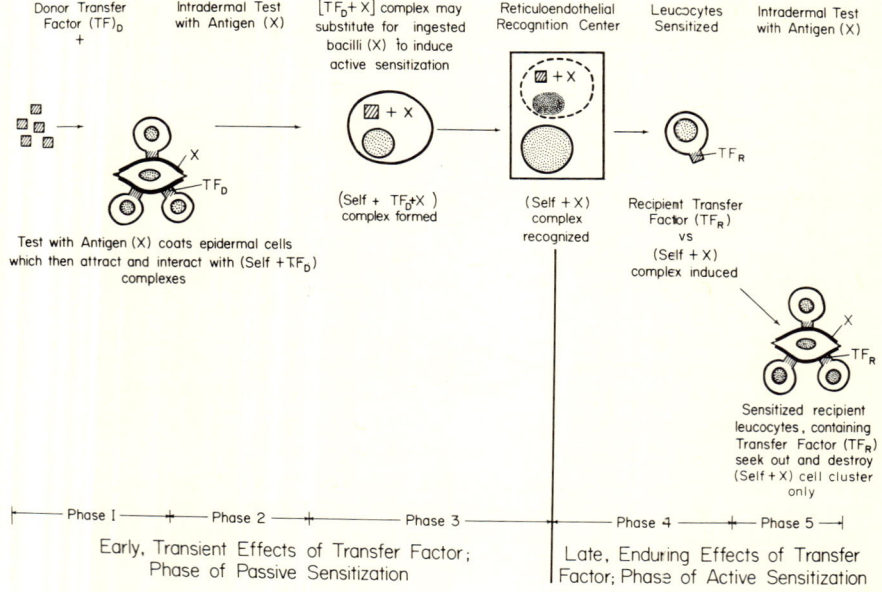

Fig. 60 Transfer of tuberculin type hypersensitivity in the context of the self + X hypothesis.

(Reproduced with permission of Physiological Reviews)

VI. MODELS FOR RECEPTOR SITES ON THYMIC LYMPHOCYTES

resultant inflammatory response and subsequent coating of host cells and/or ingestion by host macrophages (cf donor TF + tuberculin) could upon phagocytosis in turn present the host with antigenic determinants sufficiently foreign to function as an immunogen, thereby launching a phase of "active" sensitization and the generation of the recipient's own transfer factor. This last interpretation, if corroborated by experimental data would answer a critical objection to the immunogen concept - namely that transfer factor is too small a molecule to function as an antigenic determinant for delayed sensitivity. The interpretation may also provide a mechanism for Dutton's earlier suggestion of "conservation of antigen" by transfer factor (see Session III).

Of considerable interest to this issue is Burnet's recent proposal that an essential requirement for the induction of delayed sensitivity, as against humoral antibody responses, is the integration of the antigenic determinant into the surface of mobile cells (i.e., lymphocytes, monocytes). Burnet also proposed: "The hypothesis is that the antigenic determinant which confers specificity becomes incorporated in the lipoprotein on the cell surface in such a form that when the cell is autolyzed in the body or disintegrated *in vitro* the complex antigenic determinant plus cell-surface component, which we can call the immunogen, can be transferred to another cell. The immunogen incorporated in the new recipient cell surface can continue to react with immunocytes newly produced from the thymus and of appropriate avidity." (Burnet, Cellular Immunology, Cambridge University Press, p. 584-6, 1969). Burnet points out the similarities of his proposal to our self + X hypothesis detailed here, and to Pappenheimer's proposal (Harvey Lectures 52, 100, 1956), that transfer factor is passed from sensitive to non-sensitive leucocytes.

It is noteworthy that in the decade since its formulation, the self + X hypothesis has found experimental proof in the discovery that oncogenic as well as non-oncogenic viruses actually do alter host histocompatibility antigens as determined by rejection of such tissues transplanted to isogenic animals (see Rowe; also Roizman, in Cross-Reacting Antigens and Neoantigens, Ed. Trentin, Williams and Wilkins, 1967). Moreover, Mitchison's earlier suggestion of chemically induced isoantigens has also found experimental support in similar alterations of histocompatibility antigens induced by chemical carcinogens, (see Prehn, ibid).

In the context of the self + X hypothesis, I would question the ideal of absolute immunological specificity. It is disturbing to me, and I assume to others as well, that the more one sifts the information available, particularly recent studies using in vitro systems, the less one is convinced that any living creature is immunologically virginal and that in nature a zero base-line of immunological reactivity ever exists. I have already made the heretical suggestion that the homograft reaction itself may by the means of its detection only mimic an actively acquired state of sensitivity and really could result from the elevation of a latent isoimmune state (In: Histocompatibility Testing, P. 141, Nat. Res. Council, 1965). The next great thrust in immunology may very well be to seek an understanding of what isoimmunity really is, and thereby define the baseline against which we measure all of our immunologically "specific" responses.

ABBREVIATIONS

ALS	antilymphocyte serum
BCG	Bacille Calmette-Guerin
BGG	bovine gamma globulin
BSA	bovine serum albumin
CNS	central nervous system
DNCB	2,4 dinitrochlorobenzine
DNP	2,4 dinitrophenol
GVH	graft versus host
HLA	the major system of human leucocyte antigens
HSA	human serum albumin
Ig	immunoglobulin
IgA, IgG, IgM	standard nomenclature for human -globulin classes; also used here to name analogous proteins in other species
IgX	hypothetical category of imunoglobulin with affinity for thymic lymphocytes
KLH	keyhole limpet hemocyanin
LCM	lymphocytic choriomeningitis
LT	lymphotoxin
MIF	macrophage inhibitory factor
MLC	mixed leucocyte culture
OT	old tuberculin
PFC	plaque-forming cells

ABBREVIATIONS

PHA	phytohemagglutinin
PMN	polymorphonuclear
PPD	purified protein derivative
PVP	polyvinylpyrrolidone
PWM	pokeweed mitogen
sRBC	sheep red blood cells
SD	streptodornase
SK	streptokinase
TF	transfer factor

AUTHOR INDEX

A

Amos, D. B., 31

B

Bach, F. H., 197, 205, 206, 237 - 239, 240, 292 - 294, 340, 362, 390, 391
Baram, P., 181, 182, 189, 196, 210 - 213, 218, 219, 235, 242, 398, 399
Billingham, R. E., 228, 284, 315, 318, 388 - 390, 392 - 394
Bloom, B. R., 19, 144, 220, 249 - 262, 268 - 271, 274, 284, 285, 338, 443 - 445
Brandriss, M. W., 133, 191 - 195, 202, 203, 207, 208, 235, 383, 384
Braun, W., 36, 37, 43, 62, 63, 89, 92, 229 - 231, 240, 241, 292, 362, 385

C

Chase, M. W., 105, 109, 195, 217, 218, 222 - 228, 244, 245, 309, 312, 318, 397, 433, 434
Chessin, L. N., 17, 18, 21, 136, 217, 301
Cohn, M., 41, 42, 59, 62, 94, 95, 97, 110, 140, 202, 232, 284, 292, 340

D

David, J. R., 133 - 135, 176, 237, 262 - 267, 269 - 273, 278, 346
Dixon, F. J., 207, 271, 272, 404, 405
Dutton, R. W., 53, 54, 59, 61, 66, 84 - 89, 94, 176, 178, 231, 232, 274

E

Eisen, H. N., 107, 108, 206, 207, 344, 419

F

Fireman, P., 139, 140, 197, 202, 244

G

Gell, P. G. H., 13 - 15, 26, 63, 68, 80, 110, 420, 422, 423, 435 - 437
Good, R. A., 175, 189, 191, 193, 194, 207, 208, 215, 220, 229, 237, 239, 245, 277, 278, 284, 315 - 319, 386, 387, 391, 397, 401 - 403, 405, 421 - 426, 434 - 435, 442 - 443
Granger, G. A., 41, 205, 269, 299, 300, 324 - 346, 350 - 354, 363, 363 - 367, 369, 370, 397

H

Hirschhorn, K., 3 - 12, 15 - 17, 20, 21, 27, 28, 30, 31, 36, 39 - 41, 55, 64, 129, 130, 138, 139, 233, 234, 242, 284, 356, 360, 361, 363, 392, 400, 401

L

Landy, M., 16, 30, 64, 65, 69, 129, 132, 219, 220, 299, 300, 341, 365, 367 - 369, 387, 391, 397, 398

AUTHOR INDEX

Lawrence, H. S., 43, 56, 57, 111 - 120, 131, 135 - 137, 139, 145 - 175, 175 - 182, 184 - 188, 190 - 192, 194 - 197, 199, 203, 204, 210, 218, 221, 222, 229, 231 - 236, 297 - 300, 312, 313, 319, 354 - 361, 364, 385, 403, 404, 441, 442, 448 - 454

M

Mackaness, G. B., 309 - 314, 370 - 387, 391
Marshall, W. H., 31, 32, 66, 67, 199 - 201
Mitchison, N. A., 38, 58, 62, 73 - 81, 90, 93 - 95, 97, 106, 107, 140, 141, 229, 419
Moller, G., 12, 13, 16, 20, 33, 35, 37, 38, 42, 43, 50, 51, 54 - 56, 58, 59, 65 - 68, 81, 82, 91 - 93, 99, 107, 198, 216, 217, 273, 295, 296, 346 - 351, 353, 366, 368, 394, 395, 400, 424, 425, 437 - 439

O

Oppenheim, J. J., 18, 19, 21 - 26, 31, 83, 84, 107, 129, 136, 182, 295, 339, 383

R

Rosenau, W., 28 - 31, 175, 300

S

Salvin, S. B., 130, 131, 189, 190, 274 - 277, 283, 284
Schlossman, S. F., 33 - 36, 101 - 107, 110, 111, 137, 138, 216, 426, 427

Silverstein, A. M., 36, 39 - 41, 97 - 106, 139, 214, 314, 315, 323, 324, 345, 370, 383, 388, 390, 392, 393, 395, 396, 401, 404, 421, 445 - 447
Smith, R. T., 44 - 49, 68, 183, 213, 217, 239, 240, 272, 273, 385, 386

T

Thomas, L., 192, 193, 343, 344, 387, 409, 437, 447, 448
Thor, D. E., 26, 27, 93, 131, 243, 244, 285 - 292, 299
Turk, J. L., 32, 33, 38, 39, 89, 91, 98, 99, 121 - 129, 186, 187, 189, 283, 284, 291, 301 - 309, 313, 427 - 432

U

Uhr, J. W., 15, 16, 58, 60, 138, 208 - 210, 213 - 215, 219, 220, 273, 291, 292, 311, 345, 400, 401, 403, 409 - 422, 426, 432, 433

V

Valentine, F. T., 19, 20, 61, 67, 68, 131 - 133, 183, 185, 186, 197, 198, 201, 202, 205, 213, 214, 235, 294, 344, 361 - 365, 367

W

Waksman, B. H., 54, 55, 81, 90 - 96, 98, 99, 101, 111, 120, 121, 130, 132, 133, 135, 138, 140, 230, 231, 269, 278 - 283, 313, 352, 353, 395, 396, 439 - 441
Wilson, D. B., 15, 51 - 53, 55, 56, 59 - 61, 63, 64, 66, 98, 199, 234, 271, 343

SUBJECT INDEX

A

"A" band," helper cell in, 84
AB 4 system, use of, 13 - 14
Abyssinian guinea pigs, 92
n-Acetylgalactosamine, PHA attachment and, 6
Acridine orange binding test, 42 - 43
Acrylamide gel electrophoresis, 255, 262 - 265, 309, 339
Actinomycin D
  effector substance production and, 259 - 260
  skin reactive factor production and, 307
Adherence, lymphocyte fractionation by, 76 - 77
Adjuvant
  alumina as, 251
  cellular immunity and, 79, 256 - 258
Adoptive transfer, of cellular immunity, 375 - 381, 385 - 386
Agammaglobulinemia
  Bruton's, 401 - 402
  reconstitution of, 228
Allergic encephalomyelitis, cells in, 272, 396
Allogeneic inhibition, 50 - 51, 56, 393 - 395, see also Lymphotoxin, activity of
Allogeneic stimulation, 48 - 49
Allotype suppression, recovery from, 79 - 80
Alumina, as adjuvant, 251
Ampicillin, "Lupus" syndromes and, 17

Anti-allotype antibody, 13 - 14, 21 - 22, 420
Anti-complement serum, 431
Anti-immunoglobulin antibody, 13 - 14, 83, 84, 421
Anti-light chain antibody, 81 - 83, 419 - 420, 424
Anti-lymphocyte serum
  adoptive transfer and, 380 - 381
  blast transformation and, 21 - 22
  experimental leprosy and, 403
  lymphotoxin release and, 328
  thymus derived cells and, 74, 428, 431
  transfer factor and, 155
Anti-lymphotoxin antibody, 345, 352, 413
Anti-phytohemagglutinin antiserum, 18 - 19
Antibody production
  bone marrow cells and, 77
  in Hodgkin's Disease, 135, 137 - 138
  in leprosy, 135
  radioresistance of, 98 - 99
  responder cell frequency in, 52, 53, 58
  in sarcoidosis, 135, 137
  structural changes in, 414 - 416
  thymectomy and, 84, 436
Antigen-antibody complexes, migration inhibition by, 270, 431
Antigen liberated transfer factor
  dialysable transfer factor and, 171-172
  kinetics of release of, 164
  production of, 183, 198, 205
  specificity of, 184 - 185
Antigen mediated recruitment, 171, 173, 199, 201 - 202, 231 - 232, 234 - 235, 410

SUBJECT INDEX

Antigen recognition, by lymphocyte, 426 - 427
Antigen responsive cells, enumeration of, 168, 199 - 202, 205 - 206
Antigen-RNA complex, 38
Antigen route, cellular immunity and, 79
Antigen size, 102 - 111
Antigen trapping, 428
Autoallergic encephalomyelitis, 396
Autoantibody, in leprosy 123

B

Blast transformation
    anti-allotype serum and, 13 - 14
    anti-immunoglobulin antibody and, 13 - 14, 83, 84
    anti-light chain antibody and, 81 - 83, 424
    anti-PHA serum and, 18 - 19
    antibody production and, 429
    antigen mediated transfer factor in, 168 - 171, 184, 298 - 299
    blocking of, 13 - 14
    cell division and, 10 - 11, 40, 168
    clonal proliferation and, 168
    cytotoxic factor synthesis in, 10
    dialysable transfer factor and, 158 - 167
    DNA synthesis in, 14, 15, 28 - 29, 41
    dose-responses in, 238
    drug induced "Lupus" syndromes and, 17 - 18
    hapten inhibition in, 107
    histocompatibility antigens and, 46 - 49, 50 - 51
    histoplasmosis and, 130 - 131
    immune complexes and, 21 - 26
    immunocompetence and, 21 - 22
    inhibitors of, 5 - 6
    interferon synthesis in, 10
    kinetics of, 40
    in leprosy, 123, 135
    lipid turnover in, 6 - 7
    lymphotoxin release and, 327 - 329
    lysosomes and, 8, 15, 38 - 40, 44
    macrophages and, 20 - 23, 25, 38
    in measles, 139 - 140
    membrane cyclases and, 7
    MIF synthesis in, 10
    mitogenic factor synthesis in, 16 - 17
    in moniliasis, 130
    of mouse lymphocytes, 44 - 49
    nucleoprotein phosphorylation in, 8
    "piggyback" effect in, 14, 15
    pinocytosis and, 7, 15, 17, 40
    pokeweed mitogen and, 30, 429
    polysaccharide antigens and, 17 - 18
    protein synthesis in, 9 - 10, 40, 64
    recruitment in, 54, 58 - 61
    responder cells frequency in, 51 - 54, 58 - 61, 168, 199 - 202, 205 - 206
    ribosome synthesis in, 9, 40
    ribonucleic acid and production of, 243
    ribonucleic acid synthesis in, 8 - 9, 14, 15, 28 - 29, 40, 64, 233
    ribonucleic acid turnover in, 8 - 9
    in sarcoidosis, 112, 129 - 130
    stimulants of, 4 - 5, 21 - 22
    suppression by serum factors of, 129, 132 - 133
    streptococcal factor and, 31
    transfer factor and, 184
    transfer factor synthesis in, 10
    tumor specific antigens and, 47
    Wiskott-Aldrich syndrome and, 136, 138 - 139
Blastogenic factor, see Mitogenic factor
Boeck's sarcoid, see Sarcoidosis
Bone marrow derived cell, see also Lymphocyte
    antibody forming cells and, 77
    macrophage as, 250, 310
Bruton's agammaglobulinemia, 401 - 402
Bursectomy
    effect on blast transformation of, 83
    lymphocyte depletion by, 74
Butazolidine, "Lupus" syndromes and, 17

SUBJECT INDEX

C

Candidiasis
  anergy in, 237
  delayed hypersensitivity in, 118, 133 - 134
  MIF production in, 237
Carrier specificity, 33 - 36, 97 - 98, 206
Cellular immunity
  adoptive transfer of, 375 - 381, 385 - 386
  antigen concentration in, 77
  induction of, 79
Chemotactic factor
  MIF and, 271 - 272
  production of, 254
  separation from MIF, 255, 264, 266
O-Chlorobenzyl bovine gamma globulin, sensitization to, 262
Chlorpromazine, 62
Coccidioidin sensitivity, transfer of, 146, 153 - 154, 157 - 158, 189, 204, 218, 219, 236
Complement
  acute inflammation and, 323
  as effector substance, 413
  homograft reaction and, 316
  role of, 431
Contact hypersensitivity
  antibody in, 434
  carrier specificity in, 206
  cellular transfer of, 206 - 208, 222 - 228
  radioresistance of, 98 - 99
  RNA and production of, 243
  transfer factor and, 190 - 195
Cortisone
  leucocyte emigration and, 314
  lymphotoxin release and, 330
Cytotoxic factor, *see* Lymphotoxin
Cytophilic antibody
  acquisition by thymocytes of, 93
  delayed hypersensitivity and, 383
  macrophage activation and, 383
  migration inhibition by, 429

D

"D band," precursor cell in, 34
Delayed hypersensitivity
  see also Cellular immunity, Contact hypersensitivity
  acceleration of, 309 - 314
  as adjuvant, 256 - 258
  anti-complement serum and, 431
  anti-lymphocyte serum and, 431
  antigen persistence and, 384
  antigen-antibody precipitates and, 431
  cell contact in, 350, 351 - 354, 362, 412 - 413
  cell division and, 412
  chronic disease and, 258, 323, 401 - 403
  cortisone treatment and, 314
  cytophilic antibody and, 383
  desensitization of, 100
  graft-versus-host reaction as, 391
  histology of, 428 - 429, 430
  in Hodgkin's disease, 135, 137 - 138
  initiation of, 409 - 419, 427 - 432
  intracellular infection and, 370 - 383
  in leprosy, 135
  in measles, 139 - 140
  minimal antigen size in, 102 - 111
  to phytohemagglutinin, 31, 32 - 33
  plasma transfer of, 315 - 318
  radioresistance of, 98 - 99, 310
  in sarcoidosis, 111 - 117, 135, 137
  surface antibody and, 420 - 423
  vaccinia and, 118, 258 - 259, 402, 403
  viral infections and, 118, 139 - 140, 236, 256, 258 - 259, 402, 403
  X-irradiation and, 98 - 99, 310
Deoxyribonuclease, transfer factor susceptibility of, 178
Deoxyribonucleic acid
  lymphotoxin release and, 330 - 331, 348, 361
  synthesis of, 14, 15, 28 - 29, 41
Dextran sulphate, lymphocyte depletion by, 76

SUBJECT INDEX

Dialysable transfer factor
  accelerated reactions and, 312
  antigen liberated transfer factor and, 171 - 172
  blast transformation and, 158 - 167
  contact hypersensitivity and, 193 - 194, 207 - 208
  enzymatic sensitivity of, 175 - 176, 182
  heat inactivation of, 158
  interaction with lymphocytes of, 161 - 163
  interspecific activity of, 186, 239 - 241
  immunogenicity of, 230 - 233
  MIF production and, 159
  mouse lymphocytes and, 186, 239 - 240
  polynucleotide as, 181 - 182
  properties of, 172, 196
  purification of, 156 - 159
  quantitation of, 196, 197
  recruitment by, 173, 231 - 232, 234 - 235
  in sarcoidosis, 113 - 117
  separation from histocompatibility antigens of, 179 - 181
  size of, 157 - 158, 217 - 218
  specificity of, 184, 218

DiGeorge syndrome
  anergy in, 402 - 403, 436
  immunoglobulin synthesis in, 135, 137 - 138, 425 - 426, 436

Dinitrochlorobenzene
  as hapten, 109, 112, 119, 123
  sensitivity, transfer of, 193 - 195, 206 - 208

Dinitrofluorobenzene sensitivity, transfer of, 191, 194

Dinitrophenyl-oligolysine, use of, 34 - 35, 101 - 111, 243, 267, 286 - 290, 292

Diphtheria toxoid sensitivity, transfer of, 145, 153, 184, 194, 204, 210, 218, 219, 236

E

Effector substances, *see also* individual substances
  complement as, 413
  concentration of, 397
  feedback control of, 398 - 399
  as gene products, 259 - 260
  inactivation of, 398
  from macrophages, 350
  metabolic inhibitors and, 259 - 260
  production of, 397 - 398, 412
  properties of, 251 - 254, 297 - 298
  regulation by, 366 - 367
Encephalomyelitides, delayed hypersensitivity and, 258 - 259, 272, 396
Epstein-Barr virus, 11
Ethylene oxide treated human serum, 177
Euchrysine staining, 45
Experimental allergic encephalomyelitis, 272

F

Flagellin, antibody production to, 428

G

Gradient centrifugation, lymphocyte fractionation by, 76 - 77
Graft rejection, *see* Homograft reaction
Graft versus host reaction
  frequency of responder cells in, 52 - 54, 59 - 61
  lymphotoxin and, 400
  macrophage activation in, 389 - 391, 396
Guinea pig
  Abyssinian, 92
  strain 2, 105, 243, 286 - 290, 292, 389 - 390
  strain 13, 105, 243, 286 - 290, 292, 389 - 390

462

SUBJECT INDEX

H

Hapten inhibition, of blast transformation, 107
HeLa cells, lymphotoxin and, 341, 354 - 356
Heparinoids, lymphocyte depletion by, 76
Hepatitis
  in Bruton's disease, 402
  lymphocyte cell lines in, 11
Herpes simplex, lymphocyte cell lines in, 11
Herpes zoster, lymphocyte cell lines in, 11
Histocompatibility antigens
  alteration of, 449 - 454
  blast transformation and, 46 - 51
  migration inhibition and, 66 - 67
  nature of, 55, 57
  separation from transfer factor of, 156, 158, 179 - 181
  transfer factor and, 57
Histoplasmin sensitivity, transfer of, 153, 189, 219, 236
Histoplasmosis, delayed hypersensitivity in, 118, 130 - 131
Hodgkin's disease
  anergy in, 236 - 237
  delayed hypersensitivity in, 118, 135, 137 - 138
  lymphocytes in, 236 - 237
  lymphotoxin production and, 327
Homograft reaction
  as adjuvant, 79
  anti-immunoglobulin and, 421
  complement and, 316
  macrophages and, 395
  mediators in, 388 - 393
  plasma transfer of, 317
  as secondary response, 58, 62, 66 - 67
  transfer factor and, 146, 154 - 156, 178 - 180, 204, 219
Human MIF, production of, 285
Hydralazine, "Lupus" syndromes and, 17

I

Immune complexes, blast transformation and, 21 - 26
Immunoglobulin G, synthesis during transformation of, 9
"Immunoglobulin X," as receptor, 78 - 81, 97, 173
Immunological surveillance, 249, 323, 338, 403, 447 - 448
Immunosuppressive agents, see also individual agents
  transfer factor and, 155
  tumor incidence and, 249
Inflammation
  acute, complement and, 323
  chronic, delayed hypersensitivity and, 323
Interferon
  DiGeorge syndrome and, 402 - 403
  production of, 10, 254
Intracellular infection, resistance to, 370 - 383
Irradiation
  immunocompetence and, 98 - 99
  lymphocytes and, 76, 85 - 87
Isoniazid, "Lupus" syndromes and, 17

K

Keyhole limpet hemocyanin sensitivity, transfer of, 123, 210 - 213, 242

L

Leprosy
  delayed hypersensitivity in, 118, 135
  histology of, 123 - 128
  immunological state in, 121 - 128
  immunosuppression and, 403
  Liacopoulos phenomenon and, 140 - 141
  transfer factor therapy in, 119

SUBJECT INDEX

Liacopoulos phenomenon, 140 - 141
Listeriosis, resistance to, 371 - 387
LT, *see* Lymphotoxin
Lupus erythematosus cells, in leprosy, 123
Lupus syndromes, blast transformation in, 17 - 18
Lymphocyte, *see also* Bone marrow derived cell, Thymus derived cell
   anatomical origin of, 74 - 75
   antigen recognition by, 426 - 427
   cultivation *in vitro* of, 3 - 12
   depletion of, 75 - 76
   effector substances from, 251 - 254, 297 - 298
   enumeration of responder types, 51 - 54, 58 - 61, 168, 199 - 202, 205 - 206
   fractionation of, 76 - 77, 84 - 86
   in Hodgkins disease, 236 - 237
   inhibitors of, 5 - 6
   interaction with macrophage, 20 - 21, 276, 295, 398 - 399, 417 - 418
   irradiation of, 76, 85 - 87
   from lymphoproliferative diseases, 11, 18
   migration inhibition of, 81 - 82
   multi-potentiality of, 60 - 61, 63 - 64
   from normal blood, 18
   "permanent" lines of, 11 - 12, 18
   precomittment of, 73 - 79
   receptor sites on, 15, 100
   recruitment of, 171, 173, 176, 199, 231 - 232, 234 - 235, 364, 410
   replication of, 152, 184, 185
   stimulants of, 4 - 5
   transfer factor and, 152, 161 - 163, 186, 198
Lymphocyte activating material, 238 - 239, *see also* Non-dialysable transfer factor
Lymphocyte-lymphocyte interactions, 78, 84 - 88, 101
Lymphocyte-macrophage interactions, 276, 295, 398 - 399, 417 - 418

Lymphocyte-target cell interaction, 325, 429
Lymphocytic choriomeningitis, 272, 404 - 405, 410
Lymphocytic leukemia, lymphotoxin production and, 327
Lymphoproliferative diseases, lymphocytes from, 11, 18
Lymphotoxin
   activity of, 333 - 334, 338 - 339
   antibody to, 345, 352, 413
   assay of, 340 - 341, 356 - 361, 363
   cell contact and, 350 - 354, 362
   cell types affected by, 332 - 333
   hemolytic activity of, 333, 343 - 344
   inactivation of, 365
   kinetics of toxicity of, 347, 349
   as lysolecithinase, 344
   macrophages and, 333
   membrane lipids and, 361
   MIF activity of, 299 - 300, 335 - 336, 345, 346, 363 - 364
   mitogenic factor and, 362, 364
   morphological effects of, 333 - 334, 341 - 343, 355 - 361
   from murine cells, 300
   phytohemagglutinin and, 368
   polyanions and, 352
   preparation of human, 335
   production of, 10, 252, 362, 369 - 370
   properties of, 331 - 332, 334 - 335
   release of
      by antilymphocyte serum, 328
      blast transformation and, 327 - 329
      cortisone and, 330
      kinetics of, 329 - 330
      lymphoproliferative diseases and, 327
      mixed leucocyte culture and, 328
      nucleic acid synthesis and, 330 - 331, 348, 361
      by PHA, 327
      by Pokeweed mitogen, 328

SUBJECT INDEX

protein synthesis and, 330, 348, 361
by streptolysin O, 328
thymocytes and, 327, 341, 343
by tuberculin, 354 - 356
reversibility of activity of, 365
ribosomal synthesis and, 361
species differences and, 332
specificity of, 332 - 333
stimulation by, 345 - 346
target cell binding of, 364 - 365
transfer factor and, 298
ultrastructural changes and, 333 - 334, 341 - 343
Lysolecithin, incorporation of, 411
Lysolecithinase, as lymphotoxin, 344
Lysosomes, *see also* Macrophage, morphology of
blast transformation and, 8, 10, 15, 38 - 40, 44

M

Macrophage, accelerated reactions and, 309 - 314
activation of, 266, 277 - 283, 370 - 375, 381 - 384, 389, 391, 396
antigen processing by, 38
antigen trapping by, 428
autoallergic encephalomyelitis and, 396
biophysical changes in, 283 - 284
blast-transformation and, 20 - 23, 25
as bone marrow derived cell, 250, 310
cytophilic antibody and, 383
cytotoxicity of, 350, 352
effect of MIF on, 266, 277 — 286, 295
effector substances from, 350
as helper cell, 85, 90 - 91
homograft reaction and, 395
intracellular infection and, 370 - 383
lymphotoxin and, 333
lysolecithin incorporation by, 411

morphology of, 274 - 276, 277, 278 - 283
origin of, 95 - 96
Macrophage-lymphocyte interactions, 20 - 21, 276, 295, 398 - 399, 417 - 418
Measles, 139 - 140
Membrane cyclases, blast transformation and, 7
Membrane lipid, lymphotoxin and, 361
Migration inhibiting factor
in candidiasis, 133 - 134, 237
characterization of, 255, 262 - 265
chemotactic factor and, 271 - 272
cytotoxicity of, 266 - 267
dialysable transfer factor and, 159
effect on macrophage of, 266 - 267, 284 - 286, 295
feedback control by, 399
fractionation of, 255, 262 - 265
from human cells, 285
interspecific activity of, 219, 285, 314 - 315
isolation of, 262 - 265
kinetics of release of, 235
macrophage morphology and, 266 - 267, 276 - 384
mitogenic factor and, 364
production of
DNP-oligolysine and, 267, 286 - 290
genetic constitution and, 286 - 290, 292
induction by RNA of, 288 - 292
kinetics of, 252
protein synthesis and, 251, 273 - 274
RNA synthesis and, 251
purification of, 262 - 265
recruitment by, 388
release by transfer factor of, 218 - 219
RNA and production of, 243
from sea star, 314 - 315
skin reactive factor and, 268 - 269
transfer factor and, 218 - 219, 298

SUBJECT INDEX

yield of, 367
Migration inhibition, *see also* Migration inhibiting factor
   anti-light chain antibody and, 424
   antibody and, 429
   as correlate, 251 - 252
   cytophilic antibody and, 429
   histocompatibility and, 66 - 67
   histoplasmosis and, 130 - 131
   by immune complexes, 270
   by lymphotoxin, 299 - 300, 335 - 336, 345, 346, 363 - 364
   moniliasis and, 130
   poly-U and, 26 - 27
Mitogenic factor
   fractionation of, 293, 294
   lymphotoxin and, 362, 364
   MIF and, 364
   preparation of, 293
   production of, 254, 292 - 294
Mitomycin C
   effector substance production and, 225, 251, 259 - 260
   MIF production and, 251
   transfer factor production and, 225
Mixed lymphocyte culture, 50 - 54, 58 - 61, 63, 64, 66, 67, 81 - 82, 238, 292 - 294, 328, 362, 424
Moniliasis
   blast transformation in, 130
   delayed hypersensitivity in, 118
   transfer factor therapy in, 119
Mumps
   lymphocyte cell lines in, 11
   virus sensitivity, transfer of, 236

N

Non-dialysable transfer factor
   cell division and, 164 - 165
   clonal proliferation and, 164
   dose dependency and, 164, 186
Nuclease, transfer factor susceptibility to, 176

O

Orthanilic acid, as hapten, 107

P

Paraminobenzoate, as hapten, 98
Paranitrobenzene, as hapten 98
Phosphodiesterase, transfer factor susceptibility to, 175
Phytohemagglutinin
   antigenicity of, 31 - 33
   antiserum to, 18 - 19
   attachment of, 6
   cytotoxicity of, 27 - 28
   delayed hypersensitivity to, 31 - 33
   dose response of, 45
   fractionation of, 28 - 29
   immediate hypersensitivity to, 32
   lymphotoxin release by, 327, 368
   skin reactive factor production and, 309
   species variation to, 84
   variability of, 27 - 29, 84
Phytomitogens, distinguishing characteristics of, 21 - 22
Picryl chloride
   as hapten, 109
   sensitivity, transfer of, 222 - 228
"Piggyback" effect, 14, 15, 420 - 421
Pinocytosis, blast transformation and, 7, 15, 17, 40
Pneumococcal polysaccharide
   antibody production to, 428
   blast transformation and, 17 - 18, 38
Pokeweed mitogen
   blast transformation and, 429
   fractionation of, 30
   lymphotoxin release and, 328
Polyanions, lymphotoxin activity and, 352
Polynucleotide, as transfer factor, 181 - 182
Poly-U, migration inhibition and, 26 - 27

SUBJECT INDEX

Procaine amide, "Lupus" syndromes and, 17
Pronase, transfer factor susceptibility to, 176
Protein synthesis
    blast transformation and, 9 - 10, 40, 64
    effector substance production and, 251, 259 - 260, 273 - 274
    lymphotoxin release and, 330
    MIF production and, 251, 273 - 274
Puromycin
    effector substance production and, 259 - 260
    skin reactive factor production and, 307

R

Receptor sites, 100 - 111
Rhesus monkey, transfer factor from, 242
Ribonuclease, transfer factor susceptibility to, 175, 176, 181
Ribosome synthesis
    blast transformation and, 9, 40
    lymphotoxin and, 361
Ribonucleic acid
    blast transformation production and, 243
    cutaneous sensitivity production and, 243
    induction of MIF production by, 243, 288 - 292
Ribonucleic acid-antigen complex, 38
Ribonucleic acid synthesis
    blast transformation and, 8 - 9, 14, 15, 28 - 29, 40, 64
    effector substance production and, 251, 259 - 260
    lymphotoxin release and, 330 - 331, 348, 361
    MIF production and, 251
Ribonucleic acid turnover, blast transformation and, 8 - 9
RPMI 1640 medium, use of, 27, 44 - 49

S

Sarcoidosis
    blast transformation in, 112, 129 - 130, 135, 137
    delayed hypersensitivity in, 111 - 117, 129 - 130, 135, 137
    lymphocyte cell lines in, 11
    transfer factor and, 235 - 236
Scrapie, transfer factor and, 229
Sea star, MIF from, 314 - 315
Self + X hypothesis, 449 - 454
Skin reactive factor
    activity of, 301 - 309
    MIF and, 268 - 269
    production of, 254
    release by PHA of, 309
    separation from MIF, 255, 262 - 265
Strain 2 guinea pigs, 105, 243, 286 - 290, 292, 389 - 390
Strain 13 guinea pigs, 105, 243, 286 - 290, 292, 389 - 390
Streptococcal factor, purification of, 31
Streptococcal M substance, transfer of sensitivity to, 151, 153, 194, 204
Streptolysin O, lymphotoxin release and, 328
Syphilis, serum factors in, 129

T

Thoracic duct drainage, 74
Thymectomy
    antibody production and, 84, 436
    effect on blast transformation of, 83, 436
    experimental leprosy and, 403
    lymphocyte depletion by, 74
    tumor incidence and, 249
Thymus derived cell, *see also* Lymphocyte
    cellular immunity and, 74, 92, 250
    depletion of, 75 - 76
    development of, 428
    as helper, 77

SUBJECT INDEX

at local reaction site, 96
as sensitized cell, 96
specific functions of, 94
thoracic duct drainage and, 74

Transfer factor, *see also* Antigen mediated transfer factor, Dialysable transfer factor, Non-dialysable transfer factor
accelerated reactions and, 312
ac activator, 240 - 241
anergy and, 117, 133 - 134, 174, 403 - 404
anti-lymphocyte serum and, 155
blast transformation and, 184
characterization of, 181 - 182
coccidioidin sensitivity and, 146, 153 - 154, 157 - 158, 189, 204, 218, 219, 236
comparison with native sensitization of, 146
contact hypersenitivity and, 190 - 195, 206, 207
cytotoxicity of, 242
definition of, 190
dinitrochlorobenzene sensitivity and, 206 - 208
dinitrofluorobenzene sensitivity and, 191, 194
diphtheria toxoid sensitivity and, 145, 153, 184, 194, 204, 210, 218, 219, 236
dose employed of, 228
enzymatic susceptibility of, 153, 176 - 231
fractionation of, 181 - 182
histoplasmin sensitivity and, 153, 189, 219, 236
homograft reaction and, 146, 154 - 156, 177 - 181, 204, 219
histocompatibility antigens and, 57
immunogenicity of, 209 - 210, 213 - 217, 219 - 220, 236, 240, 244, 418, 452 - 453
interaction with lymphocyte of, 152
interspecific activity of, 186, 210, 222 - 228, 239 - 245

KLH sensitivity and, 210 - 213, 242
latent sensitivity and, 153 - 154, 187 - 188, 191 - 193, 196, 233
lymphotoxin and, 298
MIF and, 298
MIF release by, 218 - 219
minimal effective dose of, 203 - 204
mitomycin C and, 225
mouse lymphocytes and, 240 - 241
mumps virus sensitivity and, 236
non-human assay of, 239 - 245
nuclease sensitivity of, 176
phenomenology of, 145 - 156
picryl chloride sensitivity and, 222 - 228
production kinetics of, 233 - 234
properties of, 114 - 116, 154 - 156, 157 - 159
purification of, 156 - 159
quantitation of, 207 - 208
replication of, 152 - 153
from Rhesus monkey, 242
Rhesus monkey lymphocytes and, 186, 210 - 213
ribonuclease sensitivity of, 175, 176, 181
RNA extracts from, 418
sarcoidosis and, 235 - 236
scrapie and, 229
serial transfer of, 146 - 152
species differences and, 159, 181, 227 - 228
specificity of, 218
streptococcal sensitivity and, 151, 153, 194, 204, 218, 236
therapeutic uses of, 118, 133 - 134, 174, 403 - 404
tuberculin sensitivity and, 146, 151, 153, 161, 164, 184, 187, 191 - 192, 208, 210, 218, 219, 236
yield of, 202
Trinitrochlorobenzene, as hapten, 109
Tuberculin sensitivity, transfer of, 146, 151, 153, 161, 164, 184, 187, 191 - 192, 208, 210, 218, 219, 236

SUBJECT INDEX

Tuberculosis
    resistance to, 371 - 387
    serum factors in, 129, 132 - 133
Tumor antigens, blast transformation and, 47
Tumor development, immunocompetence and, 249

V

Vaccinia
    delayed hypersensitivity in, 118, 258 - 259, 402, 403
    DiGeorge syndrome and, 402
    transfer factor therapy in, 118, 403 - 404
Vi polysaccharide, blast transformation and, 17 - 18

Viral encephalitides, antibodies in, 272, 404 - 405
Viral infections, delayed hypersensitivity in, 118, 139 - 140, 236, 256, 258 - 259, 402, 403

W

Wiskoff-Aldrich syndrome, immune responses in, 136, 138 - 139

X

X-irradiation, delayed hypersensitivity and, 310

QR
185
C4 M4